Cross-Cultural Research in Health, Illness and Well-Being

Series editor

Pranee Liamputtong, School of Science and Health, Western Sydney University, Penrith, NSW, Australia

This new series examines determinants of health from a cross-cultural perspective. The focus of this perspective is on factors which could influence and determine the health and well-being of people. These factors include biological and genetic factors; health behaviors; socio-cultural and socio-economic factors and environment factors. This series fills a gap by including books which are research-based and contain diverse issues relevant to determinants of health including emerging health issues, such as HIV/AIDS and other infectious and non-infectious diseases/illnesses from a cross-cultural perspective. Volumes in the series will be a valuable resource for researchers and students in sociology, quality of life studies, anthropology, medicine, public health, social work and medicine.

More information about this series at http://www.springer.com/series/13178

Marisa J. Perera • Edward C. Chang
Editors

Biopsychosocial Approaches to Understanding Health in South Asian Americans

Springer

Editors
Marisa J. Perera
Department of Psychology
University of Miami
Coral Gables, Florida, USA

Edward C. Chang
Department of Psychology
University of Michigan
Ann Arbor, Michigan, USA

ISSN 2366-6056 ISSN 2366-6064 (electronic)
Cross-Cultural Research in Health, Illness and Well-Being
ISBN 978-3-319-91118-2 ISBN 978-3-319-91120-5 (eBook)
https://doi.org/10.1007/978-3-319-91120-5

Library of Congress Control Number: 2018950100

Printed on acid-free paper

This Springer imprint is published by the registered company Springer Nature Switzerland AG.
The registered company address is: Gewerbestrasse 11, 6330 Cham, Switzerland

This book is dedicated to all the individuals who have played major roles in guiding me in my scholarly pursuits, especially Dr. Edward Chang, as well as all the exceptional contributors to this book who serve as leaders in the study of South Asian American health. This book is additionally dedicated to my parents Vijayanthi and Jude Perera for cultivating in me an understanding of both South Asian and American cultures throughout my upbringing and for their endless support of my scholarly development.

Marisa J. Perera

This book is dedicated to the many wonderful individuals who have shared their passion and expertise in developing this important work, most especially to Marisa for allowing me to work together with her.

Edward C Chang

Preface

During our careers studying Asian American health outcomes, we were exposed to the practice of aggregation or compilation of group information without separation into potentially different and meaningful sublevels. We repeatedly encountered instances where data on Asian American health status and chronic disease burden (i.e., prevalence of cancers, diabetes, heart disease, etc.) was collected primarily from one subgroup of Asian ethnic origin and generalized to all individuals identifying as Asian in the USA. As Asian Americans are of different Asian origins, it was evident to us that such generalization was lacking in accuracy at times when generalized to different Asian subgroups. It was also evident that continued use of aggregation had potential to mitigate the potential risk for harmful health conditions that vary by Asian subgroup, including those conditions for which South Asians in the USA have high risk. In support of the disaggregation movement, we sought to bring together scholars devoted to various aspects of the health of South Asians in the USA in order to initiate a health conversation and scholarly space dedicated to the health needs of this Asian subgroup. This process inherently brought about an interdisciplinary effort involving scholarly contributors across the fields of medicine, psychology, public health, and health policy.

Stemming from health psychology and behavioral medicine, this handbook is committed to the incorporation of South Asian culture into the science and practice of health promotion and disease reduction in South Asians in the USA. Raised as Asian Americans, we have been exposed to beliefs about health that are rooted in South Asian culture and that possess potential to exacerbate disease risk. More often than not, effective prevention and self-management of chronic conditions obliges long-term, lifestyle changes that are predicated on the adoption of health-promoting beliefs and practices. Combining our professional experiences in health psychology with personal experiences as Asian American individuals of different Asian descent, it became evident to us that the South Asian American patient's system of beliefs about health, illness, and disease should be considered to increase effectiveness of long-term health promotion and prevention/maintenance of chronic conditions. For these reasons, the biopsychosocial model is applied throughout this handbook to consider not only biomedical aspects, but also psychological and sociocultural aspects of South Asian American conceptualizations of health that can impact the health and chronic disease status of South Asians in the USA.

A note for the reader is to exercise caution due to the nascent and emerging understanding of the health of South Asians in the USA. Although this handbook tends to take a group approach to conceptualizing health, individual differences must not be forgotten. Overall, we hope that the present work helps to facilitate discourse, research, and practice among those scholars interested in the health of South Asians in the USA.

We would like to express our gratitude to all the distinguished collaborators of the present volume for sharing their clinical insights with us and for sharing their passion to improve the health of this Asian subgroup. We hope readers from the present volume will be inspired to learn from these great contributors and gain greater appreciation for the nuanced relationship between culture and health that can guide our understanding of health by continuing to improve upon our existing models of health.

Coral Gables, FL Marisa J. Perera
Ann Arbor, MI Edward C. Chang

Contents

1 **Introduction to Biopsychosocial Approaches to Understanding Health in South Asian Americans** 1
Edward C. Chang, Marisa J. Perera, Casey N.-H. Batterbee, and Zunaira Jilani

Part I History of South Asian Americans

2 **South Asian Immigration to United States: A Brief History Within the Context of Race, Politics, and Identity** 15
Sunil Bhatia and Anjali Ram

3 **South Asian Identity in the United States** 33
Anju Kaduvettoor-Davidson and Ryan D. Weatherford

Part II Models of Health in South Asian Americans

4 **Biological Models of Health** 53
Namratha R. Kandula and Manasi A. Tirodkar

5 **Psychological Models of Health** 71
Zunaira Jilani, Edward C. Chang, Jerin Lee, and Casey N.-H. Batterbee

6 **South Asian American Health: Perspectives and Recommendations on Sociocultural Influences** 95
Riddhi Sandil and Ranjana Srinivasan

Part III Major Health Conditions in South Asian Americans

7 **Type 2 Diabetes Mellitus in South Asian Americans** 121
Suhaila Khan, Nilay Shah, Nisha Parikh, Divya Iyer, and Latha Palaniappan

8 **Cancer Risk, Risk Reduction, and Screening and Treatment Access among U.S. South Asians** 149
Francesca Gany, Anuradha Hashemi, and Jennifer Leng

9 **Mental Health Conditions among South Asians in the United States** 171
Pratyusha Tummala-Narra and Anita Deshpande

Part IV Barriers to Promoting Health in South Asian Americans

10 **Issues in Counseling South Asian Americans** 195
Farah A. Ibrahim and Jianna R. Heuer

11 **South Asian American Health Research and Policy** 215
Chandak Ghosh

Part V Conclusion

12 **A Call for Healthy South Asian Americans: Need to Shape Intervention by Providers, Policies, and Prospects** 237
Marisa J. Perera and Edward C. Chang

Chapter 1
Introduction to Biopsychosocial Approaches to Understanding Health in South Asian Americans

Edward C. Chang, Marisa J. Perera, Casey N.-H. Batterbee, and Zunaira Jilani

1.1 Introduction to Biopsychosocial Approaches to Understanding Health in South Asian Americans

The conceptualization of health has evolved throughout the centuries with emerging and modified models to account for health factors deemed important. Traditional views of health focused on the dominant model of health in the biomedical sciences: a disease-based model in which health refers to the absence of disease (Seligman and Csikszentmihalyi 2000). This model was quite successful in advancing the medical field, however, it did not acknowledge the complexities of individuals (Green et al. 2002). While the importance of both the inner mental aspects of human experience and the outer context of culture and society is undeniable, disproportionate emphasis of the biological model has persisted into the present day (e.g., Brain Initiative; National Institutes of Health 2014). For these reasons, there have been calls for interdisciplinary approaches to understanding and studying health. Indeed, recent discussions regarding health's definition center around the mind-body connection, which highlights the relationship between one's mental well-being and physical health, as well as the need to account for varied human experiences in relation to culture and society. This shift in perspective became known as the biopsychosocial model of health (Engel 1997).

E. C. Chang (✉) · C. N.-H. Batterbee
University of Michigan-Ann Arbor, Ann Arbor, MI, USA
e-mail: caseybat@umich.edu; changec@umich.edu

M. J. Perera
University of Miami-Coral Gables, Coral Gables, FL, USA
e-mail: mperera@miami.edu

Z. Jilani
Wayne State University, Detroit, MI, USA
e-mail: zunaira.jilani@wayne.edu

M. J. Perera, E. C. Chang (eds.), *Biopsychosocial Approaches to Understanding Health in South Asian Americans*, Cross-Cultural Research in Health, Illness and Well-Being, https://doi.org/10.1007/978-3-319-91120-5_1

1.2 The Importance of the Biopsychosocial Model: Moving toward a more Holistic Examination of Health

The biopsychosocial model of health (Engel 1997) has been defined as a framework that encompasses both philosophy and practicality. In philosophical terms, this model serves to create a holistic picture of the spectrum of variables that may impact a person's health, while also functioning as a practical guide for understanding a person's subjective and complex experience of both mental and physical illness (Borrell-Carrió et al. 2004). More specifically, this model aims to address health issues through a biomedical, psychological, and sociocultural lens. Prior to this model, most scientists discussed health using a biomedical model to explain behavior and mental processes. While this perspective on health led to countless important advancements throughout its history, it was deemed to have a narrow view of health maintained by the biological sciences (Borrell-Carrió et al. 2004). Indeed, when the healthcare system views a complex human being as a mere case or label, scientific advancement can come at the expense of overlooking other important health factors including emotions and mental processes (Green et al. 2002). Thus, it becomes important to be cognizant of an individual's psychological well-being (e.g., stress, anxiety, depression) in regard to the individual's physical health. Furthermore, beyond the mind and body connection, there is great value in incorporating not only the psychological perspective into medical treatment, but also the sociocultural perspective (e.g., social norms, traditional practices, cultural nuances). As such, the biopsychosocial model seeks to expand its scope to include the inner cognitive world of the mind and the outer cultural context. Indeed, as the term itself encompasses the biological, psychological, and sociocultural, it is important to consider the importance of all three aspects of the model. However, in practice, the sociocultural aspect of the biopsychosocial model has historically been undervalued. The mind-body connection has been studied for decades, addressing the biomedical and psychological aspects, while cultural/social norms have often been overlooked. It is important to understand the importance of including all aspects of the model by considering the framework in its entirety.

The biopsychosocial model represents a framework that necessitates both top-down and bottom-up perspectives for comprehensive treatment. In general, a top-down approach would utilize existing models and understanding of health previously applied to other populations, whereas a bottom-up approach involves considering important aspects that are on a small scale in order to understand a larger complex system. In other words, a bottom-up approach to the health of various groups of people involves considering each as distinct in order to examine for unique patterns of mental and physical health. Specifically, culture, or the system of meaning one develops for perceiving the world due to the circumstances of their upbringing, has been argued to be a prerequisite for an individual's experience of the world (Burkett 1991). Encompassing important aspects of human identity like race, gender, and religion, culture is a construct that encapsulates much of the vastness and complexity of life. Indeed, given the nuance, sophistication, and variation found across different cultures, it may sometimes be necessary to consider health idiomatically when studying ethnoracial groups. Indeed, culture is an important aspect of life that influences both patterns and perceptions of physical and mental health (i.e., pathology & psychopathology). Thus, given that patterns of physical and mental health may vary greatly by culture, especially between those with vastly different physical environments and sociocultural norms (e.g., United States & India), it becomes necessary to consider the idiomatic nature of the physical and mental health of various ethnoracial groups.

Despite that the United States is comprised of a multitude of different groups with various ethnoracial backgrounds, the examination of both psychological and physical health has largely been restricted to European Americans (i.e., Caucasians). Of those attempts that have been made to understand the influence that a broader range of cultures may have on health, majority have taken place among the largest minorities in the United States (e.g., African American, Hispanic, Latino/a; U.S. Census Bureau 2015). While significant research has been conducted among larger minority populations such as African Americans and Latino/a Americans, others have remained comparatively understudied. For example, although major journals of health have existed for African Americans and Latino/a Americans since the late 1970s (e.g., Journal of Black Psychology & Hispanic Journal of Behavioral Sciences), the Journal of Asian American Psychology was not established until 2009. Moreover, this journal is not specific to South Asian Americans, which has distinct patterns and perceptions of disease and health compared to other types of Asians, such as East Asians. Thus, to move toward more egalitarian research practices that are representative of the diversity of the United States, researchers must examine the physical and mental health of specific ethnoracial groups in America, including those of South Asian descent.

1.3 Diversity in Scientific Inquiry: The Importance of Developing a more Culturally Nuanced Perspective on Health in South Asians Living in the United States

As abovementioned, nuance is often sacrificed when striving for standardization in scientific inquiry. Thus, when developing a nuanced view of various ethnoracial groups in America, it is of vital importance to consider differences between cultures with the intention to holistically understand the diverse cultural landscape in the United States. In other words, it is highly necessary to consider differences between groups for the purpose of benefitting those groups, as opposed to further marginalizing them. Scholarly research in the United States has historically tended to give disproportionate attention to the majority population in a given area while neglecting the study of minorities. This represents a problematic norm in the United States, especially given that Caucasian Americans may no longer be the majority by 2020 (U.S. Census Bureau 2014). In fact, while Asia is the largest continent in the world and South Asian Americans represent one of the fastest growing minority populations in the United States (Pew Research Center 2012), this population has remained relatively understudied when compared to groups like Black/African Americans and Latino/a Americans. South Asian Americans are those individuals with ancestral roots from the geographical region of South Asia, including Bangladesh, Bhutan, India, Maldives, Nepal, Pakistan, & Sri Lanka. Afghanistan is sometimes included in this list.

Although approximately a quarter of the entire world's population resides in South Asia, little attention has been given to the differential influence that cultural background may have on the health of South Asians. More specifically, it can be problematic to implement health models tailored toward Westerners without accounting for such cultural differences for South Asians living in America. In fact, much of the research that does exist for South Asian Americans uses aggregation, which is when varying racial/ethnic backgrounds are grouped together and categorized into one group, ignoring cultural differences and making it difficult to understand health differences by group. The way that data is typically collected regarding race/ethnicity often clusters together all types of Asian Americans. Asian Americans encompass individuals from a wide range of countries from the Asian continent, often broken down into East Asian (e.g., Chinese, Japanese, Korean), South Asian (e.g., Bangladeshi, Indian, Pakistani), and Southeast Asian (e.g., Filipino, Indonesian, Vietnamese) Americans. This rather long list of countries comprises more than 25 groups and 40 distinct cultural subgroups that all embody varying beliefs, traditions, religions, languages, and norms. Yet, most research that has examined Asian Americans has tended to focus on East Asian Americans, while neglecting other subsets of the Asian American population including South Asian Americans. For example, although one of the largest surveys of minority populations in the United States was conducted in 2003 (i.e., the National Latino and Asian American Study or NLAAS), past studies using data from the NLAAS have suggested that South Asian Americans made up less than 8% of the Asian Americans sampled (Masood et al. 2009). This is especially concerning for South Asian Americans, as this population has been rapidly growing over the past few decades. According to the 2010 U.S. Bureau of Census, from 2000 to 2010 the population of South Asian Americans jumped from 1.7 million to 2.8 million (an increase of 70%), making South Asians the second fastest growing ethnic population in the U.S. (e.g., Hoeffel et al. 2012).

Amalgamating individuals with vastly differing cultural backgrounds, or aggregation, can also lead to failure to account for sociocultural context of specific populations. It seems unreasonable to lump these groups together and important to consider that perhaps members of this group should not be streamlined into one group (Futa et al. 2001). As stated previously, majority of the research on Asian Americans has studied samples typically comprised majority of East and Southeast Asian (e.g., Chinese, Japanese, Korean, Vietnamese, Filipino Americans). Therefore, there is limited data on South Asian Americans specifically. Furthermore, there are countless studies that do not specify the racial breakdown of Asian Americans, and it is unknown how many of these Asian Americans identified as South vs. East/

Southeast Asian. For example, of the data that was obtained by the National Intimate Partner and Sexual Violence Survey (Black et al. 2011), there were over 1.5 million Asian American victims of sexual violence other than rape. However, cultural background beyond "Asian American" was not identified, making it unknown how many of those victims were, for example, Indian vs. Chinese. Given that the United States' population is shifting towards being composed of mostly multiracial individuals by 2060 (as predicted by the U.S. Census Bureau; Colby and Ortman 2015), it becomes increasingly important to account for cultural background in research, particularly for South Asian Americans.

Moreover, having one or more different ethnic backgrounds may directly influence an individual's experience of life. Relatedly, significant differences in cultural practices may even exist within the same country; for example, two individuals living in separate regions of India may speak a different language (e.g., Bengali vs. Tamil), eat vastly different food (e.g., North Indian vs. South Indian cuisine), and practice a different religion (e.g., Hinduism vs. Islam). Such aspects of life may influence how each person experiences immigrating to America, and may even play a role in the family life of 2nd or 3rd generation Asian Americans. For example, South Asian Americans can experience acculturative stress upon immigrating to the United States (Bhattacharya and Schoppelrey 2004), and studies in other Western countries (e.g., Canada) have also indicated that further generations (e.g., second generation) may encounter similar challenges (Abouguendia and Noels 2001). How are these distinct unique experiences accounted for in regard to health?

Methodologies that were developed to assess more Westernized populations may not be culturally sensitive or compatible to victims with a non-Western background. It is important to be cognizant of the tools used for assessment to account for cultural nuances and include variables assessing sociocultural context (Runner et al. 2009). For these reasons, it is important to not only avoid aggregation of different cultural groups (e.g., lumping South Asian Americans within Asian Americans) in research, but to also expand research beyond the identification of an existing problem within such communities. Thus, it may be worthwhile to consider how the biopsychosocial model of health may facilitate the development of a more culturally nuanced view of health that may be beneficial in treatment and research in the U.S.

Overall, despite that the South Asian population in the United States significantly increased between 2000 and 2010 (Hoeffel et al. 2012), nationally representative research that specifically examines South Asian Americans has been scarce. Moving forward, it is imperative to continue to expand the scope of idiomatic research on South Asians in America by further examining the health of this population. Thus, the present volume seeks to outline the extant literature on South Asian Americans to strive for a more culturally conscious perspective on health in the United States. Before considering the established patterns of health among South Asian Americans, it becomes necessary to consider the ways in which researchers examine ethnoracial groups in general to understand health outcomes for these groups.

1.4 Integrating Bottom-Up and Top-Down Perspectives on Health: How should Researchers Approach Examining South Asian Americans?

It is important to specifically examine how researchers should approach the study of the mental and physical health of an understudied ethnoracial group such as South Asian Americans. As mentioned previously, existing models of health typically represent an important framework that facilitates the consideration of health from a top-down perspective. However, the study of distinct ethnoracial groups may necessitate a bottom-up approach for examining health when the mental and physical needs of groups are considered to be distinct and unique from one another. For example, while it is important to determine the generalizability of findings from studies examining the majority population of a region, restricting research on minority populations to the context of cross-cultural replication studies may obscure the important nuances that characterize various ethnoracial populations. Considering the individual needs of various cultural groups through a bottom-up approach may not only improve understanding of health outcomes for the ethnoracial group, but may even serve to communicate to such groups that their health needs are important and will not be neglected. Furthermore, given the importance of considering the specific needs of various ethnoracial populations such as South Asian Americans, any comprehensive examination of mental and physical health should also consider the importance of culture. Thus, the present work seeks to underscore the idiographic nature of the mental and physical health needs of South Asian Americans (i.e., bottom-up approach), along with considering the health of this population in relation to that of other important groups (i.e., top-down approach).

1.5 A Culturally Conscious Examination of Health: Why Are South Asian Americans Important to Study?

Even when considering only the size and population density of the region of South Asia, it is clearly incredibly vast. Indeed, the population of South Asia is greater than that of the major East Asian countries combined (e.g., China, Japan, South Korea). In fact, South Asian culture is extremely large and complex, containing hundreds of languages and religious traditions (e.g., Hinduism, Christianity, Islam, Jainism, Sikhism; Census of India 2001). Furthermore, the region of South Asia has had a diverse history of rule even prior to the infamous British Occupation. For example, even Alexander the Great conquered parts of India (Narain 1965). Indeed, the South Asian region has fluctuated greatly, and throughout its colorful history has grown profoundly diverse. Thus, as mentioned previously it is important to consider how this unique cultural background may influence the life of South Asians in the United States.

Importantly, South Asian immigration to the United States has increased significantly over the past decade (Hoeffel et al. 2012). Given that South Asia represents a vast and diverse region with a vibrant cultural history, it is important to consider the challenges that may be involved in adjusting to life in the United States. For example, a South Asian immigrant is no more immune to mental and physical health challenges than the average American, and in certain cases may even be more vulnerable (e.g., diabetes, human immunodeficiency virus infection and acquired immune deficiency syndrome [HIV/AIDS]; South Asian Americans Leading Together [SAALT] 2009; Joint United Nations Programme on HIV/AIDS [UNAIDS] 2011). Furthermore, aspects of American culture may differ significantly from South Asian culture (e.g., individualism/collectivism, gender roles, religion), and South Asian Americans may experience acculturative stress when adjusting to an unfamiliar cultural environment (Bhattacharya and Schoppelrey 2004). Indeed, while South Asians have been immigrating to America since the early 1800s, this population has remained relatively unstudied until very recently. While there historically remains a lack of nationally representative research on South Asian Americans, this population has grown significantly in recent years, and research has increased in parallel.

1.6 Patterns of Physical and Mental Health among South Asian Americans

When examining the physical health of South Asians, it is important to consider that this population commonly suffers from heart disease, diabetes, cancer, tuberculosis, and HIV/AIDS (SAALT 2009). Indeed, the prevalence rate of diabetes among South Asian Americans is nearly double that of Caucasian Americans (Barnes et al. 2008). Additionally, while HIV/AIDS is a prevalent problem among South Asian Americans, little research on HIV/AIDS has been conducted in this population. However, given that India alone accounts for more than half of all AIDS mortalities in Asia (UNAIDS 2011), HIV/AIDS is certainly an important health concern among South Asian Americans. Furthermore, South Asian Americans may face difficulties related to receiving medical care, including access to health insurance and language barriers (SAALT 2009). Thus, it becomes clear that it is particularly important to develop culturally competent healthcare in order to address these barriers and provide adequate healthcare for South Asian Americans.

In terms of mental health, South Asian Americans face a variety of physical and mental health challenges (e.g., interpersonal violence, racism and racial discrimination, suicide; SAALT 2009). In particular, it is important to consider that, despite the various mental health difficulties that may affect South Asian Americans, they often resist seeking treatment from a psychologist or social worker (Panganamala and Plummer 1998). Indeed, mental health is rarely considered in South Asian American communities often due to religious and cultural factors (Panganamala and Plummer 1998). However, given that many South Asian Americans have been victims of hate crimes in the United States, and considering the high rate of domestic violence in this population, mental health difficulties such as acculturative stress and posttraumatic stress-disorder may go largely unaddressed (Patel and Gaw 1996).

Indeed, while there are many barriers to both mental and physical care among South Asian Americans, the present volume seeks to provide accurate and culturally sensitive information on South Asians in America for the purpose of developing holistic and effective healthcare for this population. More specifically, we seek to address a major limitation in the extant literature on mental and physical healthcare, namely, the current understanding of healthcare of South Asian Americans, a population that is growing significantly in the United States.

1.7 Overview of the Present Volume

The purpose of the present work is to consider the biopsychosocial health of South Asian Americans. In particular, the authors seek to review the current literature relating to the psychological and biological health of South Asian Americans, and consider how sociocultural factors may impact and even explain various aspects of South Asian American health. Overall, we seek to emphasize the importance of considering culture in both medical and psychological healthcare. Given the vast cultural history of South Asian Americans, we have divided the present work into three chronological sections.

Part I focuses on the general history of South Asians in America. In Chap. 2, Bhatia and Ram provide a broad history of the South Asian diaspora, highlighting the varied experiences of different South Asian subgroups that have immigrated to America. More specifically, they paint a picture of the diverse history of South Asian American immigrants, highlighting both the challenges faced by certain groups, as well as the successes of others. Finally, the authors consider the present sociopolitical climate of the United States, discussing how it may shape the future of South Asians in America. In Chap. 3, Kaduvettoor-Davidson and Weatherford take a critical look at the meaning of South Asian identity. They begin by expansively reviewing the heterogeneous nature of South Asian identity, and emphasize the many countries that make up the region of South Asia. Next, building upon this broad review, the authors continue to focus on South Asian identity in America, addressing a variety of concerns and issues, ranging from conceptions about South Asian Americans as the model minority to experiences of racial prejudice and discrimination among this group. Finally, the authors conclude their chapter by looking forward and exploring the intersectionality of South Asian identity with other aspects of identity within the American context.

Part II focuses on the how the present models of health pertain to South Asian Americans. The section is divided into biological models of health, psychological models of health, and sociocultural models of health. In Chap. 4, Kandula and

Tirodkar provide an overview of the indigenous medicine systems of South Asia (e.g., Ayurveda). More specifically, they consider how South Asian Americans' perceptions of health and health behaviors may differ from those of European Americans, and discuss the importance of indigenous South Asian medicine in relation to the medical treatment in the United States for South Asian Americans. Finally, the authors emphasize the importance of holistic and culturally conscious treatment for South Asian Americans, providing some guidelines for how health providers can incorporate cultural awareness and understanding into treatment. In Chap. 5, Jilani, Chang, Lee, and Batterbee broadly discuss how the biopsychosocial model of health relates to treatment for South Asian Americans. Beginning with an overview of the currently recognized models of health, the authors then delve more specifically into the psychological aspect of the biopsychosocial model of health. They consider the importance of various forms of psychological intervention that take root in South Asia (e.g., meditation) and how they relate to the psychological health of South Asian Americans. Finally, the authors conclude by emphasizing the importance of further scientific efforts that may be beneficial in developing a more complete understanding of the South Asian American psyche. In Chap. 6, Sandil and Srinivasan broadly emphasize the importance of viewing the mental and physical health of South Asian Americans through a cultural lens by providing an overview of some important cultural factors that characterize South Asian Americans (e.g., collectivism, religious identity), as well as challenges that influence their experience in the United States (e.g., acculturative stress). The authors then give recommendations for more culturally-competent treatment among South Asian Americans, concluding with a nuanced examination of both cultural issues and patterns of physical and mental health that may be important to consider when treating this population.

Part III provides an overview of the major health conditions that affect South Asian Americans. In Chap. 7, Khan, Shah, Parikh, and Palaniappan begin to focus specifically on the physical health of South Asian Americans. Providing an overview of South Asian American mortality, the authors discuss the physical health challenges that South Asian Americans face, focusing on one of the most prevalent concerns among this population, namely, diabetes and cardiovascular health. They conclude by expanding the scope of diabetes' effects on South Asian Americans, considering its importance at a social and economic level. In Chap. 8, Gany, Hashemi, and Leng discuss the epidemiology of cancer among South Asian Americans. Specifically, the authors begin by broadly considering the various factors that may influence the risk of cancer as well as issues in screening and treatment of cancer, including genetic factors, infections and chronic inflammation, environmental pollutants, health behaviors (i.e., tobacco, diet, physical activity, etc.), and health care access and utilization. They highlight the importance of continuing to expand the limited extant literature on cancer among South Asian Americans. In Chap. 9, Tummala-Narra and Deshpande broadly discuss the difficulties faced by South Asian immigrants to America as they relate to mental health. Building on this, the authors provide a more specific consideration of the various aspects of acculturative stress, from difficulties with communication in English to direct experiences of discrimination. The authors then note the generational differences between South Asian Americans, and conclude with an examination of various challenges to culturally informed mental health care.

Part IV addresses the barriers to health promotion among South Asian Americans. In Chap. 10, Ibrahim and Heuer provide a general overview of the challenges involved in health promotion among South Asian Americans. The authors begin by summarizing both the common medical conditions for which South Asian Americans are at risk, as well as the common risk factors for mental disorders among this population. Overall, they seek to emphasize the cultural factors that play a role in medical and psychological treatment, and to provide guidance for healthcare providers when working with South Asian American patients. In Chap. 11, Ghosh discusses the representation of South Asian Americans in institutionalized healthcare. Specifically, the author discusses the underrepresentation of South Asian Americans in health policy and provides a detailed plan that addresses this issue.

The present volume concludes by taking a prospective view of South Asian American health. In Chap. 12, the first and second authors call for the improvement of the study and treatment of chronic health conditions in South Asian Americans and proffer recommendations for providers working with this subset of the U.S. population. The chapter ends with emphasis placed on use of both top-down and bottom-up approaches for conceptualizing the health of South Asians in the U.S. to promote culturally-conscious physical and mental healthcare.

1.8 Final Thoughts

Above all else, the present volume seeks to emphasize the importance of culture in healthcare. Through the development of culturally-conscious and holistic models of mental and physical healthcare, practitioners can not only create a comfortable and understanding environment in which patients receive care, but they may be able to directly validate the humanity and dignity of the populations which they serve. Indeed, while some of the present paradigms of healthcare in the United States address a range of challenges faced by the general population, they may fall short in addressing the unique needs of various ethnoracial groups, such as South Asian Americans. Thus, a more culturally nuanced approach to healthcare must be taken: In short, culture does matter.

References

Abouguendia, M., & Noels, K. A. (2001). General and acculturation-related daily hassles and psychological adjustment in first- and second-generation south Asian immigrants to Canada. *International Journal of Psychology, 36*, 163–173.

Barnes, P. M., Adams, P. F., & Powell-Griner, E. (2008). Health characteristics of the Asian adult population: United States, 2004–2006. *Advance Data from Vital and Health Statistics, 394*, 1–24.

Bhattacharya, G., & Schoppelrey, S. L. (2004). Preimmigration beliefs of life success, postimmigration experiences, and acculturative stress: South Asian immigrants in the United States. *Journal of Immigrant Health, 6*, 83–92.

Black, M. C., Basile, K. C., Breiding, M. J., Smith, S. G., Walters, M. L., Merrick, M. T., & Stevens, M. R. (2011). *The National Intimate Partner and sexual violence survey (NISVS): 2010 summary report*. Atlanta: National Center for Injury Prevention and Control, Centers for Disease Control and Prevention.

Borrell-Carrió, F., Suchman, A. L., & Epstein, R. M. (2004). The biopsychosocial model 25 years later: Principles, practice, and scientific inquiry. *Annals of Family Medicine, 2*, 576–582.

Burkett, G. L. (1991). Culture, illness, and the biopsychosocial model. *Family Medicine, 23*, 287–291.

Census of India. (2001). *Religion*. Retrieved December 1, 2016 from http://censusindia.gov.in/Census_And_You/religion.aspx

Colby, S. L., & Ortman, J. M. (2015). Projections of the size and composition of the U.S. population: 2014 to 2060. *U.S. Census Bureau, 9*, 1–13.

Engel, G. L. (1997). From biomedical to biopsychosocial. *Psychotherapy and Psychosomatics, 66*, 57–62.

Futa, K. T., Hsu, E., & Hansen, D. J. (2001). Child sexual abuse in Asian American families: An examination of cultural factors that influence prevalence, identification, and treatment. *Clinical Psychology: Science and Practice, 8*(2), 189–209.

Green, A. R., Carrillo, J. E., & Betancourt, J. R. (2002). Why the disease-based model of medicine fails our patients. *Western Journal of Medicine, 176*, 141–143.

Hoeffel, E. M., Rastogi, S., Kim, M. O., & Shahid, H. (2012). The Asian Population: 2010. 2010 Census Briefs issued *March 2012*. Washington. Census Bureau.

Joint United Nations Programme on HIV/AIDS [UNAIDS]. (2011). *The Gap Report*. Retrieved November 17, 2016 from http://files.unaids.org/en/media/unaids/contentassets/documents/unaidspublication/2014/UNAIDS_Gap_report_en.pdf

Masood, N., Okazaki, S., & Takeuchi, D. T. (2009). Gender, family, and community correlates of mental health in south Asian Americans. *Cultural Diversity & Ethnic Minority Psychology, 15*, 265–274.

Narain, A. K. (1965). *Alexander and India*. Greece & Rome, *12*(2), 155–165.

National Institutes of Health [NIH]. (2014). *Brain Research through Advancing Innovative Neurotechnologies (BRAIN) Initiative*. Retrieved October 5, 2016 from https://braininitiative.nih.gov/pdf/BRAIN_brochure_508C.pdf

Panganamala, N. R., & Plummer, D. L. (1998). Attitudes toward counseling among Asian Indians in the United States. *Cultural Diversity and Mental Health, 4*, 55–63.

Patel, S. P., & Gaw, A. C. (1996). Suicide among immigrants from the Indian subcontinent: A review. *Psychiatric Services, 47*, 517–521.

Pew Research Center. (2012). *Asian Americans*. Retrieved November 15, 2016 from http://www.pewsocialtrends.org/asianamericans-graphics/

Runner, M., Novick, S., & Yoshihama, M. (2009). Intimate partner violence in immigrant and refugee communities: Challenges, promising practices and recommendations. Retrieved August 15, 2016 from https://folio.iupui.edu/bitstream/handle/10244/788/ipvreport20090331.pdf?sequence=1

South Asian Americans Leading Together [SAALT]. (2009). *Healthcare issues affecting South Asians in the United States*. Retrieved November 17, 2016 from http://saalt.org/wp-content/uploads/2012/09/Health-Care-Issues-Affecting-South-Asians-in-the-United-States.pdf

Seligman, M. E.-P., & Csikszentmihalyi, M. (2000). Positive psychology: An introduction. *American Psychologist, 55*, 5–14.

U.S. Census Bureau. (2015, July 1). *Annual Estimates of the Resident Population by Sex, Race, and Hispanic Origin for the United States, States, and Counties.* Retrieved October 11, 2016 from https://factfinder.census.gov/faces/tableservices/jsf/pages/productview.xhtml?src=bkmk
U.S. Census Bureau. (2014). *Projections of the Size and Composition of the U.S. Population: 2014 to 2060.* Retrieved November 29, 2016 from https://www.census.gov/content/dam/Census/library/publications/2015/demo/p25-1143.pdf.

Part I
History of South Asian Americans

Chapter 2
South Asian Immigration to United States: A Brief History Within the Context of Race, Politics, and Identity

Sunil Bhatia and Anjali Ram

2.1 Introduction

In late spring, the Scripps National Spelling Bee holds its championship finals. Since 1999, the children of South Asian immigrants have led the contest, prompting news headlines such as "Indian Americans dominate the National Spelling Bee" and "Why Indian-Americans dominate spelling bees" (Helm 2015; Hannun 2013), These news stories conjure up images of high achieving, model minority students who seem to be innately primed for success. Alternatively, in post 9/11 America with its increased vigilance and suspicion of what is constructed as foreign, threatening, and "the other," stories of bullying, discrimination, racial profiling, state surveillance, and hate crimes are proliferating in South Asian communities but rarely reach the orbit of mainstream news. Consider the violent attack that left people six people dead and several injured in a Sikh temple in Oak Creek, Wisconsin and the story of the young 12-year old boy of South Asian heritage in Texas who was arrested and detained without his family's knowledge because he was falsely accused of carrying a bomb (Romell 2012; Young Lee 2015). Both these discourses, one that highlights achievement and success and the other that alerts us to the experience of systematic and pervasive racism have contributed to the historical formation of identity in the South Asian diaspora. In this chapter, we draw on our previous scholarship on diaspora and identity (Bhatia 2007, 2010, 2011; Bhatia and Ram

S. Bhatia (✉)
Connecticut College, New London, CT, USA
e-mail: ssbha@conncoll.edu

A. Ram
Roger Williams University, Bristol, RI, USA
e-mail: aram@rwu.edu

M. J. Perera, E. C. Chang (eds.), *Biopsychosocial Approaches to Understanding Health in South Asian Americans*, Cross-Cultural Research in Health, Illness and Well-Being, https://doi.org/10.1007/978-3-319-91120-5_2

2001, 2004; Ram 2014) to chart out a brief history of South Asian migration to the United States.

From a geographic perspective, South Asian migrants living in the United States originate from South Asia which includes Bangladesh, Bhutan, India, Nepal, Pakistan and Sri Lanka (Schmidt 2015). However, in the context of the diaspora, the term "South Asian" is not always meaningful. Diasporic organizations are typically named "Indian American" or "Pakistani American," and so on, indicating that South Asia is a vast and varied terrain with durable and indelible cultural, religious, and political divisions. Moreover, for first generation immigrants, their identities are clearly related to their homeland nation-state and sometimes even more specifically to their local region identity (Gujarati, Bengali, Tamil, etc.). Yet the economics of the diaspora has sometimes entailed a more universal South Asian approach as Khandelwal (2002) notes that, "out of commercial necessity, grocery stores were perhaps the most powerful promoters of pan-Indian and pan-South Asian unity; a jar of pickles or a bag of rice might be used by immigrants from India, Bangladesh, Pakistan or Sri Lanka," (p. 40).

For the second generation, the label South Asian has been adopted as a marker of solidarity. Prashad (2012) points out that the term "South Asian American" refers less to a place and more to "a sense of community among children of parents from various countries of South Asia. These parents might not have that much in common . . . but their children saw the connections intuitively." (p. 13). Given these variations and ambivalences, the label South Asian needs to be employed with care. It is important to recognize and respect the differences between what it means to be Indian American vs. Bangladeshi American and not engage in homogenizing generalizations. However, in the context of the United States, South Asians as a group are often ascribed by the white majority as a racial "other" and are not always distinguished in terms of their specific regional identity or culture. Indeed, the misrecognition of Sikhs as Muslims is an example of how religious bigotry intersects with a more generalized racism aimed at South Asians. This ascription along with the fact that South Asians share many cultural values, norms and practices means that it is possible to talk about a greater South Asian diaspora that encompasses immigrants who trace their heritage to the subcontinent of South Asia and those who are considered "twice migrants" as they and their ancestors migrated from South Asian countries to Africa, the Caribbean, Europe and the Middle East (Bhachu 1985). Immigrants of Indian descent form the largest South Asian group in the United States and much of the research literature and documentation focuses on the lives of Indian Americans. Consequently, in this chapter, while we inevitably draw upon this existing research on the Indian American diaspora, we focus on key themes that impact South Asian diasporic communities in general. First, we briefly examine South Asian immigrant journeys to the U.S. that occurred during the height of British colonization and were mainly composed of labor migration before the partition of the Indian subcontinent. In particular, we examine the migrant journeys undertaken by South Asians after the Immigration and Nationality Act/Hart-Celler Act of 1965, when they primarily arrived in the U.S. as students and highly educated professionals, working as doctors, engineers and computer scientists. Second, we examine how South Asian immigrants have deployed and internalized a model minority discourse to succeed and assimilate in the U.S. In this section, we also analyze the experiences of racism and discrimination experienced by South Asian immigrants particularly in the context of post 9/11 America. Finally, we conclude by looking at some of the ways in which first, second and subsequent generations in the South Asian diaspora creatively and politically engaged with their identity.

2.2 Early South Asian Immigration Journeys

In the mid-1800s the oriental imagination of the West resulted in a circuit of a small number of Indians coming to the United States as cultural ambassadors. The fascination with Indian mysticism and spirituality encouraged students and academics in a cultural exchange (Shukla 2003; Bald 2013, 2015). Perhaps the most venerated visitor from South Asia was Swami Vivekananda who visited Chicago in 1983 and ushered in the trend of adopting Indian spiritual practices in the United States that continues today. According to Bald (2015), American marketers used:

> …ideas and images of "India"—largely blurred together with the Middle East and North Africa—to make their goods and entertainments more alluring. Consuming goods, reading stories, watching performances, and witnessing "natives" from "the East" gave ordinary Americans access to something that was simultaneously exotic and sophisticated. Silks, perfumes, rugs, and hookahs, along with yoga, mystic philosophies, and tales of far off colonies, deserts, and jungles, all connected Americans to a world they imagined as adventurous, magical, spiritual, free from constraints, and ripe with possibility for refashioning themselves and their relation to the world (p. 28–29).

Despite this trend of consuming goods from India and seeking spiritual enlightenment by upper-and middle-class Americans, South Asian migrants who arrived on American shores to toil in the lumberyards and railroads were not welcomed in the United States. This rejection of South Asians manifested itself in exclusionary immigration policies, persecution, and violent acts of racism towards South Asian workers.

West Coast Immigration At the turn of the twentieth century, one of the first significant groups of South Asian migrants to settle in North America arrived on the Pacific coast. Between 1905 and 1912, several thousand South Asian male labourers migrated to the West coast ports in North America (Rangaswamy 2000). Many worked on the railroad construction and the lumber mills of Bellingham, Washington near the Canadian border. During this time, the larger Indian sub-continent was under British Imperial rule and immigrants from British India were categorized as "other Asians." A substantial number of these first South Asian workers in North America were Punjabi Sikhs, and were mostly young farmers and experienced soldiers who had fought in the British army (Bhatia 2007). Punjabi soldiers travelled across East Asia and into North America finding employment in the lumber and agricultural industries (Sohi 2014). On the other hand, Punjabi farmers faced high taxation and rural indebtedness in British India. Such economic hardships were exacerbated by population expansion and social factors, such as inheritance by male heirs, that led to unsustainable fragmented land holdings. Furthermore, population expansion and famines and epidemics such as cholera, plague, and smallpox added to the devastation and male family members were pressed to seek out sources to support their families (Sohi 2014). They then migrated from Washington and Vancouver to California which was followed by an increase in the direct immigration of the Sikh farmers from Punjab to California in the early 1900s. The young Sikh men who worked in the cotton farms and orchards of California were mostly in their early twenties and came from the Hoshiarpur and Jullundur districts of Punjab. These Punjabi men working in the agriculture areas of Sacramento and San Joaquin Valley soon distinguished themselves as good workers (Jensen 1988; Leonard 1992). Through hard work and thrift and with a tight community network, the farmers rapidly moved from being labourers to leasing land from the local banks. In a few years, the Punjabi diaspora began to grow in the agricultural areas of Sacramento, San Joaquin Valley, and the Imperial Valley, and the Sikh migrants began to form small residential communities in many parts of California. By 1912 many of the farmers began to pool their assets and money to lease large acres of agricultural land (Jensen 1988). They conducted their agriculture business as a collective unit and divided their costs and profits between themselves. The Sikh migrants' business meetings with the bankers usually occurred through a spokesperson, and soon they earned reputations as excellent negotiators. Some of the Sikh farmers also earned the title of the "Rice Kings of Colusa County" (Jensen 1988, p. 39).

Although the Punjabi migrants experienced success, incidents of prejudice and racial discrimination from Americans occurred. In 1910, *The Holtville Tribune* printed an article on barring Hindus from settling in California (Leonard 1992). Both the people and the press often referred to the Sikh migrants as the "Hindu undesirable," "menace to the whole valley" and "ragheads" (Leonard 1992, pp. 45–49). When the Punjabi men gained reputations as good farmers, the attitudes of banks and government officials generally changed. Over time, the incidents of overt racism, harassment and prejudice against the Sikhs lessened, and they were perceived as "dependable" neighbours. (Leonard 1992, p. 59).

The Alien Land Law of California, passed in 1913, disqualified all foreigners and non-citizens from owning or leasing land. Most Sikh farmers were able to overcome the law by forming business partnerships with Anglo lawyers and judges in California and Arizona. Verbal understandings were also often formed between Anglo farmers, bankers, and lawyers, who held land in their own names for Punjabi farmers. For example, Holtville Bank earned the name "Hindu Bank" (Leonard 1992 p. 52). Furthermore, due to miscegenation laws in most states in the U.S., Sikh men were barred from marrying white women. Subsequently, Punjabi men married Mexican women, who had often been uprooted by the Mexican revolution and worked in the cotton fields of Southern California. The Punjabi-Mexican marriage alliance developed rapidly and expanded into a complex network of relationships.

Overwhelmingly, the wives of Punjabi men in Imperial Valley were Hispanic. Leonard (1992) writes that most of these marriages involved some courtship, and women had some choice about whom they wanted to marry. As the Punjabi-Mexican diaspora expanded, the Mexican women played a role in arranging marriages for their friends with eligible Punjabi men (Leonard 1992). The marriage between Punjabi men and Mexican women were shaped by love, convenience, loyalty, familial ties and by religious, linguistic and cultural differences.

East Coast Immigration A lesser-known trajectory of early South Asian migration was the arrival of small groups of Muslim traders from Bengal at Ellis Island. Bald (2013) has documented this arduous and relatively invisible migrant journey of these traders that has contributed to the formation of the South Asian diaspora in his recent book *Bengali Harlem.* In contrast to the South Asian diaspora on the West Coast of the country, the groups of Bengali Muslim peddlers responded to the American demand for silk and other "oriental" goods and made their way through Ellis Island in the 1880s. Later on, beginning around the time of World War I, hundreds of Indian maritime workers escaped into the East coast waterfronts. They had been working as indentured labourers at the mercy of British sea captains and took the opportunity of docking at American ports to free themselves of their brutal work conditions. Like the Punjabi immigrants on the West coast, these Indian Muslim traders married women of other ethnicities, such as Creole, Puerto Rican, and African American. They adapted and integrated themselves with the communities of color in the United States. Unfortunately, most of the migrants who arrived after 1917 were undocumented and there is limited archival data on them. Yet, as Bald asserts, their presence is chronicled in the many oral histories in working class migrant communities.

The immigration and citizenship policies of the U.S. in the past 200 years fostered "racial regimes" that were intended to keep "slaves," "indentured laborers," and non-European "foreigners" as aliens and outsiders (Mohanty 1991). In 1917, South Asian immigrants were restricted by the Asiatic Barred Zone Act. In 1924, the Oriental Exclusion Act suspended labor immigration from mainland Asia. In 1934, the Tydings-McDuffie Act restricted Filipino immigration to the U.S. (Mohanty 1991). Citizenship through naturalization was denied to all individuals of Asian descent from 1924 to 1943. Such Exclusion Acts sought to ensure that the flow of non-European immigration was contained, and that these immigrants were allowed only to meet the demands of the fluctuating U.S. labor markets. Consequently, South Asian migration to the U.S. came to a nearly complete halt. For instance, by the 1930s, Indians in the U.S. were mostly Pacific coast farmers, numbering roughly 3000 (Rangaswamy 2000). There were approximately another 1000 South Asian skilled workers, merchants, and traders in the U.S. Others in the South Asian immigrant category included about five hundred students scattered throughout the U.S., and approximately 30 *swamis*, or holy men.

2.3 The Immigration and Nationality Act of 1965

After the passage of the Immigration Act of 1965, South Asian immigrants were predominantly students and professional and technical workers. This group of South Asian professionals quickly obtained prominent positions in many areas of U.S. culture, including positions in the medical, engineering, scientific, and other professional fields. For instance, within business enterprise, Asian Indians operated 28% of U.S. motels and hotels in the U.S. (Helweg and Helweg 1990).

At least two fundamental reasons for the immigration reform of 1965 have been noted (Prashad 2000). First, President Kennedy sought to increase the number of highly skilled immigrants in order to use their technical expertise and provide the U.S. with a competitive edge against the technological advances being made by the USSR at the time. The second reason for this reform was to reverse the belief that the U.S. was a racist nation. Under this new immigration law, the primary group of South Asians came from India, and these post-1965 immigrants were trained as medical doctors, engineers, scientists, university professors, and doctoral and post-doctoral students in science-related disciplines including chemistry, biochemistry, mathematics, physics, biology, and medicine. Between 1966 and 1977, 83% of Indians who migrated to the U.S. were highly skilled professionals and were comprised of approximately 20,000 scientists with Ph.D.'s, 40,000 engineers, and 25,000 doctors, and transitioned to elite (Prashad 2000; Rangaswamy 2000). This wave of professional Indians immigrants settled in suburban diasporas in towns and cites all across the U.S.

Subsequently, under the family reunification provisions of the immigration policies, family members from the South Asian sub-continent also started arriving. This pattern of relationship-driven migration expanded the demographic profile of South Asian migrants. By the 1980s, the technically educated class of migrants decreased and was complemented by South Asians who invested in motels, worked in family business, the service sector, and other low-wage jobs (Prashad 2000). For instance, in the 1990s, there was a surge in Bangladeshi immigrants who were less educated and settled in cities such as New York, Boston, Dallas, and Houston (Rahman 2010). Using the 2000 census data, Dutta and Jamil (2013) state that the highest concentration of Bangladeshis living in the United States is in New York City. Of this population in the city, 44% live on less than $35,000 and 22% live below the U.S. declared poverty line. Further, Dutta and Jamil (2013, p. 172), maintain that, "among the low-income Bangladeshis in New York City, most work as restaurant workers, as cab drivers, in convenience stores, and in service industries such as hotels." The preponderance of South Asians working as taxi drivers in New York City is another example that belies the notion that the South Asian diaspora in the U.S. is solely composed of a professional class (Das Gupta 2006; Matthew 2008). More recently, the increasing presence of older adults who are immigrating through the family reunification provision, has added another demographic layer to the community. Bhattacharya and Shibusawa (2009), state that "between 1990 and 2000, Asian Indians aged 65 and older increased by 169% (from 23,004 to 62,089) in the total

U.S. population" (p. 447–448). Research examining the vulnerabilities, stresses, and coping mechanisms of older South Asians point to the unique challenges both for the immigrant families themselves and for public health policy as a whole (Tummala-Narra et al. 2013).

The South Asian American diaspora today includes both educated upwardly mobile professionals and an increasing number of people from the working class. They are also a multi-generational group that encounters the racialized hierarchy that is deeply embedded in U.S. society. Yet, the success stories of the post-1965 migrants who arrived to the U.S. as students and professionals has contributed to an enduring discourse of the South Asian diaspora as a model minority group. Much of this narrative glides over the difficulties of surviving and coping as a non-white immigrant community. The following section examines how these ideas of success and achievement persist to create powerful mythology for thc construction of identity in the South Asian diaspora.

2.4 Model Minority Discourse

Racial identity development in middle-class South Asian communities in the U.S. reveals that they express an ambivalence towards their racial identity and this point has been well documented by several scholars (George 1997; Koshy 1998; Mahalingam 2012, Maira 2004; Prashad 2000). By employing and constantly reproducing the model minority discourse, post-1965 immigrants who are part of the professional class make attempts to reposition their difference as being the same or equal to the dominant majority. This effort to establish sameness by using a model minority discourse also means that many participants are reluctant to see themselves as a racially distinct community that is different from white America. Koshy (1998) observes, "The model minority position has increasingly come to define the racial identity of a significant number of South Asian Americans; it depends on the intermediary location of a group between black and white and holds a particularly powerful appeal for immigrant groups" (p. 287). The model minority discourse provided the interpretive arc across which the post-1965 immigrants inscribed their sense of self, their constructions of culture, and their aspirations for future generations.

In their book, *The Myth of Model Minority: Asian Americans Facing Racism*, Rosalind Chou and Joe Feagin (2008) write about a young Chinese American woman named R.W.– who murdered her mother by strangling her. R.W was a school valedictorian, a talented musician and was studying at prestigious Ivy League university. The authors note that her crime received little attention from the press, but the incident deeply unsettled the Asian American community in which R.W. and her parents lived. Chou and Feagin further write that R.W.'s failure to complete her degree at the Ivy League school may have provoked her to commit suicide on several occasions and may have also compelled her to murder her mother. Chou and Feagin (2008) observe that R.W.'s "demeanor was quiet, which likely suggested to white outsiders only a stereotyped Asian passivity. The white-created 'successful model minority' stereotype made it difficult for non-Asians around her to see her illness and encouraged silence among the Asian Americans who knew her" (p. 1). The authors argue that many Asian American immigrants view their acculturation within the United States through a strong "white racial frame" (Chou and Feagin 2008, p. 4). The white racial frame positions Asian Americans as high achievers, model minorities, with special aptitude for math, science, and engineering. An important part of this racial framing is the view that Asian Americans don't experience racism or racial barriers in the American society. Chou and Feagin explain:

> "… such analyses may be correct in regard to a certain type of success measured by particular socioeconomic indicators for Asian American groups as a whole, but not in regard to the socio-economic problems faced by large segments within these groups or in regard to the various forms of racial discrimination that most Asian Americans still face in their daily lives" (p. 12).

The model minority myth described by Chou and Feagin is applicable to the collective mindset of the post-1965 Indian diaspora. Both professional and non-professional Indian immigrants tend to be ambivalent about the racial and ethnic discrimination they face at work and in their daily lives. The model minority myth was first created in the 1960s as a response to the introduction of the civil rights movement, and the larger demands from the African American and Mexican Americans to end discrimination and be treated as equal citizens. As a response to the demands, several white scholars, politicians, and journalists conceived the model minority myth in order to "allege that all Americans of color could achieve the American dream—and not by protesting discrimination in the stores and streets as African Americans and Mexican Americans were doing, but by working as 'hard and quietly' as Japanese and Chinese Americans supposedly did" (Chou and Feagin 2008, p. 12).

The South Asian American diaspora adopted this version of this assimilation narrative and conformed to the model of acculturation that did not interrogate the systemic racism on which this model is based. Once professional South Asian migrants were in American universities, they began to rely on their advanced education, educational competence, professional networks, strong work ethic and savings to build their economic and cultural capital. Prashad (2000) notes that the members of the post-1965 migration "came without access to or holdings of large amounts of capital (in dollars), thereby ensuring that their place in the middle class was to be secured entirely by current income (and the moderate savings from that income)" (p. 101).

The first author, in his book *American Karma: Race, Culture, and Identity in the Indian Diaspora*, outlines three important facets of the model minority myth (Bhatia 2007). First, many South Asian immigrants, such as Pakistani-Americans, Bangladeshi-Americans, Indian Americans and Sikh Americans believe that they are talented, work hard, and have made it in America solely on their merit. The idea here is that through hard work and cultural values, model or "good" minority communities can rise above their difficult circumstances. Consequently, minority communities that may not have a plethora of success stories are simply seen as lazy, lacking in the right cultural values, not naturally bright, and enjoy being dependent on welfare. Many South Asian immigrants in America neglect to acknowledge that back home they were part of an educated middle class and that they were cherry picked by the state to gain entry in the U.S. (Bhatia and Ram 2001, Prashad 2012). They then furthered their advantages by acquiring a world-class education subsidized by university scholarships. This largely "free" education then propelled them into a professional well-paying, white-collar class, along with other symbols of success such as fancy cars and palatial houses in exclusive suburbs. Educated, professional Indian immigrants, for example, have a different economic and educational starting point than many other low-income, working class minorities in the U.S. It is inappropriate to compare the achievements of a small group of selective, elite professionals to the educational and economic attainments of other underrepresented minority groups who have been oppressed and marginalized for centuries.

Second, the model minority myth perpetuates the idea that Asian migrants, irrespective of their individual aptitude and social class origins, have it in their cultural DNA to become highly accomplished, doctors, engineers, mathematicians, scientists, and business executives (Chou and Feagin 2008). For example, by stubbornly clinging to the model minority myth, what is not recognized by the larger Indian "middle class" diaspora is that there are thousands of working class Indian immigrants in the U.S. who are working as janitors, gas-station workers, taxi-cab drivers, motel maids, and as undocumented workers in Indian restaurants.

Third, adopting the model minority myth also implies being silent about experiences of color, class, sexuality, race and racism (Mazumdar 1989; Mahalingam et al. 2006). Despite achieving tremendous economic success in the United States, South Asian professionals experience varying levels of racism and discrimination in their workplace and their suburban communities. For instance, the skin color, *bindi*, sari, food, gods and goddesses and "thick accents" of professional Indians invite racial attacks. Indian migrants interviewed by the first author spoke about their encounters with racism, but then deflected it by giving the following reasons: "every culture discriminates," "look, Indians are racists as well," and "it is human nature to marginalize others" (Bhatia 2007). Following the model minority myth also involves shunning any attempt to form political alliances with other "unmodel" minorities such as Blacks and Hispanics. Instead model minority groups often seek alliances with the dominant white, upper-class majority. Being a model minority thus presents a complex paradox where you are required to negotiate your identity as being both a "model citizen" and as a cultural and racial "minority." Muninder Ahluwalia (2011), a Sikh American woman raised in the U.S., describes the paradox of being a model minority:

> In the predominantly White suburbs where I was raised, I saw myself as an American girl and kept the Indian and Sikh cultural aspects of my identity hidden from those around me. Still, due to my appearance, I was subjected to insults, being afraid for myself and my family. I was treated like a perpetual foreigner, despite being born in the United States. In the school, by all outward appearances, I was the model Asian student who was academically successful, well behaved, and excelled at playing the violin (p. 42).

Mahalingam (2012) points out that model minorities usually internalize their sense of ethnic pride and this feeling of being successful in a foreign country becomes a source of resilience and also gives migrant groups legitimacy in the eyes of the dominant groups. However, if they experience discrimination on an everyday basis, "despite being model minorities, the impact of such treatment on the psychological and physical well-being could be severe" (p. 301).

2.5 South Asians and the Politics of Race in a Post 9/11 America

Prior to 9/11 there were many upper-class, privileged South Asian immigrants who had believed that they had achieved full "cultural citizenship" and "integration" in America. There is no doubt that racist rhetoric, abuse and attack have always been directed at South Asians. An early example is the horrific attacks on South Asian migrants in 1907 by white workers who felt threatened that the former were taking away their jobs generated the following statement in the local newspaper editorial, "The Hindu is not a good citizen. It would require centuries to assimilate him, and this country need not take the trouble" (cited in Lee 2015, p. 79). A more recent example of racist attacks on the South Asian community can be seen in the violence perpetrated against women and girls wearing *bindis* by the hate group, Dotbusters in the late 1980s. However, by and large, the status of the South Asian diaspora as a model minority eventually ensured a sizable proportion of them a slice of the American dream with homes in suburban enclaves and the requisite middle-class material comforts to send their children to college.

Yet, the single, cataclysmic, political event of 9/11 upturned their taken-for-granted acculturation process and migrant identity. Suddenly and quite dramatically, they moved from a relatively comfortable sense of belonging to an uneasy state of being an outsider, and a threatening one at that. South Asians with their diverse religious and cultural identities such as Muslim and Sikh and their racial and ethnic positioning as non-white minorities have become increasingly vulnerable to baseless suspicion, bigotry, and xenophobia. Their claim to citizenship has been called into question provoking everything from stereotyping and social exclusion to state-sponsored surveillance and violent hate crimes.

Citizenship as a legal concept has typically been formulated in political and civic terms and guarantees individuals certain constitutional rights and protections from the nation state. As Maira (2009) notes:

> The state defines the "citizen" as someone who embodies values central to the national social order and economic system; for example, as productive, consuming individuals who subscribe to a capitalist ethos of work and meritocracy, as loyal subjects willing to bear arms for the nation, and as heterosexuals who will marry and reproduce the family as a unit. (p. 84).

Cultural citizenship, on the other hand is anchored in perceptions about outsiders and insiders, patriots and terrorists, safe and dangerous spaces, and so on. Particular historical and social forces have shaped the practices and performances of citizenship, and norms about appropriate citizenship are often determined by groups that are in power (Bhatia 2011; Flores, 2003; Isin and Turner 2007; Maira 2009; Mohanty 1991; Rosaldo 1994). Siu (2001) describes cultural citizenship as the "behaviors, discourses, and practices that give meaning to citizenship as lived experience" within an "uneven and complex field of structural inequalities and webs of power relations" (p. 83). Cultural citizenship, then, is both normative and exclusionary and designed to marginalize, disregard, and even punish groups who are seen as racially and culturally different. Historically, within the U.S. context, the idea of a "good citizen" has been used to refer to individuals who belonged to upper class, White, and Euro-American backgrounds. Miller (2001, p. 2) argues that "Cultural citizenship concerns the maintenance and development of cultural lineage through education, custom, language, and religion and the positive acknowledgment of difference in and by the mainstream." The consequences of not having proper and normative cultural lineage during times of political crisis can be deadly for immigrants and minorities (Bhatia 2011). The post-9/11 spotlight and media coverage had suddenly framed many South Asian male adults as being part of the terrorist/enemy camp. Their physical resemblance corresponded to a generic idea in the American imaginary of "Muslim/Arab/Middle Eastern" and had made them vulnerable to discrimination and attack.

The Sikh American community and Muslim South Asians have borne the brunt of this heightened racial profiling violence. Writing about the physical and psychological terror that was unleashed on South Asians immediately after 9/11, Prashad (2012, p. 4) states that "mistaken identity was the order of the day." He elaborates that:

> . . .the bulk of the attacks took place against not only those who are of West and South Asian descent, but against small merchants and workers, those who work the lonely, long-hour jobs at kiosks or in taxis, and those who live in minority neighborhoods. . . . Anthropological and geopolitical distinctions seemed to make no difference. It was sufficient if you resembled a terrorist: olive skin, turbans, head scarves, facial hair, and other such tokens were the markers of danger. (p. 5–8).

9/11 intensified the rhetoric against Muslims, Arabs and, Middle Easterners. Maira (2011) argues that after the 9/11 attacks, "questions of religion, racialization, national identification, and citizenship have taken on new, urgent meanings for Muslims living in the United States and Arab and Middle Eastern Americans more generally, as well as South Asians and others mistakenly profiled in the post-9/11 backlash, particularly (turbaned, male) Sikh Americans, some of who were attacked or killed for 'looking Muslim'" (Maira 2011, p. 111). For example, some members of the Muslim community were subjected to wiretapping and spying in the privacy of their homes. Sikh men became highly visible because of their turban and beards and were associated with images of Arabs, Taliban, and Osama Bin Laden. After 9/11, many South Asians, including Sikhs, were also mistakenly perceived as Arabs and ascribed as being non-patriotic, belonging in the enemy camp, and non-Americans (Verma 2006; Ahluwalia 2011, Purkayastha (2005). On the surface, it would appear that these professional South Asians have "made it" in America and ultimately are structurally integrated within the larger society. Their experiences with fear, alienation and racism after 9/11, however, have forced them to reanalyze their identities as assimilated citizens of America (Bhatia 2007; Rahman 2010).

2.6 Reactions, Remixes and Resistances

Scholars have noted stressors specific to the different generations within various diasporic communities. For the first generation, the trauma due to migration is a notable stressor. For the second generation, negotiating identity and developing a bicultural or multicultural identity can be a significant stressor. For all generations, some common stressors include acculturative stress, loss of interpersonal and familial support, and racial/ethnic discrimination. Here we consider some of the ways that different generations of South Asians have responded to some of these stressors.

Cultural Belonging and Preservation For many first generation immigrant South Asian communities, cultural associations provide social support, sustain cultural belonging, and preserve cultural tradition and heritage. Both regionally- and religiously-based community associations have been formed, such as Gujarati, Pakistani, and Sri Lankan associations and Sikh associations, respectively. Typically, these community and cultural organizations have eschewed political participation in favour of cultural consolidation and celebration. For instance, Bhattacharjee (1992) reported on how the prominent Indian women's organization, *Sakhi*, which focuses on domestic violence, was not allowed to participate in an annual Diwali celebrations of the New York Indian immigrant community in the early 1990s. The play that *Sakhi* wished to stage was considered by the organizers of the commemoration as "too political and [having] no place in this exclusively cultural celebration" (p. 29). Rudrappa (2004) documented how the Indo American Center in Chicago strove towards maintaining what they considered a "non-political' image" (p. 102). Rather, they focused on fostering a sense of community among Indian Americans, helping new Indian immigrants adapt, and "enabling mainstream America to recognize Indian immigrants' potential as good citizens" (p. 108). Other well established organizations such as the North South Foundation vigorously promote educational contests including spelling and geographic bees for the Indian diaspora. Additionally, community based professional networking organizations that provide support abound. Afzal (2015) details the networking practices in the South Asian Ismaili diaspora as an example of community engagement in the diaspora that provides support to "mediate periods of risk, crises, and uncertainty" experienced by professionals in the Ismaili Muslim diaspora (p. 93). For South Asians who adopt and internalize the rhetoric of the model minority there is an "ambivalent desire to seek proximity to white culture because it signifies success and represents the norm"

(Bhatia 2007, p. 225). These various cultural and professional organizations in the diaspora enable ways in which diasporic subjectivity is formed more in cultural terms and less in racial terms. By promoting belonging and identity and providing affiliation and support they rhetorically construct and reify cultural ideas. The discourse of diaspora, as Raghuram and Sahoo (2008, p. 1) note, rejects the notion of culture as "dwelling" in favour of culture as "multilocale." George (1997) writes that most South Asians have been reluctant to cast their identities in racial terms and have instead adopted the discourse of culture to explain their model minority identities. By situating and reframing their identities through the lens of culture, most South Asians have been able to assert their identities as "Indian-American" or "Pakistani-American" and have thus formed their diasporic identities around practices and rituals of their culture from their homeland.

Diasporic journeys are about travelling elsewhere and putting up roots. They are about arriving at a new location, settling down, and having a memory and longing for "elsewhere" or another place. This longing to be at "home" or in another "homeland" is not just based on the power of nostalgia but rather is spurred by notions of belonging, inclusion, and exclusions (Brah, 1996). Diasporic movements are about border crossings, traversing across cultural spaces, but they also create "multiple identifications," "contested affiliations," and political alliances and collusions around vectors of race, ethnicity, and class (Raghu and Sahoo 2008, p. 5). Werbner (2007) argues what makes a diasporic community different from an ethnic community is that members of the diaspora communities have to be involved in collective displays of mobilizing cultural and material goods for their homeland by carrying out fundraising activities, engaging in political lobbying and participating in enactments of religious rituals, arts, and dances. The activities in the diasporas, Werbner further notes, are achieved through ritual, reinvention, and performance. For the South Asian diaspora, particularly the first generation, such activities reinforce cultural and ethnic identity at the cost of recognizing their racial positioning (George 1997).

Acknowledging Race and Reframing Identity The children of the post 1965 South Asian immigrant generation became adults in the 1980s onward and they have reshaped South Asian diaspora politics by shifting their discourse from culture to race and reframing their identities through the language of "Brown Skins," "Brown Bodies" and "Being Brown." Since then, a solidarity and a common youth culture have been forming among the second and third generations of the South Asian diaspora. For example, Maira (2002) documents the ways in which the "*desi* club culture" in New York city has created an aesthetic that sits between cultural nostalgia and urban cool (p. 190). Her research explores the ways in which *Bhangra* remix music is hybridized with hip-hop to create a popular cultural space that holds appeal for South Asian American youth. The term *desi* itself is worth examining here as it has become a commonly and variously used term to refer to people of South Asian origin. However, it has morphed and is used as an endonym or self-appellation, sometimes tongue in-cheek, to refer to people of South Asian origin both in South Asia and in the diaspora (Ram 2014). Maira (2002) notes that for second generation youth this term has crossed national boundaries. For many South Asian Americans this term has been collectively embraced to designate a collective identity. The use of *desi* popular culture as an expressive space for South Asian youth is not limited to the New York club scene and can be seen from other versions of *desi* club scenes in all the major metropolitan areas to Bhangra- and Bollywood-inspired dance shows and competitions across the United States. This kind of creative cultural appropriation and remixing plays a powerful role in how second generation South Asian Americans are forming and developing an identity that departs from the more culturally-essentialized versions of their parents.

Activism Then and Now Political activism in the South Asian diaspora is not just the purview of the second generation. Rather, accounts of activism date back to the mobilization of the *Ghadar* Party, which was started by the Sikhs in 1913 to oppose the British rule in India. The *Ghadar Party*, a revolutionary party, was inspired by the 1857 Sepoy Mutiny against the British.[1] The purpose of the party and the newspaper, *Ghadar*, was articulated in the following slogans, "Today in a foreign country, but in the language of our own country, we start a war against the British Raj. What is our name? *Ghadar*. What is our work *Ghadar*. Where will *Ghadar* break out? In India. The time will come when rifles and blood will take place of pen and ink." (Prashad 2000, p. 127). There were several courageous Punjabi migrants who played an important role in keeping the *Ghadar* party alive and functioning. Prashad (2000) writes that one important member of the party was Baba Sohan Singh. Upon arriving in Seattle from Punjab, an immigration officer questioned Sohan Singh about the cultural practices of polygamy and polyandry that existed in some parts of Punjab. In his response, Sohan Singh did not offer a straightforward denial of the existence of these kinds of cultural practices in Punjab. The officer directly confronted, asking how he could deny the belief in such marital practices if they existed in his village (Bhatia 2007). To this, Sohan Singh remarked, "Everyone has the right to reject a particular tradition or custom which he does not like" (Prashad 2000, p. 127). Prashad argues that Sohan Singh's statement is testimony to the bravery and the radical culture that existed among the *Ghadar* party.

In post 9/11 America, as mentioned above, Sikh and Muslim South Asians have been rendered particularly vulnerable. Rahman (2010), in his study of Bangladeshi Americans, talks about a "forced Muslim identity." He discusses the crises that had been created for many of the Bangladeshi Americans that he interviewed where there was a dissonance in terms of how they thought of themselves vs. how they are viewed in mainstream America. Talking about a young woman, Naseema, he writes, "for the first time in her life she had to think intensely about a part of her life and identity that she had never thought about before. The issue was so strong that Naseema could not escape the thought of it" (p. 64). Thus, after 9/11 many South

[1] Sepoy or *Sipahi* was the rank given to native Indian soldiers who were recruited to fight for the British army in India. In 1857, the sepoys, who belonged to Hindu, Muslim and Sikh religion, initiated one of the first social uprising against the British colonial government.

Asian Muslims and Sikhs, who were exposed to racial attacks and suspicion, sought to further reconstruct their "cultural citizenship" by being with family, travelling to their homes in South Asia, and forging bonds in the community by attending religious events in the mosque or the *Gurudwara* (Sikh religious temple). Sikh men became highly visible because of their turbans and beards and were associated with images of Arabs, the Taliban, and Osama bin Laden. The presence of diverse religious and cultural identities such as Muslims and Sikhs in Western societies touches on important issues of cultural citizenship and "questions of national belonging, linking it to issues of race, religion, ethnicity, labor, and particularly to the War on Terror." (Maira 2009, p. 80).

Second and third generation South Asian Americans, who have grown up in a multicultural America, have sought to create a new political identity that tackles issues of racism, xenophobia, profiling, that many "Brown" men and women face particularly in the post-9/11 climate. They are active in progressive South Asian organizations as Manavi, SAALT (South Asians Leading Together), South Asian Journalist Association (SAJA), South Asian Women's Creative Collective (SAWCC), Youth Solidarity Summer (YSS), South Asian Action and Advocacy Collective (SAAAC), South Asian Youth Action (SAYA!), Sikh Media Watch and Resource Task Force (SMART). These organizations have provided South Asian Americans with a new space to cultivate a new language of racial belonging that is largely based on political goals and a shared solidarity about being a part of a larger minority group in the United States (Prashad 2012). These new South Asian organizations are less focussed on acquiring social mobility, assimilation, and more interested in recognizing how racial politics is linked to the role of imperialism in American's empire building activities. Prashad (2012) explains: "This ideology was an invaluable resource after 9/11, and it provided the courage among some of the South Asian American groups to openly confront both the outrages of racism and the horizon of wars that emerged from Washington" (p. 19).

2.7 Place, Space, and the South Asian Diaspora

It is important to explore further how new generations of South Asian Americans can create an alternative space to reconfigure their longings, fears, and aspirations in a demographically changing America. The politics of the South Asian immigrants who adopt an assimilationist discourse are emblematic of what Monisha Das Gupta (2006) in her book, *Unruly Immigrants*, characterizes as "place-taking politics"—a type of politics that does not acknowledge or address problems such as poverty, domestic violence, racism, homophobia and xenophobia in the larger South Asian migrant community. This type of politics is largely concerned with embracing the model minority discourse, succeeding in America, and finding ways to assimilate and adapt to the larger structures of the system.

In contrast, Das Gupta (2006, p. 11) argues for formulating a stance of dissenting citizenship that she characterizes as, "space-making politics" – a type of politics that believes in social reforms that create "structures and resources that transform daily life into an arena of political contest." These contested practices of citizenship provide social and economic support to marginalized men and women of the South Asian comminutes while simultaneously working to bring change within larger American institutions such as legal and social services, law enforcement and immigration agencies and public policy workers.

In 2016, the United States elects a new president. As we complete the writing of this chapter, the political rhetoric of exclusion is heightening. The leading Republican candidate, Donald Trump has called for a ban on all Muslim immigration and suggested the creation of a national registry to track Muslims. Such xenophobic rhetoric is reminiscent of the calls to ban and expel "Hindoos" in the turn of the last century. South Asian Muslims may be the direct and immediate target of this exclusion and scrutiny. However, all South Asians, regardless of their religious affiliation, are invoked through such messages of ostracism and retribution. As "brown bodies," South Asian Americans continue to be viewed as "forever foreign." Recognizing how the South Asian diaspora is racialized allows us to better understand the constant process of contradiction, negotiation, intervention, and mediation that is connected to a larger set of political and historical practices that continue to be part of the South Asian diasporic experience.

References

Afzal, A. (2015). *Lone star Muslims: Transnational lives and the south Asian experience in Texas*. New York: New York University Press.

Ahluwalia, M. K. (2011). Holding my breath: The experience of being Sikh after 9/11. *Traumatology, 17*(3), 41–46. https://doi.org/10.1177/1534765611421962.

Bald, V. (2013). *Bengali Harlem and the lost histories of South Asian Americans*. Cambridge: Harvard University Press.

Bald, V. (2015). American orientalism. *Dissent, 62*(2), 23–34.

Bhachu, P. (1985). *Twice migrants: East African Sikh settlers in Britain*. London/New York: Tavistock Publications.

Bhatia, S. (2007). *American karma: Race, culture, and identity in the Indian diaspora*. New York: New York University Press.

Bhatia, S. (2010). Interpreting the meanings of schooling, hybridity, and multicultural citizenship in diaspora communities. *Yearbook of the National Society for the Student of Education, 109*(1), 66–81.

Bhatia, S. (2011). Lost in translation: Cultural hybridity, acculturation, and human development. *Human Development, 54*(6), 400–407. https://doi.org/10.1159/000334730.

Bhatia, S., & Ram, A. (2001). Rethinking "acculturation" in relation to diasporic cultures and postcolonial identities. *Human Development, 44*(1), 1–17. https://doi.org/10.1159/000057036.

Bhatia, S., & Ram, A. (2004). Culture, hybridity and the dialogical self: Cases from the south Asian-American diaspora. *Mind, Culture, and Activity, 11*, 224–240. https://doi.org/10.1207/s15327884mca1103_4.

Bhattacharjee, A. (1992). The habit of ex-nomination: Nation, woman and the Indian immigrant bourgeoisie. *Public Culture, 5*(1), 19–44.

Bhattacharya, G., & Tazuko, S. (2009). Experiences of aging among immigrants from India to the United States: Social work practice in a global context. *Journal of Gerontological Social Work, 52*(5), 445–462. https://doi.org/10.1080/01634370902983112.

Brah, A. (1996). *Cartographies of diaspora: Contesting identities*. London: Routledge.

Chou, R. S., & Feagin, J. R. (2008). *The myth of model minority: Asian Americans facing racism*. Boulder: Paradigm Publishers.

Das Gupta, M. (2006). *Unruly immigrants: Rights, activism, and transnational south Asian politics in the United States*. Durham: Duke University Press.

Dutta, M. J., & Jamil, R. (2013). Health at the Margins of Migration: Culture-Centered Co-Constructions Among Bangladeshi Immigrants. *Health Communication, 28*(2), 170–182.

Flores, W. V. (2003). New Citizens, New Rights. *Latin American Perspectives, 30*(2), 295–308.

George, R. M. (1997). "From expatriate aristocrat to immigrant nobody": South Asian racial strategies in the southern Californian context. *Diaspora, 6*(1), 27–59. https://doi.org/10.1353/dsp.1997.0017.

Hannun, J. (2013, May 30). Why Indian Americans d-o-m-i-n-a-t-e spelling bees. *Foreign Policy*. Retrieved from http://foreignpolicy.com/2013/05/30/why-indian-americans-d-o-m-i-n-a-t-e-spelling-bees/

Helm, J. (2015, May 25). Indian Americans dominate national spelling bees then slurred on internet. *The Washington Post*. Retrieved from https:// www.washingtonpost.com/local/indian-americans-dominate-national-spelling-bee-then-slurred-on-internet/2015/05/25/8ec01098-f414-11e4-bcc4-e8141e5eb0c9_story.html.

Helweg, A. W., & Helweg, U. (1990). *An immigrant success story: East Indians in America*. Philadelphia: University of Pennsylvania Press.

Isin, E. F., & Turner, B. S. (2007). Investigating citizenship: An agenda for citizenship studies. *Citizenship Studies, 11*, 5–17. https://doi.org/10.1080/13621020601099773.

Jensen, J. M. (1988). *Passage from India: Asian Indian immigrants in North America*. New Haven: Yale University Press.

Khandelwal, M. S. (2002). *Becoming American, being Indian: An immigrant community in*. New York City/Ithaca: Cornell University Press.

Koshy, S. (1998). Category crisis: South Asian Americans and questions of race and ethnicity. *Diaspora, 7*(3), 285–319. https://doi.org/10.1353/dsp.1998.0013.

Lee, J. H. X. (2015). *History of Asian Americans: Exploring diverse roots*. Santa Barbara: Greenwood Press.

Leonard, K. I. (1992). *Making ethnic choices: California's Punjabi Mexican Americans*. Philadelphia: Temple University Press.

Mahalingam, R. (2012). Misidentification, misembodiment and the paradox of being a model minority. *Sikh Formations: Religion, Culture, Theory, 8*(3), 299–304. https://doi.org/10.1080/17448727.2012.752679.

Mahalingam, R., Philip, C., & Balan, S. (2006). Cultural psychology of marginality: Exploring the immigrant psychology of Indian diaspora. In R. Mahalingam (Ed.), *Cultural psychology of immigrants* (pp. 151–168). Mahwah: Lawrence Erlbaum.

Maira, S. M. (2002). *Desis in the house: Indian American youth culture in*. New York City/Philadelphia: Temple University Press.

Maira, S. (2004). Imperial feelings: Youth culture, citizenship, and globalization. In M. Suárez-Orozco & D. Qin-Hilliard (Eds.), *Globalization: Culture and education in the new millennium* (pp. 203–234). Berkeley: University of California Press.

Maira, S. (2009). *Missing: Youth, citizenship, and empire after 9/11*. Durham: Duke University Press.

Maira, S. (2011). Islamophobia and the war on terror. Youth, citizenship, and dissent. In L. Esposito & I. Kalin (Eds.), *Islamophobia: The challenge of pluralism in the 21st century* (pp. 109–126). Oxford: Oxford University Press.

Mathew, B. (2008). *Taxi! Cabs and capitalism in*. New York City/Ithaca: Cornell University Press.

Mazumdar, S. (1989). Racist responses to racism: The Aryan myth and south Asians in the United States. *South Asia Bulletin, 9*(1), 47–55.

Miller, T. (2001). Introducing cultural citizenship. *Social Text, 19*(4), 1–7. https://doi.org/10.1215/01642472-19-4_69-1.

Mohanty, C. T. (1991). Cartographies of struggle. Third world women and the politics of feminism. In C. T. Mohanty, A. Russo, & L. Torres (Eds.), *Third world women and the politics of feminism* (pp. 2–47). Bloomington: Indiana University Press.

Prashad, V. (2000). *The karma of brown folk*. Minneapolis: University of Minnesota Press.

Prashad, V. (2012). *Uncle swami: South Asians in America today*. New York: The New Press.

Purkayastha, B. (2005). *Negotiating ethnicity: Second-generation south Asian Americans Traverse a Transnational World*. New Brunswick: Rutgers University Press.

Raghuram, P., & Sahoo, A. J. (2008). Thinking "Indian diaspora" for our time. In P. Raghuram, A. K. Sahoo, B. Maharaj, & D. Sangha (Eds.), *Tracing the Indian diaspora: Contexts, memories and representations* (pp. 1–20). New Delhi: Sage Publications.

Rahman, S. (2010). Imagining life under the long shadow of 9/11: Backlash, media discourse, identity and citizenship of the Bangladeshi diaspora in the United States. *Cultural Dynamics, 22*(1), 49–72. https://doi.org/10.1177/0921374010366782.

Ram, A. (2014). *Consuming Bollywood: Gender, globalization and media in the Indian diaspora*. New York: Peter Lang International Academic Publishers.

Rangaswamy, P. (2000). *Namaste America: Indian immigrants in an American metropolis*. Pennsylvania: Pennsylvania State University Press.

Romell, R. (2012, Auguest, 06). 7 killed, including shooter, at Sikh temple in Oak Creek. Milwaukee-Wisconsin Journal Sentinel. Retrieved from http://archive.jsonline.com/news/crime/reports-of-people-shot-at-sikh-temple-in-oak-creek-qc6cgc0-165059506.html.

Rosaldo, R. (1994). Cultural citizenship and educational democracy. *Cultural Anthropology, 9*(3), 402–411.

Rudurappa, S. (2004). *Ethnic routes to becoming American: Indian immigrants and the culture of citizenship*. New Brunswick: Rutgers University Press.

Schmidt, K. J. (2015). *An atlas and survey of south Asian history*. Armonk: M.E. Sharpe Publishers.

Shukla, S. R. (2003). *India Abroad: Diasporic cultures of postwar America and England*. Princeton: Princeton University Press.

Siu, L. (2001). Diasporic cultural citizenship: Chineseness and belonging in central America and Panama. *Social Text, 19*(4), 7–28. https://doi.org/10.1215/01642472-19-4_69-7.

Sohi, S. (2014). *Echoes of mutiny: Race, surveillance, and Indian anticolonialism in North America*. Oxford: Oxford University Press.

Tummala-Narra, P., Sathasivam-Rueckert, N., & Sundaram, S. (2013). Voices of older Asian Indian immigrants: Mewwntal health implications. *Professional Psychology: Research and Practice, 44*(1), 1–10.

Verma, R. (2006). Trauma, cultural survival and identity politics in a post 9/11 era: Reflections by Sikh youth. *Sikh Formations: Religion, Culture, Theory, 2*(1), 89–101. https://doi.org/10.1080/17448720600779877.

Werbner, P. (2007). The place which is diaspora: Citizenship religion, and gender in the making of chaordic transnationalism. In A. K. Sahoo & B. Maharaj (Eds.), *Sociology of diaspora: A reader* (Vol. 2, pp. 643–662). Jaipur: Rawat Publication.

Young Lee, P. (2015, December 18). Arman Singh Sarai. *Salon*. Retrieved from http://www.salon.com/topic/armaan_singh_sarai/.

Chapter 3
South Asian Identity in the United States

Anju Kaduvettoor-Davidson and Ryan D. Weatherford

3.1 South Asian Identity in the United States

3.1.1 Background

South Asian Americans are a diverse group and come from a number of countries including India, Pakistan, Nepal, Bangladesh, Sri Lanka, Bhutan and the Maldives (Shankar and Sikanth 1998). The 2010 U.S. Census Bureau reflects a huge increase in South Asian Americans in the United States over the past decade. There are 3.4 million South Asian Americans living in the United States, comprising about 20% of the total Asian American population. In 2010, the South Asian American population had nearly doubled (>80% increase) from the past decade (SAALT and Asian American Federation 2012). The South Asian Americans Leading Together (SAALT) and the Asian American Federation organizations (2012) report that South Asians are the fastest growing Asian American group in the United States. They are most heavily concentrated in five U.S. states: California, New York, New Jersey, Texas, and Illinois.

Broadly speaking and as discussed in the prior chapter, South Asian Americans immigrated to the United States in two waves. In the first wave, wealthier farmers, mostly from the Punjab territory in India, moved to the United States in the early twentieth century. They settled primarily on the West Coast for agricultural opportunities. U.S. immigration laws in 1917 and 1924 created stricter quotas for immigrants from the Asian continent, which halted the flow of South Asian immi-

A. Kaduvettoor-Davidson (✉)
University of Florida, Gainesville, FL, USA

R. D. Weatherford
West Chester University, West Chester, PA, USA

M. J. Perera, E. C. Chang (eds.), *Biopsychosocial Approaches to Understanding Health in South Asian Americans*, Cross-Cultural Research in Health, Illness and Well-Being, https://doi.org/10.1007/978-3-319-91120-5_3

grants. In the second large wave, a more diverse group of South Asian families entered the United States from India, Pakistan, Bangladesh, Nepal, and Sri Lanka after the passing of the Immigration and Nationality Act of 1965, which loosened quotas and requisite work skills for immigrants (Leonard 1997). There has also been a greater increase in South Asian immigrants in the United States over the past 15 years due to the spike in high-skilled science, engineering, medicine and finance job opportunities (Pew Research Center 2012).

South Asian Americans have been labeled “South Asian American” or “Asian American” in the United States, but many do not resonate with the latter term (Shankar and Sikanth 1998). Rather, many find their ethnic or religious group identity more salient (Jacob 1998) and often identity with their state of origin (e.g., Gujarat). Some South Asians identify with the term “*Desi*” meaning “one from our country” in Sanskrit (Park 2010). Shankar and Srikanth (1998) note that the label South Asian implies that there are common ties between the groups. Yet, many differences exist between South Asian communities.

Ibrahim et al. (1997) note that although South Asians are often categorized as one group in the United States, South Asians are a heterogeneous group with diverse languages (originating from Indo-Aryan and Dravidian language roots; Leonard 1997), including Hindi, Bengali, Gujarati, Marathi, Tamil, Telugu, Urdu, Punjabi, Malayalam, and dozens of other languages and dialects (Park 2010). Many South Asians also come to the United States speaking English.

Ibrahim et al. (1997) also state that South Asians have diverse religions, food and cultural practices. Many South Asians identify with religious identities, most commonly Hinduism (Pew Research Center n.d.), though Islam, Sikhism, Buddhism, and Christianity are also common depending on the origin in South Asia. Organized religion has been particularly important for South Asian American community connections and organizations. The Asian Women in Business (n.d) list a number of South Asian cultural centers state-by-state, such as the *India Cultural Association of Central Jersey*. These types of cultural organizations provide social support and a connection to traditional values for many South Asian Americans living in the United States.

With such varying identities and cultural practices among South Asian Americans, we start with a brief background and description of each of the major South Asian subgroups.

3.1.2 India

Asian Indian Americans are the largest South Asian American group, with 2.8 million living in the United States in 2010 (SAALT and Asian American Federation 2012). They make up a diverse group of individuals, coming from 29 states and 7 territories in India (ProximityOne 2015). There are significant differences between Asian Indian immigrants in the last half-century and the first wave immigrants in the early 1900s. The first wave immigrants, mostly from the Punjabi region of India, held a wide range of agricultural jobs from laborers to land operators. They faced discrimination and financial hardship as the cost of farming increased through the twentieth century. Despite these barriers, early Asian Indian Americans quickly established important status in their communities, and established strong ties to financial and political institutions at the time. Many Asian Indian Americans in the early 1900s also blended cultures with Mexican/Mexican American families (Leonard 1997).

Following the passage of new immigration legislation in 1965, Asian Indians from all states and territories and from varying socioeconomic classes came to the United States. Given expertise in industrial and service professions, this group of Asian Indian Americans settled in the leading states for industry including New York, California, New Jersey, Texas, and Pennsylvania (closely followed by Illinois). Also, a high volume of "international" undergraduate and graduate students have come to the United States from India in the past half-century.

South Asian Indians have been very prosperous in the United States. They hold the highest income and tend to hold higher job positions (e.g., high-skilled work, managerial positions) among foreign-born residents. However, a major tension for Asian Indian Americans in the late twentieth century was the issue of dual citizenship; India did not allow nationals to claim citizenship in the United States. This placed considerable pressure on families that eventually wanted to return to India, while also navigating the work force in the United States. Despite this conflict, many Asian Indians have become U.S. citizens (Park 2010).

Regarding religious identity, Hinduism is the dominant religion among Asian Indian Americans (Pew Research Center 2015). The Hindu religion originated in the "Indus Valley" (includes present day India and surrounding South Asian countries) around the sixth century B.C., though the original founders of the religion and the specific date of origin is unclear. The word, Hindu, was used historically to describe both the religion and people from India. Many people who identify as Hindu do not subscribe to a particular religious or spiritual belief system. Hinduism is the world's 3rd largest religion after Christianity and Islam. There are many theological belief systems within the Hindu religion; followers range from polytheistic to monotheistic to atheistic belief systems. The prominent religious beliefs in Hinduism are found in ancient Sanskrit texts and include the beliefs of dharma (rules for behavior), karma (good acts or cause/effect), samsara (reincarnation), and moksha (release from reincarnation). Many of the rules involved in the dharma also historically informed societal norms in India, including the caste system and the role of women. These religious beliefs and customs may play a role in Asian Indian health care utilization. For example, Asian Indians may believe that they are ailing due to karma and may not want to seek out health care providers.

American Hindus vary significantly in their practice. Followers often engage in traditional rituals and celebrate annual dedications to prominent gods (e.g., Diwali), though South Asian Americans experience some confusion regarding the "right" way to practice. South Asian Americans also experience significant pressure to define their religious practice compared to the prominent U.S. religion of Christianity (Leonard 1997).

3.1.3 Pakistan

Pakistani Americans are the second largest South Asian American and seventh largest Asian American group, with more than 363,000 living in the United States in 2010 (SAALT and Asian American Federation 2012). Though, Pakistani Americans are also often inaccurately categorized under the ethnic group Arab American. There are four provincial languages and one national language (i.e., Urdu) in Pakistan (Ibrahim et al. 1997). Seventy-two percent of Pakistani Americans report speaking Urdu, with many other languages spoken among the ethnic group including Punjabi (6%) and Hindi (2%) (Migration Policy Institute 2008).

Pakistan was first established as an independent country from English colonial rule in 1947–1948. With diverse influence from Asian, South Asian, and Middle Eastern cultures, the country of Pakistan was eventually the result of a struggle for an independent Muslim nation in the South Asian subcontinent; it is currently an Islamic Republic. Greater numbers of Pakistani immigrants started coming to the United States in the 1990s (Leonard 1997).

While Islam is the 3rd largest major religion in the United States, South Asian Americans only make up 25% of the U.S. Muslim population. All three major sects of Islam - Sunni, Shi'ite and Suff - are represented among South Asian Americans; however, South Asian American Muslims (predominantly those from Pakistan) make up some of the most conservative religious practice in the United States (i.e., adherence to Quran instruction for clothing, food, and commerce) and experience some of the worst anti-Muslim discrimination. Muslim cultural practice is significantly influenced by their religion, since the Five Pillars of Islam speak directly to societal practices including finances, health, family life, diet, and ways of treating people.

3.1.4 Bangladesh

129,000 Bangladeshi Americans lived in the United States in 2010 (SAALT and Asian American Federation 2012). Bangladesh was originally a part of the country of Pakistan and was established as an independent country after a civil war in 1971. It is currently a parliamentary democracy. Bangladesh is the 8th most populated country in the world but only the 93rd largest, so Bangladeshi Americans move to the United States from a densely populated country to a substantially different landscape (even in populated cities). The dominant religion among Bangladeshi Americans is Muslim, many from the Sunni sect. Bangladeshi Americans started moving to the United States in larger numbers in the 1970s and most live in New York, California, or Florida. Bengali is the prominent language spoken among Bangladeshi Americans (British Broadcasting Corporation (BBC) 2016a, b, c, d, e).

3.1.5 *Nepal*

Nepali Americans are one of the fastest growing South Asian American groups in the United States, with 51,000+ living in the United States in 2010 (SAALT and Asian American Federation 2012). Nepal was a royal kingdom between 1768 and 2008. Nepal's king was supported by India in the 1950s to withhold Chinese movement into the region; therefore, they share a close cultural relationship with India. Nepal became a Federal Republic after years of pressure toward a democratic movement in 2008. Nepali Americans have immigrated to the United States in greater numbers since the 1990s (British Broadcasting Corporation (BBC) 2016a, b, c, d, e).

As a relatively smaller group of South Asian Americans, Nepali Americans do not have nearly the political and social influence of Asian Indian or Pakistani Americans. As a result, many Nepali Americans identify with Asian Indian American groups or are, in some cases, marginalized. Hinduism is the most prominent religion among Nepali Americans (though some may identify as both Hindu and Buddhist; BBC, British Broadcasting Corporation (BBC) 2016a, b, c, d, e).

3.1.6 *Sri Lanka*

Sri Lankan Americans are a smaller, but culturally diverse, South Asian American group, with 38,000+ living in the United States in 2010 (SAALT and Asian American Federation 2012). Sri Lanka became an independent democratic socialist republic in 1948; it is the oldest democracy in Asia. Sri Lanka has a robust economic, health, and educational system. Sri Lankan Americans started immigrating in greater numbers to the United States in the 1950s. Like Nepali Americans, Sri Lankan Americans are more politically and socially isolated than larger South Asian American groups. Buddhism is the prominent religion in Sri Lanka and Sri Lankan American Buddhism is a prominent presence on the U.S. west coast (British Broadcasting Corporation (BBC) 2016a, b, c, d, e). Buddhists share many beliefs with Hinduism, including reincarnation and karma as well as a similar belief in an escape from the cycle of suffering. An important tenant of Buddhism is the practice of living correctly through the Noble Eightfold Path, which is developed most powerfully through meditative practice.

3.1.7 *Bhutan and the Maldives*

Finally, the country of Bhutan and the Maldives islands are sometimes considered a part of the South Asian group. A small country in the Himalayan Mountains, Bhutan is located between and influenced by East Asian and South Asian countries. Bhutan's government is a constitutional monarchy, with a king and Prime Minister and two-party parliament. The country has only recently opened themselves to outside tourists in 1974. The primary religion in Bhutan is Buddhism (British Broadcasting Corporation (BBC) 2016a, b, c, d, e). As of 2010, 19,439 U.S. citizens identified as Bhutanese-American. Though, there may be another 28,000 individuals from Bhutan living in the United States, having emigrated from Nepal as political refugees.

The Maldives, or Islamic Republic of Maldives, is a South Asian country in the Indian Ocean south of India and Sri Lanka. It comprises 1192 coral islands or 26 atolls spread over a large geographic area (35,000+ square miles). The government is a presidential republic. The primary religion of the Maldives is Islam (British Broadcasting Corporation (BBC) 2016a, b, c, d, e). Population numbers in the United States are often folded into population statistics for Sri Lanka; therefore, the population of people living in the United States is not officially known.

3.2 Perceptions of South Asian Americans

Despite the diverse and rich culture South Asians bring to the United States, South Asian groups may have similar personal and professional experiences in the United States that can contribute to stress and health and health care utilization. For example, narrow perceptions, stereotypes, identity, conflict, and pressure can negatively contribute to South Asian American's psychological and physical well-being (Kaduvettoor-Davidson and Inman 2013). South Asian Americans face a number of unique stressors, including dealing with external and internal stereotypes and expectations of South Asian Americans (and related experiences of discrimination), and navigating a bicultural and/or multicultural identity. These psychosocial experiences and conflicts impact the health of South Asian Americans in various ways. We first discuss the impact of common perceptions/stereotypes of South Asian Americans in this section, followed by identity pressures in the next section.

3.2.1 Model Minority Myth

South Asian Americans have been successful (e.g., occupationally and socially) immigrants in the United States (Park 2010) and many have talked about this group as an immigrant group to look to as an example or role model of success in the United States. Poon et al. (2015) describe a long history of Asian Americans being labeled as the "model minority" to discount claims of institutional and systemic racism toward other racial minority groups (e.g., primarily African Americans). This description of Asian Americans, and specifically South Asian Americans, presents them as a monolithic racial group. Researchers for years have produced research counter to the model minority myth, stating how the myth ignores the diversity within Asian Americans, the hardships they face, and the pressures this myth can put on young Asian Americans. The idea of South Asian Americans as a model minority also leads to tension and discrimination from White Americans (e.g., igniting isolationist beliefs about immigration and jobs), thus causing further experiences of alienation among South Asian Americans in the United States (Ng et al. 2007). Mukherjea (2010) notes that a view of South Asians as "model minority" is related to them being a low priority for public health and social services. She notes that there is a clear lack of attention on this group within the public health field. Chen and Hawks (1995) state that there is a stereotype of Asian American/Pacific Islander groups as being perceived as healthy and note that this is a myth with data that show higher rates of multiple illnesses within this population. Perceptions of South Asians as a model minority have negative impact on their health in direct (e.g., increased levels of stress) and indirect ways (e.g., lack of attention in health research).

3.2.2 *Navigating Experiences of Discrimination*

A common part of the South Asian American identity has been navigating experiences of discrimination in the United States. Inman et al. (2015) found that first generation Asian Indian participants experience individual, cultural and institutional forms of discrimination in the United States. These participants handled and coped with discrimination in varying ways, including avoidance and disengagement, and many participants described not being taught how to handle racism and discrimination. South Asians have a history of discrimination experiences in the United States (Park 2010), but have faced increased discrimination after September 11, 2001. Muslim Americans have been targeted and other South Asian groups (e.g., Sikhs) have been stereotyped and victimized (Kaduvettoor-Davidson and Inman 2013). In their meta-analysis of 293 studies, Paradies et al. (2015) found significantly stronger relationships between racism and negative mental health for Asian Americans and Latinos compared with African Americans. They also found that racism was significantly related to poorer mental health, general health and physical health. In their review of literature, Gee et al. (2009) found that in most studies, discrimination was related to poorer health and more consistently, discrimination was negatively related to mental health outcomes. South Asian Americans describe feeling like "perpetual foreigners" in the United States (Ng et al. 2007) and often describe feeling separate or "other." They often hear questions like, "Where are you really from?" even though they were born in the United States. Huynh et al. (2011) found that after controlling for perceived discrimination, awareness of the perpetual foreigner stereotype predicted identity conflict and lower sense of belonging to American culture for Asian Americans. They also found that awareness of the perpetual foreigner stereotype significantly predicted lower hope and life satisfaction for this group. Lower sense of belonging, hope and life satisfaction can have an impact on South Asian Americans' health.

Nadimpalli et al. (2016) found that Sikh Asian Indians who wore turbans/scarves reported higher levels of discrimination than those who did not wear turbans/scarves. They also found that discrimination is significantly related to poorer self-reported physical and mental health. In their meta-analysis, Pascoe and Richman (2009) found that perceived discrimination has a significant negative effect on both physical and mental health and produces significantly heightened stress responses. They note that higher levels of perceived discrimination are related to participation in unhealthy behaviors and nonparticipation in healthy behaviors. Carter (2007) proposes that racism and race-based traumatic stress is related to emotional trauma (Carter and Sant-Barket 2015). In summary, negative perceptions and overt discrimination of South Asian Americans contribute to poorer physical and mental health outcomes.

3.3 South Asian American Identity

3.3.1 Navigating a Bicultural and Multicultural Identity

South Asian Americans growing up in the United States navigate a bicultural identity. They develop a racial and ethnic identity and may also have other demographic influences on their identity development (e.g., gender, sexual orientation). Level of acculturation, despite immigration status, may also influence one's identity.

Ibrahim et al. (1997) describe person of color identity development models that can be applied to South Asian Americans. They note that American-born and immigrant-born South Asians may have different factors impacting their identity (e.g., immigrants may have colonization history that impact their identity). Ethnic identity describes how connected one feels to his or her country of origin, while racial identity is related to feelings of connection with the social construct of race.

Ethnic and racial identity develops over time and may be influenced by place and experiences. Many ethnic identity models begin with a Pre-encounter or Conformity Stage in which an individual blindly accepts the dominant culture. Ibrahim et al. (1997) note that South Asian immigrants may be more accepting of cultural differences and the "American dream" than other groups and they may not experience a Pre-encounter or Conformity Stage as outlined by other ethnic identity models. In this way, South Asians may have an idealized sense of the United States. In the Dissonance Stage, the immigrant generation may have experiences that hinder their success and acceptance into American culture. These type of experiences and awareness may make South Asian Americans question more of the dominant culture than previously. Ibrahim et al. (1997) describe the next stage, the Resistance and Immersion Stage, and note that in this stage, the South Asian immigrant may experience a crisis. They may go back to their South Asian values and experiences and reject the "mainstream" American values in a recommitment to their South Asian roots. Following this, in an "Introspection Stage," South Asians may reflect on their traditional South Asian beliefs and values and may start recognizing positive elements of the dominant culture. In this stage, South Asians may reach out to other Americans and begin to build bonds with them. In the final stage of internalization and commitment (or synergistic articulation and awareness; Atkinson et al. 1998), South Asians may have concerns for their South Asian group as a whole and others as well.

Kim (1981, 2001) describes a five-stage racial identity development from an Asian American perspective. In the case of South Asian Americans, individuals would form an ethical awareness and identity through their family of origin. Next, a South Asian American would identify more with the dominant White group and actively try to conform and assimilate to this identity. Following this, individuals may awaken to social political consciousness through realization of discrimination experiences. In this phase, South Asians may begin to align with and cooperate with other marginalized groups in the United States. Next, there is a redirection to Asian American consciousness. In this stage, a sense of pride for the South Asian identity is developed within. Finally, in the Incorporation stage, South Asian Americans, develop a "healthy self-concept," which helps them interact with others both within and outside of their own race.

It is common for people to go back and forth and experience different identity stages based on experiences. South Asians who immigrate to the United States and who are born in the United States go through racial and ethnic identity development as they encounter the dominant culture in the United States and navigate their own feelings and identity. Navigating racial identity can be a stressful experience and related to negative health outcomes.

Traditional South Asian culture is typically community focused and hierarchical in nature (Hofstede et al. 2010; Deepak 2005). U.S. culture is typically more individualistic, causing conflict in different areas of South Asian Americans' lives. South Asian Americans may struggle with individualistic choices and family and community expectations and desires. This can be a struggle in a number of areas including career choice and relationship choices (Kaduvettoor 2010). Iwamoto et al. (2013) note that discrimination, community factors, and parental factors all played a significant role in Asian Indian's identity development. They found that Asian Indians' context during multiple developmental time periods (e.g., emerging adulthood) impacted their racial and ethnic identity development and continued to impact them throughout their lifetimes as new challenges emerged (e.g., how to raise third-generation children). In their content analysis of research on South Asians in the United States over the last 30 years, Inman et al. (2014) note challenges experienced by this group related to cultural values and intergenerational conflict, workplace discrimination, acculturative stress, ethnic-racial identity, domestic violence, substance abuse, mental health, and racial discrimination.

South Asian immigrants often worry about their children's upbringing, loss of culture, and their bicultural experience (Inman et al. 2015). Deepak (2005) notes that parenting is impacted by the migration experience and South Asian identity. For example, rigid or narrow parenting can be related to intergenerational conflict for South Asians in the United States partly because of lack of communication and parental control over issues including education, dating, marriage and sexuality. South Asian families may be more nuclear in the United States than in South Asia and parents are confronted with many different cultural and social norms in the United States. South Asian American families have to navigate a new context as they raise families in the United States.

South Asian Americans may also have multiple minority identities that may contribute to stress. For example, for South Asian Lesbian, Gay, Bisexual, or Queer (LGBQ) individuals, heterosexist discrimination, racist events, and internalized heterosexism were correlated positively with psychological distress (Sandil et al. 2015).

3.3.2 Gender

Gender roles are clearly defined in South Asian culture, with the most strict gender role expectations for the migrating or immigrating generation (Ibrahim et al. 1997). South Asian culture is traditionally patriarchal, with expectations for women to be subordinate to first their fathers, then husbands, and then sons (Ibrahim et al. 1997). Kaduvettoor-Davidson and Inman (2012) found that South Asian Indian American women perceiving supportive family environments had less sex role conflict. Specifically, they found that families who supported the personal growth, independence, and educational achievement of their daughters contributed to less gender role stress.

Fikree and Pasha (2004) note that South Asian women and girls face gender-related discrimination at every stage of their life that contributes to health disparities in South Asian females. These stressors may also be applicable to South Asians in the United States (e.g., neglect of girls, poor access to healthcare for South Asian females, sexual violence against girls). Raj and Silverman (2003) found that South Asian female immigrants are at risk for increased levels of injury from intimate partner violence. They note that lack of social support (e.g., women's family) and lack of awareness of intimate partner violence services may contribute to increased risk of injury related to domestic violence in the United States.

South Asian American women's style of coping in relationships can also predict gender-role conflict/stress (Kaduvettoor-Davidson and Inman 2012). When women restrained their emotions or avoided conflicts in intimate partner relationships, they experienced greater gender-role stress. Family conflict is also related to higher levels of psychological distress among South Asian American women, and lower family support is related to higher 12-month prevalence of psychiatric disorders, especially anxiety (Masood et al. 2009). This study also found that South Asian American women had higher lifetime rates of anxiety than South Asian American males, while women had higher levels of psychological distress than men due to lower levels of social support outside the family.

Patel (2007) also highlights the gender role double-bind South Asian American women face between U.S. racial/gender expectations and their family/community's traditional ethnic values. The author describes how South Asian American women can be stereotypically viewed as meek/passive, exotic, and submissive. Meanwhile, there may be pressure on South Asian American women to be dutiful to their family, and assimilation to mainstream U.S. culture can be seen as becoming "too American" to family. Patel argues that this can create pressure for South Asian American women to live up to two extremes that they cannot actualize. The author conversely points to the strength of South Asian American women (e.g., sensitive, inclusive, resilient, spiritual/religious) in their relationships, which helps them navigate both the family and the U.S. cultural environment.

3.3.3 South Asian American Careers

The South Asian American community includes many highly skilled professionals including doctors and engineers (Park 2010). South Asian American students tend to study science, technology, engineering, and math (STEM) (Le and Gardner 2010; Poon 2014). This may be partly due to the high emphasis on educational and professional attainment and the immigration requirements of the 1965 Immigration Act. South Asians who come to the United States are often well educated and speak English. These factors can lead to South Asian professional success in the United States, though South Asians also continue to experience difficulties in the workplace.

South Asians who pursue non-traditionally accepted careers and courses of study may experience stress related to family pressures and identity. Compared to white students in a qualitative study, Asian American (including South Asian American) students had greater worry about living up to family expectations (Saw et al. 2013). Poon (2014) found that family desire created stress and confusion among Asian American students choosing their major. These students particularly worried about not being hired in non-traditional careers due to racial stereotypes and the potential to be isolated from peers outside STEM majors. Similarly, Shen et al. (2014) found that parent pressure was related to poorer self-efficacy, interest, and expectation for traditional careers among Asian American (including South Asian American) college students. They suggested this reaction to parent pressure may be due to feeling overwhelmed or feeling the need to rebel against parents. However, a student's sense that they are living up to their parents' expectations mediated the relationship between parent pressure and positive perception of traditional careers.

Ma and colleagues (2014) expanded on the experience of Asian American students that face approval or disapproval for their major choice. In a qualitative interview that included South Asian Indian participants, students that experienced disapproval from their family experienced guilt and utilized avoidance as a coping strategy. Conversely, students that experienced approval by family typically reached a compromise with their parents by educating them about the major choice and their decision process, and they made sure to listen to and integrate their parents input into their decision.

Family and cultural values along with interests and strengths may influence South Asian Americans' career choices. Kantamneni and Fouad (2012) found that for South Asian Americans, acculturation, cultural values, and gender predicted vocational interest areas on Holland's Strong Interest Inventory. South Asian American men are more likely to choose realistic professions, especially at lower levels of acculturation. They explain that this finding is consistent with U.S. Census data that shows that Asian Americans are overrepresented in technology fields in the United States. South Asian American women, meanwhile, were more likely to choose social professions. Leong (2001) also found that lower levels of acculturation among Asian Americans (including South Asian Americans) were related to occupational stress including role insufficiency. Asian Americans with higher levels of acculturation demonstrated greater job ratings by supervisors.

Furthermore, Shen (2015) found that the more involved/supportive parents were of Asian American (including South Asian American) student's major choice, the more likely the student was to seek STEM majors. When Asian American students were focused on academic success, they were more likely to choose physical/biological science majors. When they were more focused on career prestige, they were more likely to choose business and economic majors. South Asian parents and families often have an influence on their children's career choice or may put pressure on them to go into specific professional fields.

Despite having highly skilled, professional jobs and access to health care, many South Asian Americans experience chronic health problems including diabetes and cardiovascular disease at higher rates than other groups in the United States (Misra 2013). In the next section, we will briefly discuss health care service utilization and factors related to this.

3.3.4 Health or Health Service Utilization

External and internal factors that impact South Asian American identity and contribute to increased levels of stress may impact South Asian American health or health service utilization. For example, experiences of discrimination or cultural value conflicts related to career choices, gender role expectations, marriage and family conflicts, may contribute to health concerns. Ebreo et al. (2007) state that an increasing number of researchers have noted the importance of contextual factors in ethnic minority individual's health concerns. Patel and Islam (2013) note that it is important to look at culture-specific data to understand health issues within the South Asian American community.

Conducting a three-decade content review of literature on South Asian American mental health, Inman et al. (2014) discovered specific cultural factors related to mental health and help-seeking. They found that English proficiency and number of years in the United States affected levels of depression, with newer immigrants possessing poorer English proficiency experiencing greater levels of depression. Years in the United States may also be related to health behaviors. Though South Asian

Americans already smoke less than other Asian American groups, An et al. (2008) found longer stay in the United States was related to even lower smoking rates. Relatedly, higher levels of acculturation have been related to better psychological help-seeking attitudes (Inman et al. 2014).

Inman and Yeh (2007) note that acculturative stress from the immigration process can have an impact on one's health. The process of immigration may lead to familial and intergenerational stress that may negatively impact the health of the South Asian American family. Changes in family roles, language barriers, drop in career status and earnings for some South Asian men in the United States, pressure to transmit cultural values, and differing rates of familial acculturation can all contribute to stress within the family (Inman and Yeh 2007).

Inman and colleagues (2014) also found that South Asian American women experienced greater levels of somatic (physical) psychological manifestation with higher levels of family/marital conflict and higher domestic responsibility. Similarly, Karasz et al. (2007) found South Asian American women experienced more somatic complaints than white women. For instance, they experienced more hot/cold sensation, worry about physical illness, and body pain not explained by a medical condition. The researchers found South Asian American women minimized the importance or likelihood of psychological distress.

Hahm et al. (2010) found that a high level of discrimination (e.g., name-calling, threats) was associated with negative mental and physical health outcomes for both Asian American women and men, but women had more negative mental and physical health outcomes when exposed to a lower threshold of discrimination than men. Specifically, higher levels of discrimination were associated with higher levels of depression, suicidal ideation, externalized anger, and chronic headaches. Furthermore, South Asian Americans reported higher domestic violence rates in some samples (Inman et al. 2014). As with many other victim populations, South Asian American victims of domestic violence were found at greater risk for depression, suicidal ideation, self-blame, and poor physical health.

Among indicators of psychological health, Nguyen et al. (2015) demonstrated the relationship between family promotion of cultural tradition and ethnic identity and their impact on psychological well-being for Asian Americans. With a sample of Asian Americans that was a quarter South Asian American, they found men and women experienced greater psychological well-being (i.e., purpose, personal expression, engagement) with higher family ethnic tradition. Furthermore, South Asian American women's level of ethnic identity played a role in the relationship between family tradition and well-being.

3.4 Conclusions

South Asian Americans are a very diverse group and are rapidly growing in number in the United States. Each South Asian country shares a unique history with varying languages, religions and cultural practices. Further, there are significant regional differences within South Asian countries. South Asian groups also experience the collective influence of U.S. perceptions and stereotypes as well as identity conflict and pressure. They experience internal racial and ethnic identity development and external pressures that influence their health in the United States. For example, they can face discrimination and stereotyping across multiple identities and areas of their lives, including gender role conflict and career identity. South Asian Americans also experience pressure from traditional family cultural influences and dominant U.S. cultural socialization. Evidence clearly suggests that these challenges affect South Asian American mental and physical health and health service utilization. South Asian Americans deserve greater appreciation for their cultural diversity as well as greater cultural competence among health care professionals.

References

An, N., Cochran, S. D., Mays, V. M., & McCarthy, W. J. (2008). Influence of American acculturation on cigarette smoking behaviors among Asian American subpopulations in California. *Nicotine & Tobacco Research, 10*, 579–587. https://doi.org/10.1080/14622200801979126.

Asian Women in Business. (n.d.). Retrieved December 16, 2016 from http://www.awib.org/index.cfm?fuseaction=page.viewpage&pageid=816.

Atkinson, D. R., Morten, G., & Sue, D. W. (1998). *Counseling American minorities* (5th ed.). New York: McGraw-Hill.

British Broadcasting Corporation (BBC). (September, 2016a). *Bangladesh country profile*. Available online at http://www.bbc.com/news/world-south-asia-12650940.

British Broadcasting Corporation (BBC). (August, 2016b). *Bhutan country profile*. Available online at http://www.bbc.com/news/world-south-asia-12480707.

British Broadcasting Corporation (BBC). (September, 2016c). *Maldives country profile*. Available online at http://www.bbc.com/news/world-south-asia-12651486.

British Broadcasting Corporation (BBC). (August, 2016d). *Nepal country profile*. Available online at http://www.bbc.com/news/world-south-asia-12511455.

British Broadcasting Corporation (BBC). (September, 2016e). *Sri Lanka country profile*. Available online at http://www.bbc.com/news/world-south-asia-11999611.

Carter, R. T. (2007). Racism and psychological and emotional injury: Recognizing and assessing race-based traumatic stress. *The Counseling Psychologist, 35*(1), 13–105.

Carter, R. T., & Sant-Barket, S. M. (2015). Assessment of the impact of racial discrimination and racism: How to use the race-based traumatic stress symptom scale in practice. *Traumatology, 21*(1), 32.

Chen, M. S., Jr., & Hawks, B. L. (1995). A debunking of the myth of healthy Asian Americans and Pacific islanders. *American Journal of Health Promotion, 9*(4), 261–268. https://doi.org/10.4278/0890-1171-9.4.261.

Deepak, A. C. (2005). Parenting and the process of migration: Possibilities within south Asian families. *Child Welfare, 84*(5), 585–606.

Ebreo, S., Leung, & Yi. (2007). In Leong, Inman, Ebreo, Yang, Kinoshita and Fu (Ed.), *Health psychology and Asian Pacific Islanders: Learning from cardiovascular disease, Handbook of Asian American Psychology* (2nd ed.). Sage Publications: Thousand Oaks.

Fikree, F. F., & Pasha, O. (2004). Role of gender in health disparity: The South Asian context. *BMJ, 328*(7443), 823–826.

Gee, G. C., Ro, A., Shariff-Marco, S., & Chae, D. (2009). Racial discrimination and health among Asian Americans: Evidence, assessment, and directions for future research. *Epidemiologic Reviews, 31*(1), 130–151. https://doi.org/10.1093/epirev/mxp009.

Hahm, H. C., Ozonoff, A., Gaumond, J., & Sue, S. (2010). Perceived discrimination and health outcomes: A gender comparison among Asian-Americans nationwide. *Women's Health, 20*(5), 350–358. https://doi.org/10.1016/j.whi.2010.05.002.

Hofstede, G., Hofstede, G. J., & Minkov, M. (2010). *Cultures and organizations: Software of the mind* (3rd ed.). USA: McGraw-Hill.

Huynh, Q.-L., Devos, T., & Smalarz, L. (2011). Perpetual foreigner in one's own land: Potential implications for identity and psychological adjustment. *Journal of Social and Clinical Psychology, 30*(2), 133–162.

Ibrahim, F., Ohnishi, H., & Daya, S. S. (1997). Asian American identity development: A culture specific model for South Asian Americans. *Journal of Multicultural Counseling and Development, 25*(1), 34 Retrieved from http://search.proquest.com/docview/235905903?accountid=10920.

Inman, A. G., & Yeh, C. J. (2007). Asian American Stress and Coping. In F. T. L. Leong, A. Ebreo, L. Kinoshita, A. G. Inman, L. H. Yang, & M. Fu (Eds.), *Handbook of Asian American psychology* (pp. 323–339). Thousand Oaks: Sage Publications, Inc.

Inman, A. G., Devdas, L., Spektor, V., & Pendse, A. (2014). Psychological research on south Asian Americans: A three-decade content analysis. *Asian American Journal of Psychology, 5*(4), 364.

Inman, A. G., Tummala-Narra, P., Kaduvettoor-Davidson, A., Alvarez, A. N., & Yeh, C. J. (2015). Perceptions of race-based discrimination among first-generation Asian Indians in the United States. *The Counseling Psychologist, 43*(2), 217–247.

Iwamoto, D. K., Negi, N. J., Partiali, R. N., & Creswell, J. W. (2013). The racial and ethnic identity formation process of second-generation Asian Indian Americans: A phenomenological study. *Journal of Multicultural Counseling & Development, 41*, 224–239. https://doi.org/10.1002/j.2161-1912.2013.00038.x.

Kaduvettoor, A. (2010). South Asian Americans: Perceived discrimination, stress and well-being (Doctoral dissertation). Retrieved from ProQuest Dissertations Publishing. UMI Number: 3419366.

Kaduvettoor-Davidson, A., & Inman, A. G. (2012). Predictors of cultural values conflict for Asian Indian women. *Journal of Multicultural Counseling & Development, 40*, 2–10. https://doi.org/10.1111/j.2161-1912.2012.00001.x.

Kaduvettoor-Davidson, A., & Inman, A. G. (2013). South Asian Americans: Perceived discrimination, stress, and well-being. *Asian American Journal of Psychology, 4*(3), 155–165. https://doi.org/10.1037/a0030634.

Kantamneni, N., & Fouad, N. A. (2012). Contextual factors and vocational interests in south Asian Americans' vocational development. *Journal of Career Assessment*. https://doi.org/10.1177/1069072712454699.

Karasz, A., Dempsey, K., & Fallek, R. (2007). Cultural differences in the experience of everyday symptoms: A comparative study of south asian and european american women. *Culture, Medicine, and Psychiatry, 31*, 473–497. https://doi.org/10.1007/s11013-007-9066-y.

Kim, J. (1981). The process of Asian American identity development from Sue, et al. (1998). In *Multicultural counseling competencies: Individual and organizational development*. Thousand Oaks: Sage Productions.

Le, T., & Gardner, S. K. (2010). Understanding the doctoral experience of Asian international students in the science, technology, engineering, and mathematics (STEM) fields: An exploration of one institutional context. *Journal of College Student Development, 51*, 252–264. https://doi.org/10.1353/csd.0.0127.

Leonard, K. I. (1997). *The New Americans: The South Asian Americans*. CT: Greenwood Press.

Leong, F. T. L. (2001). The role of acculturation in the career adjustment of Asian American workers: A test of Leong and Chou's (1994) formulations. *Cultural Diversity and Ethnic Minority Psychology, 7*, 262–273.

Ma, P. W., Desai, U., George, L. S., San Filipo, A. A., & Varon, S. (2014). Managing family conflict over career decisions: The experience of asian americans. *Journal of Career Development, 41*, 487–506. https://doi.org/10.1177/0894845313512898.

Masood, N., Okazaki, S., & Takeuchi, D. T. (2009). Gender, family, and community correlates of mental health in south asian americans. *Cultural Diversity and Ethnic Minority Psychology, 15*, 265–274. https://doi.org/10.1037/a0014301.

Migration Policy Institute. (February, 2008). *Spotlight on the foreign born of Pakistani origin in the United States*. Available online: http://www.migrationpolicy.org/article/spotlight-foreign-born-pakistani-origin-united-states/.

Misra, R. (2013). *Critical Health Issues Impacting Asian Indian Americans*. In G. J. Yoo et al. (Eds.), *Handbook of Asian American Health*. https://doi.org/10.1007/978-1-4614-2227-3_2.

Mukherjea, Arnab. (2010). A critical examination and revisioning of minority health frameworks, research methodologies, and intervention models addressing South Asian American health disparities. UC Berkeley: Public Health. Retrieved from: http://escholarship.org/uc/item/3q52x0n7

Nadimpalli, S. B., Cleland, C. M., Hutchinson, M. K., Islam, N., Barnes, L. L., & Van Devanter, N. (2016). The association between discrimination and the health of Sikh Asian Indians. *Health Psychology, 35*(4), 351–355. https://doi.org/10.1037/hea0000268.

Ng, J. C., Lee, S. S., & Pak, Y. K. (2007). Contesting the model minority and perpetual foreigner stereotypes: A critical review of literature on Asian Americans in education. *Review of Research in Education, 31*(1), 95–130.

Nguyen, C. P., Wong, Y. J., Juang, L. P., & Park, I. J. K. (2015). Pathways among asian americans' family ethnic socialization, ethnic identity, and psychological Well-being: A multigroup mediation model. *Asian American Journal of Psychology, 6*, 273–280. https://doi.org/10.1037/aap0000026.

Paradies, Y., Ben, J., Denson, N., Elias, A., Priest, N., et al. (2015). Racism as a determinant of health: A systematic review and meta-analysis. *PLoS One, 10*(9), e0138511. https://doi.org/10.1371/journal.pone.0138511.

Park, K. (2010). *Americans from India and other south Asian countries*. New York: Marshall Cavendish Benchmark.

Pascoe, E. A., & Smart Richman, L. (2009). Perceived discrimination and health: A meta-analytic review. *Psychological Bulletin, 135*(4), 531.

Patel, N. R. (2007). The construction of south-Asian-American womanhood. *Women & Therapy, 30*, 51–61. https://doi.org/10.1300/J015v30n03_05.

Patel, S., & Islam, N. (2013). *Emerging South Asian Americans and Health*. In G. J. Yoo et al. (Eds.), *Handbook of Asian American Health*. https://doi.org/10.1007/978-1-4614-2227-3_8.

Pew Research Center. (June, 2012). *The rise of Asian Americans*. Available online: http://www.pewsocialtrends.org/2012/06/19/the-rise-of-asian-americans/.

Pew Research Center. (2015). *5 facts about Indian Americans*. Retrieved online at: http://www.pewresearch.org/fact-tank/2014/09/30/5-facts-about-indian-americans/.

Pew Research Center. (n.d.). *Religion in America*. Available online: http://www.pewforum.org/religious-landscape-study/.

Poon, O. (2014). "The land of opportunity doesn't apply to everyone": The immigration experience, race and asian American career choices. *Journal of College Student Development, 55*, 499–514. https://doi.org/10.1353/csd.2014.0056.

Poon, O., Squire, D., Kodama, C., Byrd, A., Chan, J., Manzano, L., & Bishundat, D. (2015). A critical review of the model minority myth in selected literature on Asian Americans and Pacific Islanders in higher education. *Review of Educational Research*. https://doi.org/10.3102/0034654315612205.

ProximityOne. (2015). *America's Asian population demographic patterns and trends*. Available online: http://proximityone.com/asian_demographics.htm.

Raj, A., & Silverman, J. G. (2003). Immigrant south Asian women at greater risk for injury from intimate partner violence. *American Journal of Public Health, 93*(3), 435–437. https://doi.org/10.2105/AJPH.93.3.435.

Sandil, R., Robinson, M., Brewster, M. E., Wong, S., & Geiger, E. (2015). Negotiating multiple marginalizations: Experiences of south Asian LGBQ individuals. *Cultural Diversity and Ethnic Minority Psychology, 21*(1), 76–88. https://doi.org/10.1037/a0037070.

Saw, A., Berenbaum, H., & Okazaki, S. (2013). Influences of personal standards and perceived parental expectations on worry for asian american and white american college students. *Anxiety, Stress, & Coping, 26*, 187–202. https://doi.org/10.1080/10615806.2012.668536.

Shankar, L. D., & Sikanth, R. (1998). *A part, yet apart: South Asians in Asian America*. Philadelphia: Temple University Press.

Shen, F. C. (2015). The role of internalized stereotyping, parental pressure, and parental support on asian americans' choice of college major. *Journal of Multicultural Counseling & Development, 43*, 58–73. https://doi.org/10.1002/j.2161-1912.2015.00064.x.

Shen, F. C., Liao, K. Y., Abraham, W. T., & Weng, C. (2014). Parental pressure and support toward asian americans' self-efficacy, outcome expectations, and interests in stereotypical occupations: Living up to parental expectations and internalized stereotyping as mediators. *Journal of Counseling Psychology, 61*, 241–252. https://doi.org/10.1037/a0036219.

South Asian Americans Leading Together [SAALT] & Asian American Federation. (2012). A Demographic Snapshot of South Asians in the United States: July 2012 Update. Retried December 16, 2016 from http://saalt.org/wp-content/uploads/2012/09/Demographic-Snapshot-Asian-American-Foundation-2012.pdf

Part II
Models of Health in South Asian Americans

Chapter 4
Biological Models of Health

Namratha R. Kandula and Manasi A. Tirodkar

4.1 Medical History in South Asia and Native Medical Systems

4.1.1 Introduction of Western Medicine

Western medicine was introduced to the Indian subcontinent around 1750 along with the British colonizers. Hospitals were initially set up primarily for the care of Europeans and for some categories of "natives," mainly military personnel. However, by the mid-1850s, more hospitals and dispensaries were established for general use. Much of the work of Western medicine in the latter half of the nineteenth century was focused on preventive medicine in the form of vaccination campaigns for small pox, plague and cholera as well as sanitary management to reduce malaria (Bhattacharya 2009). At first there was much resistance to adopting public health and medical practices disseminated by colonizers but gradually, by the twentieth century, this became the norm and coexisted with traditional medical systems.

Practitioners of traditional medicine have seen the legitimacy of their knowledge challenged by biomedicine. A major issue facing traditional practitioners is whether these medical systems should be independent and self-sufficient or whether they should be supplemented by or integrated into biomedical practice. Traditional practices are distinct and are often delineated along linguistic lines – Sanskrit for

N. R. Kandula (✉)
Division of General Internal Medicine, Northwestern University Feinberg School of Medicine, Chicago, IL, USA
e-mail: nkandula@nm.org

M. A. Tirodkar
National Committee for Quality Assurance, Washington, DC, USA
e-mail: tirodkar@ncqa.org

M. J. Perera, E. C. Chang (eds.), *Biopsychosocial Approaches to Understanding Health in South Asian Americans*, Cross-Cultural Research in Health, Illness and Well-Being, https://doi.org/10.1007/978-3-319-91120-5_4

Ayurveda, Tamil for Siddha, and Arabic and Urdu for Unani. Yet, these systems were unified in their opposition to the universalizing goals of biomedicine because the status of indigenous medicine as a local tradition, not a universal science, was central in the policy decisions of the British administration. During British rule, few educational centers of indigenous systems were permitted to be established, and the push for vaccination and sanitation as public health campaigns were seen to be in opposition to the indigenous medical systems. This was primarily because preventive and sanitary measures were implemented for European troops and populations, significantly before being implemented in the mass populations, and the policies came with a systematic derision of local culture and medical systems. Thus these campaigns were seen as yet another means for political control of local populations rather than a means to health (Arnold 1993; Jeffery 1988).

4.1.1.1 Interoperability of Medical Systems Today

In the healthcare field, allopathy, or Western biomedicine (also known as evidence-based medicine), has been the norm in South Asia for the past hundred years due to colonial influence. Allopathy is regarded as modern treatment that acts fast and is convenient. Most medicines are available as pills or capsules and they act immediately.

Prior work (Tirodkar 2005) has shown that many patients turn to Ayurveda after they have exhausted all allopathic options. Some have even tried other non-allopathic options such as homeopathy and naturopathy before trying Ayurveda. Patients' anxiety about Ayurveda stemmed from their fear of being restricted from their pleasures such as meat,[1] alcohol, cigarettes, and sweet and fatty and spicy foods, all of which are considered detrimental indulgences and are characteristic of many upper-middle class and upper class individuals that live in urban areas.

Figures 4.1 and 4.2 depict the hierarchies of resort to the different medical alternatives based on perceived need and severity of illness (Rao 2006).

For minor illnesses such as cold, cough and headache, people tend to resort to home remedies before turning to allopathic or non-drug alternatives such as yoga, acupuncture, chiropractic therapy, meditation or *reiki*. For major illnesses, people usually resorted first to allopathic treatment and then used traditional medical systems or non-drug alternatives as either supportive therapy (i.e. in addition to allopathy) or instead of it if the allopathy did not work. For example, one patient observed in a traditional Ayurvedic clinic had been diagnosed with metastatic bone cancer. He was receiving radiation therapy after a course of chemotherapy at the time of his consultation and was seeking Ayurvedic medicine to alleviate adverse symptoms such as lack of appetite, nausea, and fatigue (Tirodkar 2005). The Ayurvedic practi-

[1] Ayurveda does not advocate complete vegetarianism, however more often than not, meat is restricted because it is considered to be difficult to digest.

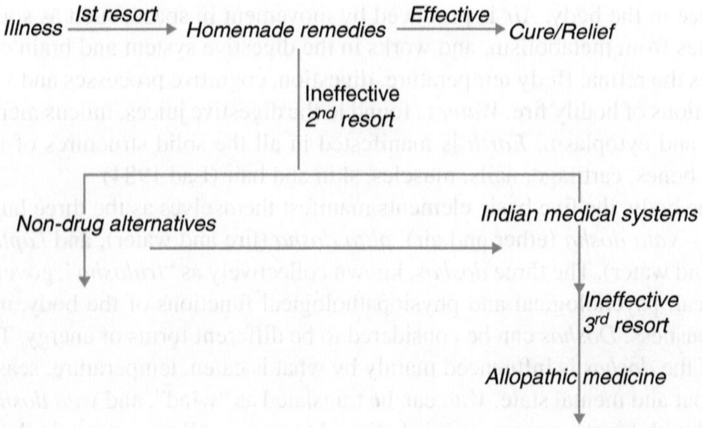

Fig. 4.1 Chart showing the pathways for hierarchy of resort for minor illness (Rao 2006). Taylor and Francis Ltd. http://www.tandfonline.com

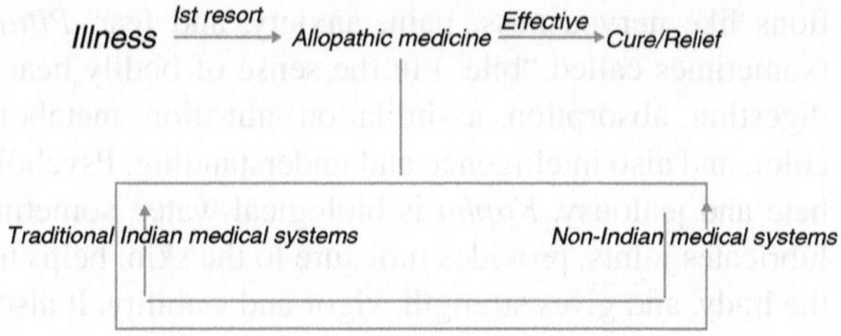

Fig. 4.2 Chart showing the pathways for hierarchy of resort for major illness (Rao 2006). Taylor and Francis Ltd. http://www.tandfonline.com

tioner prescribed a specific diet to help alleviate the symptoms in addition to Ayurvedic medicines.

4.1.2 Ayurveda

According to Caraka (2001), the purpose of practicing Ayurveda is to achieve longevity, rejuvenate the body, and maintain one's physical and mental health through use of natural substances (i.e., plants, herbs, and minerals) and regulation of lifestyle (Caraka 2001; Lad 1984). In Ayurvedic medicine, a whole person is considered to be composed of the body, mind and spirit (Caraka 2001; Frawley 1997; Larson 1993). The internal environment of the body is believed to be constantly reacting to the external environment. Disorder occurs when the internal and external environments are out of balance. The basic principle of Ayurveda is that balance in one's internal forces can be achieved by altering the diet and lifestyle habits to counteract changes in one's external environment.

In the universe and human body, there are five basic principles or elements (*panchamahabhootas*) – ether (space), air, fire, water and earth. *Ether* is constituted by any space in the body. *Air* is produced by movement in space, such as sound. *Fire* originates from metabolism, and works in the digestive system and brain cells, and activates the retina. Body temperature, digestion, cognitive processes and vision are all functions of bodily fire. *Water* is found in the digestive juices, mucus membranes, plasma and cytoplasm. *Earth* is manifested in all the solid structures of the body such as bones, cartilage, nails, muscles, skin and hair (Lad 1984).

In the body, the five basic elements manifest themselves as the three humors, or *dosha*s – *vata dosha* (ether and air), *pitta dosha* (fire and water), and *kapha dosha* (earth and water). The three *dosha*s, known collectively as "*tridosha*", govern all the biological, psychological and physiopathological functions of the body, mind and consciousness. *Dosha*s can be considered to be different forms of energy. The character of the *dosha*s is influenced mainly by what is eaten, temperature, season, sensory input and mental state. *Vata* can be translated as "wind", and *vata dosha* can be equated with kinetic energy as it is believed to govern all movement in the body. It governs breathing, blinking of the eyelids, movements in the muscles and tissues, pulsation in the heart, expansion, contraction, movement of cytoplasm and cell membranes, and single impulses in nerve cells. *Vata* also governs feelings and emotions like nervousness, pain, anxiety, and fear. *Pitta* can be translated as "fire" (sometimes called "bile") in the sense of bodily heat energy. *Pitta dosha* governs digestion, absorption, assimilation, nutrition, metabolism, body temperature, skin color, and also intelligence and understanding. Psychologically, *pitta* arouses anger, hate and jealousy. *Kapha* is biological water, sometimes called "phlegm". *Kapha* lubricates joints, provides moisture to the skin, helps to heal wounds, fills spaces in the body, and gives strength, vigor and stability. It also supports memory retention, gives energy to the heart and lungs and maintains immunity. *Kapha* is present in the chest, throat, head, sinuses, nose, mouth, stomach, joints, cytoplasm, plasma and liquid secretions of the body such as mucus. Psychologically, *kapha* is responsible for attachment, greed, envy and also calmness, forgiveness and love. Every individual has a unique constitution, *prakruti*, or proportion of the humors, which is determined at conception. The basic constitution of a person remains unchanged over the lifetime but the combination of elements that governs the continuous physiopathological changes in the body alters in response to changes in the environment.

When the humors are out of balance, they contribute to disease processes in the body and mind (Lad 1984). Diagnosis in Ayurveda revolves around accurately assessing the location and degree of imbalance between humors, tissues and wastes (internal factors), in relation to the external environment. Humoral imbalances are assessed by observing a patient's pulse, tongue, face, eyes, nails and lips. A patient is also examined by listening to sounds, lightly pressing the surface, and tapping various parts of the body. A patient is also asked several questions about the way his or her dietary habits, moods, affective reactions, memory and well-being may differ during different seasons of the year.

Treatments attempt to establish a balance between the bodily humors by elimination and neutralization of toxins in the body at both emotional and physical levels. One way an Ayurvedic practitioner treats diseases is to prescribe certain foods and liquids in accordance with the individual's humoral constitution, and the degree and nature of the imbalance. Dietary recommendations are often accompanied by the prescription of natural medicines. Medicinal substances are all natural and consist of plants, herbs, spices, minerals and stones. Ayurvedic practitioners also prescribe herbal oil massages and *panchakarma,* which is five specific procedures to cleanse the body, mind and emotions. Yoga postures and meditation techniques are often taught to a patient for spiritual development and the maintenance of mental and physical health (Frawley 1997; Lad 1984; Shanbag 1994). Sometimes a practitioner may also refer a patient to an astrologer, who will recommend the patient to wear certain gems and colors to aid in bringing about humoral balance and well-being (Lad 2002).

4.1.3 Introduction of Homeopathy

Homeopathy, or homeopathic medicine, is a medical philosophy and practice based on the idea that the body has the ability to heal itself. Homeopathy was founded in the late 1700s in Germany and has been widely practiced throughout Europe. Homeopathic medicine views symptoms of illness as normal responses of the body as it attempts to regain health. Homeopathy was introduced to India in 1839 and became popular later in the nineteenth century. There was no government control on homeopathic training and practice during the colonial period, and homeopathy was initially practiced by amateurs in the civil and military services. In 1973, the Government of India recognized homeopathy as one of the national systems of medicine and set up the Central Council of Homeopathy (CCH) to regulate its education and practice. At present, only qualified registered homeopaths can practice homeopathy in India, and homeopathy is the third most popular method of medical treatment after allopathy and Ayurveda in India. In India, there are over 200,000 registered homeopathic doctors currently, with approximately 12,000 more being added every year. The prevalence of homeopathic treatment is greater in India than in any other country (Ghosh 2010).

The concept of health and disease in homeopathy more closely aligns with the philosophies on which traditional medical systems are based in that the source of health and disease is not material but spiritual. The material life principle posits that anything which affects life morbidly must do so qualitatively and the medicine which cures diseases also does the same. Homeopathic drugs are extremely diluted substances and are not known to produce any side effects. The treatments are also very affordable and these two factors have contributed to the popularity of homeopathy (Ghosh 2010).

4.1.4 Siddha

Siddha medicine originates in South India. Texts are written in Tamil, rather than Sanskrit which is the language of Ayurvedic texts. Practitioners of Siddha medicine are called "siddhars." The basic concepts of the Siddha medicine are similar to Ayurveda, and Siddha medicine also accepts the principles of *vata*, *pitta* and *kapha*. One of the main differences is that Siddha medicine recognizes predominance of *vatham*, *pitham* and *kapam* in childhood, adulthood and old age, respectively, whereas in Ayurveda it is reversed: *kapam* is dominant in childhood, *vatham* in old age and *pitham* in adults. In the Siddha system, psychological and physiological functions of the body are attributed to the combination of seven elements:

1. *Saram* (digestive juice) *Saram* means *Prana vayu* (oxygen) responsible for growth, development and nourishment;
2. *Cheneer* (blood) responsible for nourishing muscles, imparting color and improving intellect;
3. *Ooun* (muscle) responsible for shape of the body;
4. *Kollzuppu* (fatty tissue) responsible for oil balance and lubricating joints;
5. *Enbu* (bone) responsible for body structure and posture and movement;
6. *Moolai* (bone marrow) responsible for the production of red blood cells, etc.
7. *Sukila* (semen) responsible for reproduction.

Diagnosis in Siddha is done primarily by examination of the pulse, or *nadi*, to determine the disposition of the three humors. Examination of urine is another diagnostic method and the intensity of disease is determined on the basis of urine color. If the urine is red or milky white, the disease is said to be incurable. If the urine is yellow of honey-colored, the disease is considered curable.

Siddha relies heavily on alchemy, and most prescribed medicines are metallic or mineral in nature. They are processed in specific ways to be fit for human consumption and are prescribed in minute quantities along with an adjuvant or carrier substances such as honey, clarified butter (ghee), milk, herbal extracts, ginger juice, betel leaf juice, and hot water. The adjuvant prescribed can vary by season and can modify the potency of the drug prescribed. Siddhars also believe in the influence of planetary positions and astrological calculations to assess the nature of disease and treatment regimens. Religious chants can also be prescribed in order to invoke divine blessings for the cure of diseases and to overcome the distressing effects of evil deeds in one's previous births.

4.1.5 Unani

The origins of Unani lie in ancient Greek, Arabic, and Persian medicine. Unani Tibb is also a humoral medical system and presents causes, explanations, and treatments of disease based on the balance or imbalance of four humors (*akhlaat*) in the body:

blood (*khun*), mucus (*bulghum*), yellow bile (*safra*), and black bile (*sauda*). The four humors combine with four basic qualities (*quwaat*): heat (*garmi*), cold (*sardi*), moisture (*rutubaat*), and dryness (*yabis*) (M. Shah 1966). Dominance of one of the humors in the body gives each person his or her individual temperament (*mizaj*)-sanguine (*dumwi*), phlegmatic (*balghumi*), choleric (*safravi*), and melancholic (*saudawi*) (Burgel 1976).

A practitioner of Unani is called a "hakim". Diagnosis is determined by evaluating the patient's temperament (*mizaj*); gender and age; the climate and season; the location in which he or she lives (both the geographic terrain and the specific house); and the activities in which he or she engages (type of work, type of sleep, exercise, sexual activity, diet). Specific physical diagnostic procedures accompany the discussion with the hakim regarding the patient's concerning attributes and habits. Therapy may include changes to the patient's habits and activities in order to restore balance and health in the body. Interventions by medications, massage, or surgery may be prescribed, and are discussed below.

Concern for preventive health measures are central in the Unani medical system, and there are efforts to preserve the natural healthy state of the body that exists when the humors are balanced. When the person is sick, the humors are imbalanced, and the task of the hakim is to take appropriate measures to restore balance. A hakim will observe the signs and symptoms of the imbalance, palpate the pulse, and inspect the urine and stool of the patient. A hakim will also consider the patient's age, gender, type of occupation, and habits of sleeping, diet, and exercise. The hakim also elicits the patient's description of the illness, including time of onset; changes in urination, bowel movements, eating and sleeping patterns; and any interference in normal activities, including the patient's job and/or household tasks.

Depending on the diagnosis, treatments include regimental therapy (*ilaj bitadir*): venesection (*fasad*), cupping (*mohajim*), diaphoresis (*tareeq*), diuresis (*idrar baol*), Turkish bath (*hammam*), massage (*dalak*), cauterization (*kai*), counterirritation (*imala*), vomiting (*qai*), purging (*ishaal*), leeching (*taaleeq*), exercise (*riyazat*). Other treatment options include diet therapy (*ilaaj bil ghiza*), pharmaceutical or drug therapy (*ilaaj bidawa*), and surgery (*ilaajbilyad*).

4.2 Behavioral and Clinical Implications

4.2.1 Influence of Indigenous Medical Systems on Explanatory Models

4.2.1.1 Biopsychosocial and Holistic Models

There is evidence that indigenous medical systems influence South Asians' beliefs about health and illness causation. Kleinman's (Kleinman 1980) theory of explanatory models proposes that individuals and groups can have vastly different notions about an episode of sickness and its treatment health and disease. In Ayurveda,

Siddha, and Unani, health is conceptualized as a state of balance and disease is considered a state of imbalance. While the taxonomy of balance and imbalance differ by medical system, a common explanatory principle is that balance (health) and imbalance (illness) are created by environmental, physical, psychosocial and/or spiritual factors (Andrews 2005).

Many individuals, especially those from non-Western cultures, endorse a "holistic" explanatory model of health and disease that includes biological, psychological, and social components of disease etiology, including spiritual components (Shweder et al. 1997). Ethnographic work in South Asia suggests that many communities are embedded in holistic explanatory models of health, illness, and natural processes such as childbirth and aging (Cohen 1998; Desjarlais 1992; Kakar 1982; Kurtz 1992; Lamb 2000; Obeyesekere 1981; Van Hollen 2003). For example, the process of pregnancy and childbirth are often governed by beliefs that women and their unborn children are to be treated as auspicious and are therefore treated with care and given gifts and blessings through religious ceremonies. Even among the poor, a pregnant woman should be provided with costly ceremonies to satisfy her cravings, to celebrate her fertility, and to ensure an easy delivery and birth of a healthy baby. The bio-medicalization of birth in medical facilities has been accompanied by the intensification of birth-related ceremonies, even in modern day India. Women have many dietary restrictions during pregnancy and in the post-partum period that are related to whether foods are considered to be "hot" or "cold", or have the possibility of "purgation", meaning a food that carries the risk of causing a miscarriage (Van Hollen 2003). Cohen's (Cohen 1998) work demonstrates how contemporary society in India frames cognitive decline in old age not just in terms of biology and as a natural part of the life cycle, but also as a marker of the decline of mental faculties and the joint family. Dementia is understood locally as being "hot-minded," or "weak-brained," and can transpire when an old person does not receive familial support, service (*seva*), and respect.

It is unclear if these holistic explanatory models persist after South Asians immigrate to Western countries. However, a qualitative study of South Asian immigrants in Chicago found that South Asians largely conceptualized health as a biopsychosocial process, with an emphasis on behaviors (diet), psychosocial factors (positive attitude, lack of stress), and function (lack of symptoms, ability to perform home/work duties) (Tirodkar et al. 2011). The major emphasis on diet in concepts of health is not surprising given the importance of dietary principles in preventing and treating illnesses in indigenous systems of health, such as Ayurveda and Unani, in South Asia (Andrews 2005). This same study (Tirodkar et al. 2011) also found that a subset of South Asians (20%) endorsed a holistic model of health that also included a spiritual component, such as beliefs that prayer or religious rituals help preserve health. The explanatory models of health held by South Asians appear to differ from what was found in a national U.S. survey, where only 5% of respondents mentioned psychosocial factors and even fewer (1%) mentioned spiritual factors in their concepts of health (Makoul et al. 2009).

Interestingly, South Asians' explanatory models of chronic disease, in particular coronary heart disease, diverged from their explanatory models of health; spiritual factors were rarely mentioned in disease causation. Rather, concepts about cause of chronic disease were largely thought to be stress, diet, lack of exercise, and lack of personal responsibility for one's own health (Tirodkar et al. 2011). The emphasis on stress in the explanatory models of South Asians is notable: South Asian immigrants described social isolation, intergenerational conflict, acculturative stress, and job insecurity as common sources of stress leading to chronic disease and to unhealthy behaviors (Patel et al. 2014).

4.2.1.2 Concepts of Hot and Cold

The concepts of hot and cold are also important to South Asians' beliefs about disease. Foods, bodily states and diseases are classified as being "hot" or "cold," and diseases are believed to be caused by excess heat or cold in the body. In these systems, "hot" and "cold" typically do not refer to temperature states of the food but rather to abstract qualities (Pool 1987). Certain foods, such as chicken, garlic, and cloves, are considered "hot" because they create substances in the body (such as digestive fluids) that increase the "heat" in the body. Other foods, such as yogurt, oranges, and rice, are "cold" because they dampen the digestive fire and make the body "cold." In Ayurvedic concepts, consuming certain foods can lead to a loss of balance in the humors (wind, bile, and phlegm) and cause illness. While it is overly simplistic to link hot-cold concepts to a particular condition and its treatment, it is important to recognize that this is one of the reasons that South Asians place importance not only on the nutritional value of the food, but also on its inherent nature as "hot" or "cold" (Lambert 1992). Other similar beliefs about the attributes or properties of certain foods may lead South Asian patients to follow specific dietary therapies and/or food restrictions (Mukherjea et al. 2013).

Ideas about "hot" and "cold" may influence beliefs about disease causation and dietary patterns along with aforementioned behavioral, psychosocial, and spiritual causal elements. Clinicians and health educators should elicit South Asian patients' explanatory models (i.e., "What caused your illness", "How do you think your illness should be treated"), understand how these models influence treatment options a patient may be considering, and incorporate this information into the treatment plan. This approach may improve patient-provider communication and clinical care for South Asian patients.

4.2.2 Influence of Indigenous Indian Medical Systems on Health Behaviors

India has a large number of highly trained and skilled health professionals working both within India and in other countries. Western technology and biomedical practice are trusted and widely adopted among many South Asians. However, the traditional systems of medicine are also often used, either complementarily or in preference to Western medicine. The Indian health system is characterized as "medical pluralism" where indigenous, folk and well–developed Indian and Western health systems and models co–exist (Chacko 2003; Rao 2006). Studies show that medical pluralism continues to be practiced and influences health behaviors in South Asian migrants (Rao 2006; Rhodes et al. 2008; Satow et al. 2008).

4.2.2.1 Diet

Indigenous medical systems strongly influence the food-related behaviors of South Asian immigrants (Lone et al. 2012; Mukherjea et al. 2013). There is the strongly held belief that a South Asian vegetarian diet is healthy, even though these diets have been found to be high in refined carbohydrates and saturated fat (Gadgil et al. 2015). Diet-based therapy, which means that foods have medicinal value and impact the body's physiology, draws on indigenous medical systems and is common among South Asians; a survey of U.S. South Asians found that 50% reported using diet-based therapy to improve health or treat symptoms (Misra et al. 2010; Mukherjea et al. 2013). Specific foods and spices are ascribed medicinal value and other properties (i.e. see "hot", "cold" above). Karella (also known as 'Momordica charanita', or 'bitter melon') is commonly used for treating diabetes, usually in conjunction with Western medicine (Chacko 2003; N. R. Patel et al. 2015). Spices, which are used in everyday cooking, are also used as home remedies to treat minor illnesses. A common practice is to use a pinch of turmeric in milk to fend off a cold (Krishnaswamy 2008) or *tulsi* (basil) leaves boiled in water to reduce the body's temperature if someone has a fever. Turmeric has antibiotic properties, and because turmeric by itself is extremely potent and acidic, it is consumed in milk which is an alkali medium (Lodha and Bagga 2000). Although there are no prevalence data on use of turmeric for chronic disease prevention among South Asians migrants, it is widely used in South Asian cooking and is growing in popularity as a supplement in the U.S. More recently, turmeric has garnered interest for suppression of breast cancer cells (Zhou et al. 2015) and diabetes prevention (Chuengsamarn et al. 2012).

Health care providers should recognize that South Asians place high value on many of the staple components of a South Asian diet, such as spices, vegetables, grains, and lentils, not only because of connection to cultural identity, but also for health reasons (Mukherjea et al. 2013). It may be important to explore the South Asian patient's diet-related beliefs and assess if they are using specific foods or spices for prevention or treatment or observing fasting practices for religious reasons. Because many foods are consumed as part of a staple diet, South Asians may not think of certain foods or spices as a "treatment;" thus, open-ended questions may be more fruitful. e.g. "What types of foods or spices help you control your …… (e.g. blood sugar, cholesterol, blood pressure)?" In addition, studies suggest that South Asian immigrants integrate their understanding of the medicinal value of food and spices with a Western biomedical model of "healthy" foods (Mukherjea et al. 2013). Thus, acknowledging the diversity in a South Asian immigrant diet and using both South Asian and Western dietary principles in lifestyle counseling might ultimately result in a more positive outcome.

A large number of South Asians will fast, either on a regular basis (for example, many Hindu people may fast 1 day each week) or as part of a religious observance (for example, Muslim people during Ramadan). The health implications of fasting are unclear, with some studies showing potential metabolic benefits (Shah et al. 2015) and others suggesting detrimental (Hui and Devendra 2010) or no health effects (Trepanowski and Bloomer 2010; Hui and Devendra 2010).

It has been indicated that fasting has significant meaning to patients, and an important consideration for clinicians is how to care for patients with diabetes who may be fasting for the month of Ramadan (Hui and Devendra 2010). Abstinence from food and liquid during daylight hours is observed by Muslim individuals during the month of Ramadan. Fasting can lead to hypo- or hyperglycemia and dehydration; in addition, some patients may not want to take oral medications during a fast. It is important to counsel patients with diabetes who intend to fast about how to fast safely and to adjust their diabetes medication prior to beginning any fast. Structured educational sessions specific to Ramadan have been shown to be effective. In an observational study, patients who fasted without attending a structured education session had a fourfold increase in hypoglycemic events, whereas those who attended a Ramadan-focused education program had a significant decrease in hypoglycemic events (Bravis et al. 2010). Fasting is not recommended for patients with poorly controlled type I diabetes or pregnant women with diabetes (Hui and Devendra 2010; Alkandari et al. 2012) Resources for practitioners and patients are available through the American Diabetes Association (Al-Arouj et al. 2010).

4.2.2.2 Physical Activity

The practice of yoga is predicated on equilibrium, mind–body harmony, and meditative states, and is considered a spiritual means to enlightenment in India (Andrews 2005). Yoga is central to Ayurvedic and Siddha conceptualizations of well-being and prevention, and it has also been used as a treatment for a range of acute and chronic illnesses such as musculoskeletal pain (Cramer et al. 2013) and cardiovascular diseases (Mamtani and Mamtani 2005). Unlike the Western biomedical model, which encourages moderate and vigorous intensity aerobic physical activity, most indigenous South Asian medical systems suggest that breathlessness and overexertion from exercise are to be avoided (Caperchione et al. 2009). There is also some evidence that South Asian Muslims consider the daily prayer or *namaaz* to be a form of exercise that promotes health (Tirodkar et al. 2011). Studies of South Asian immigrants have found that they have significantly lower levels of moderate and vigorous intensity physical activity than other racial/ethnic groups, (M. Patel et al. 2012; Williams et al. 2011) which may be partly driven by the idea that physical activity should be gentle and fluid and should not put too much stress or strain on the body. These beliefs may not be congruent with physical activity guidelines (Centers for Disease Control and Prevention 2015) in the U.S., leading to a mismatch between physical activity counseling and South Asians' concepts of physical activity (Dave et al. 2015).

4.2.2.3 Tobacco

Small, community-based surveys suggest that smokeless tobacco and areca nut are commonly used in some South Asian immigrant groups (Changrani et al. 2006). Oral smokeless tobacco products are strongly associated with oral cancers and cardiovascular disease. There are many types of culturally-specific tobacco products available in the United States, including *tambaku paan* (betel quid with tobacco), *gutka* (sun-dried finely chopped tobacco, areca nut, slaked lime, catechu, flavorings and sweeteners), and *zarda* (boiled and dried tobacco leaves with lime and spices, colorings, areca nut, and flavorings). Betel leaves and areca nut have been described in Ayurveda as stimulating the central nervous system, relieving pain, stomach ailments, gynecological disorders and a sore throats. Recent qualitative studies have also identified socio-cultural factors as contributing to smokeless tobacco use in South Asians in the U.S. For instance, (Mukherjea et al. 2012) reported that use of smokeless tobacco products was expressed as a symbolic behavior to maintain culture and was an expression of South Asian ethnic identity in a new dominant culture. Importantly, the harmful health effects of smokeless tobacco were not always recognized, and instead, some South Asian immigrants believed there were some beneficial health effects of these products. Similar to what is found in Ayurveda, South Asians described "constipation relief," "improvement in stamina," and stress relief from these products (Banerjee et al. 2014).

4.2.2.4 Use of Indigenous Therapies and Medicines

Studies of South Asian immigrants have described the belief that Western medications may be effective, but have more side effects and do not address the root cause of disease (Rao 2006; Rhodes et al. 2008). In addition, in South Asia there is a considerable preference and usage of Ayurvedic and plant-based therapies as these treatments are believed to be effective and considerably safer than Western medication (Chacko 2003). Because immigrants of South Asian background may have both a Western and traditional South Asian medical understanding of health and illness, multiple practices may be employed, including home remedies and treatments routinely used in Ayurveda, Siddha, Unani, homeopathy, and naturopathy. For example, in a study of Muslim immigrants to the U.S. (Alrawi et al. 2012), a participant discussed how turmeric in food can help heal plantar fasciitis in addition to the pills a doctor recommended. It is also not uncommon for South Asian immigrants to consult traditional practitioners and purchase South Asian medicines when travelling back to South Asia (Mehta 2010).

There is limited information on use of traditional South Asian therapies and medicines by South Asians living in the U.S. A national survey among Asian Indians in the U.S. found that 12% reported using Ayurveda and/or homeopathic treatments (Misra et al. 2010). A much smaller survey of a convenience sample of South Asians in California found that 59% of respondents reported past or current use of Ayurvedic treatments and that only 18% had informed their allopathic doctor (Satow et al. 2008).

One significant area of concern relates to reports of heavy metal poisoning (lead, mercury and arsenic) caused by some Ayurvedic medicines. These medicines are made from metal ashes, and are called *rasa shastra* products (Ernst 2002). Most Ayurvedic medicine preparations are not supervised, controlled, inspected, or evaluated using any official procedures or standards established by regulatory agencies. This is compounded by the fact that individuals may purchase such products over the Internet or from ethnic markets without consultation from an Ayurvedic specialist. A 2007 U.S. study found that onc-fifth of both US-manufactured and Indian-manufactured Ayurvedic medicines purchased via the Internet contained detectable lead, mercury, or arsenic (Saper et al. 2008). All metal-containing products exceeded 1 or more standards for acceptable daily intake of toxic metals. More recently, researchers reported that among 115 people tested who were using Ayurvedic medicines, 40% had lead poisoning (Breeher et al. 2015).

Taken as a whole, these findings suggest the need to educate health care providers who work with South Asian populations to solicit information about use of Ayurvedic products. It is important to recognize that Ayurvedic and other traditional medications are often perceived as less toxic than Western medicines, are deeply rooted in indigenous medical systems, and have been widely used for thousands of years. Concerns about the potential toxicity of these medications should be presented to patients in a non-judgmental way.

4.2.3 For Clinicians

Several arguments have been advanced as to why clinicians should be interested in traditional South Asian medical systems and treatments. First, traditional South Asian medical systems continue to influence South Asian patients' explanatory models of health and illness, which in turn affect health care seeking and treatment adherence. Many South Asians endorse a holistic model of health where disease is a result of an imbalance between physical, psychosocial, behavioral, and spiritual aspects of health. A critical finding in several research studies of South Asian immigrant health is that they are simultaneously using Western biomedicine and traditional South Asian medical systems; these systems are neither exclusive nor are they always contradictory. Clinicians should ask all patients about their explanatory models of health and disease and use this information to build rapport and trust, and engage in collaborative decision making. There are several ways to elicit explanatory models of health, including Kleinman's questions:

1. What do you think caused your problem?
2. Why do you think it started when it did?
3. What do you think your sickness does to you?
4. How severe is your sickness? Do you think it will last a long time, or will it be better soon in your opinion?
5. What are the chief problems your sickness has caused for you?
6. What do you fear most about your sickness?
7. What kind of treatment do you think you should receive?
8. What are the most important results you hope to get from treatment?

Another simplified approach is to use two questions (Kandula 2014): "How is your health," followed by, "How do you know (or, why do you think that)?" Depending on the answers to these questions and the reason for the visit, the clinician can then use the Kleinman questions to further explore the patient's beliefs.

Second, clinicians should be aware of the value that South Asians place on a traditional diet and/or certain foods and spices for wellness, and also for disease treatment. Before making dietary recommendations to South Asian patients, it is important to understand how the patient may value the foods being recommended or eliminated. In addition, it is important to ask if patients are using any spices or foods to treat symptoms or disease. Third, South Asian health beliefs related to diet, physical activity, and smokeless tobacco are rooted in indigenous medical systems and may not always be congruent with Western concepts of health behaviors. As a result, behavior change interventions for South Asians may be more effective if they incorporate and acknowledge deeply rooted health beliefs. Fourth, clinicians need to be aware that diet-based therapies, non-medication based therapies (e.g. yoga), and traditional medications may be among the options being actively considered by South Asian patients. Because some indigenous medicines have been found to be harmful on their own and in interaction with other drugs, greater clinical awareness can prevent adverse interactions. Clinicians should ask patients about the use of Ayurvedic medicines, plant-based medicines, other traditional medicines, and dietary treatments. Lastly, many South Asian immigrants maintain ties to South Asia and may be consulting traditional practitioners when traveling to South Asia or through family and friends living in South Asia (Mehta 2010). Older South Asian immigrants, retirees in particular, may be spending significant time in South Asia. Clinicians should ask South Asian patients about travel to South Asia, and if the patient consults traditional practitioners or gets medications in South Asia.

It is essential to recognize the heterogeneity of the U.S. South Asian community as all individuals of South Asian ancestry will not follow or share the health belief systems and behaviors discussed in this chapter. Immigrants' health belief systems are not static, but rather, evolving and fluid. At the same time, we are witnessing greater interest in and use of indigenous South Asian health models and treatments among the general American public. With globalization, increased transnational migration, and cultural exchange, it is likely that health care practitioners will continue to see increasing influence and practice of beliefs and treatments drawing on indigenous South Asian medical systems. A better understanding of how best to integrate South Asian medical systems and beliefs into clinical care and interventions is needed to help South Asians achieve optimal health.

Acknowledgements The authors thank Shinu Mammen for assistance with research and referencing this chapter.

Dr. Kandula is supported by grants #R01HL120725 and #R01 HL09009 from the National Institutes of Health.

References

Al-Arouj, M., Assaad-Khalil, S., Buse, J., Fahdil, I., Fahmy, M., Hafez, S., et al. (2010). Recommendations for management of diabetes during Ramadan: Update 2010. *Diabetes Care, 33*(8), 1895–1902. https://doi.org/10.2337/dc10-0896.

Alkandari, J. R., Maughan, R. J., Roky, R., Aziz, A. R., & Karli, U. (2012). The implications of Ramadan fasting for human health and Well-being. *Journal of Sports Sciences, 30*(sup1), S9–S19. https://doi.org/10.1080/02640414.2012.698298.

Alrawi, S., Fetters, M. D., Killawi, A., Hammad, A., & Padela, A. (2012). Traditional healing practices among American Muslims: Perceptions of community leaders in Southeast Michigan. *Journal of Immigrant and Minority Health, 14*(3), 489–496. https://doi.org/10.1007/s10903-011-9495-0.

Andrews, J. (2005). *Hinduism cultural, ethnic, and religious reference manual for health care providers*. Winston-Salem/North Carolina: JAMARDA Resources, Inc.

Arnold, D. (1993). *Colonizing the body: state medicine and epidemic disease in nineteenth-centry India*. Berkeley: Univeristy of California Press.

Banerjee, S. C., Ostroff, J. S., Bari, S., D'Agostino, T. A., Khera, M., Acharya, S., et al. (2014). Gutka and Tambaku Paan use among south Asian immigrants: A focus group study. *Journal of Immigrant and Minority Health, 16*(3), 531–539. https://doi.org/10.1007/s10903-013-9826-4.

Bhattacharya, S. (2009). *The introduction of Western medicine in India*. London: University College London.

Bravis, V., Hui, E., Salih, S., Mehar, S., Hassanein, M., & Devendra, D. (2010). Ramadan education and awareness in diabetes (READ) programme for Muslims with type 2 diabetes who fast during Ramadan. *Diabetic Medicine, 27*(3), 327–331. https://doi.org/10.1111/j.1464-5491.2010.02948.x.

Breeher, L., Mikulski, M. A., Czeczok, T., Leinenkugel, K., & Fuortes, L. J. (2015). A cwluster of lead poisoning among consumers of Ayurvedic medicine. *International Journal of Occupational and Environmental Health*. https://doi.org/10.1179/2049396715Y.0000000009.

Burgel, J. C. (1976). Secular and religious features of medieval Arabic medicine. In C. Leslie (Ed.), *Asian medical systems: a comparative study*. Bekeley: University of California Press.

Caperchione, C. M., Kolt, G. S., & Mummery, W. K. (2009). Physical activity in culturally and linguistically diverse migrant groups to western society: A review of barriers, enablers and experiences. *Sports Medicine, 39*(3), 167–177. https://doi.org/10.2165/00007256-200939030-00001.

Caraka, S. (2001). *Agnivesa's Caraka Samhita* (Vol. 1, 7th ed.). Varanasi: Sutra Sthana.

Centers for Disease Control and Prevention. (2015). *How much physical activity do adults need?* http://www.cdc.gov/physicalactivity/basics/adults/index.htm. Accessed May 11, 2016 2016.

Chacko, E. (2003). Culture and therapy: Complementary strategies for the treatment of type-2 diabetes in an urban setting in Kerala, India. *Social Science & Medicine, 56*(5), 1087–1098.

Changrani, J., Gany, F. M., Cruz, G., Kerr, R., & Katz, R. (2006). Paan and Gutka use in the United States: A pilot study in Bangladeshi and Indian-Gujarati immigrants in new York City. *Journal of Immigrant Refugee Studies, 4*(1), 99–110. https://doi.org/10.1300/J500v04n01_07.

Chuengsamarn, S., Rattanamongkolgul, S., Luechapudiporn, R., Phisalaphong, C., & Jirawatnotai, S. (2012). Curcumin extract for prevention of type 2 diabetes. *Diabetes Care, 35*(11), 2121–2127. https://doi.org/10.2337/dc12-0116.

Cohen, L. (1998). *No aging in India: Alzheimer's, the bad family and other modern things*. Berekely: University of California Press.

Cramer, H., Lauche, R., Hohmann, C., Langhorst, J., & Dobos, G. (2013). Yoga for chronic neck pain: A 12-month follow-up. *Pain Medicine, 14*(4), 541–548. https://doi.org/10.1111/pme.12053.

Dave, S. S., Craft, L. L., Mehta, P., Naval, S., Kumar, S., & Kandula, N. R. (2015). Life stage influences on U.S. South Asian women's physical activity. *American Journal of Health Promotion, 29*(3), e100–e108. https://doi.org/10.4278/ajhp.130415-QUAL-175.

Desjarlais, R. (1992). *Body and emotion: the aesthetics of illness and healing in the Nepal Himalayas*. Philadelphia: University of Pennsylvannia Press.

Ernst, E. (2002). Heavy metals in traditional Indian remedies. *European Journal of Clinical Pharmacology, 57*(12), 891–896.

Frawley, D. (1997). *Ayurveda and the mind: The healing of consciousness*. Delhi: Motilal Banarsidass Publishers.

Gadgil, M. D., Anderson, C. A., Kandula, N. R., & Kanaya, A. M. (2015). Dietary patterns are associated with metabolic risk factors in South Asians living in the United States. *The Journal of Nutrition, 145*(6), 1211–1217. https://doi.org/10.3945/jn.114.207753.

Ghosh, A. K. (2010). A short history of the development of homeopathy in India. *Homeopathy, 99*(2), 130–136. https://doi.org/10.1016/j.homp.2009.10.001.

Hui, E., & Devendra, D. (2010). Diabetes and fasting during Ramadan. *Diabetes/Metabolism Research and Reviews, 26*(8), 606–610. https://doi.org/10.1002/dmrr.1137.

Jeffery, R. (1988). *The politics of health in India*. Berkeley: University of Califonia Press.

Kakar, S. (1982). *Shaman, mystics and doctors*. Chicago: University of Chicago Press.

Kandula, N. R. (2014). A better way to know what patients believe and value about health. *Journal of General Internal Medicine, 29*(4), 560–561. https://doi.org/10.1007/s11606-013-2714-8.

Kleinman, A. (1980). *Patients and healers in the context of culture: An exploration of the borderland between anthropology, medicine, and psychiatry*. Berkley: University of California Press.

Krishnaswamy, K. (2008). Traditional Indian spices and their health significance. *Asia Pacific Journal of Clinical Nutrition, 17*(Suppl 1), 265–268.

Kurtz, S. (1992). All the mothers are one: Hindu India and the cultural reshaping of psychoanalysis. In *New York: Columbia University press*.

Lad, V. (1984). *Ayurveda: The science of self-healing*. Wilmot: Lotus Press.

Lad, V. (2002). *Textbook of Ayurveda: Fundamental principles*. Albuquerque: They Ayurvedic Press.

Lamb, S. (2000). *White saris and sweet mangoes*. Berkeley: University of California Press.

Lambert, H. (1992). The cultural logic of Indian medicine: Prognosis and etiology in Rajasthani popular therapeutics. *Social Science & Medicine, 34*(10), 1069–1076.

Larson, G. (1993). *Self as body in asian theory and practice*. Albany: State University of New York.

Lodha, R., & Bagga, A. (2000). Traditional Indian systems of medicine. *Annals of the Academy of Medicine, Singapore, 29*(1), 37–41.

Lone, A. H., Ahmad, T., Anwar, M., Sofi, G., Imam, H., & Habib, S. (2012). Perception of health promotion in Unani herbal medicine. *Journal of Herbal Medicine, 2*(1), 1–5. https://doi.org/10.1016/j.hermed.2012.02.003.

Makoul, G., Clayman, M. L., Lynch, E. B., & Thompson, J. A. (2009). Four concepts of health in America: Results of national surveys. *Journal of Health Communication, 14*(1), 3–14. https://doi.org/10.1080/10810730802592213.

Mamtani, R., & Mamtani, R. (2005). Ayurveda and yoga in cardiovascular diseases. *Cardiology in Review, 13*(3), 155–162.

Mehta, K. B. (2010). *Borders and barriers: Perspectives on aging and alternative medicine among transnational north Indian immigrants*. Amherst: Georgia State University.

Misra, R., Balagopal, P., Klatt, M., & Geraghty, M. (2010). Complementary and alternative medicine use among Asian Indians in the United States: A national study. *Journal of Alternative and Complementary Medicine, 16*(8), 843–852. https://doi.org/10.1089/acm.2009.0517.

Mukherjea, A., Morgan, P. A., Snowden, L. R., Ling, P. M., & Ivey, S. L. (2012). Social and cultural influences on tobacco-related health disparities among south Asians in the USA. *Tobacco Control, 21*(4), 422–428. https://doi.org/10.1136/tc.2010.042309.

Mukherjea, A., Underwood, K. C., Stewart, A. L., Ivey, S. L., & Kanaya, A. M. (2013). Asian Indian views on diet and health in the United States: Importance of understanding cultural and social factors to address disparities. *Family & Community Health, 36*(4), 311–323. https://doi.org/10.1097/FCH.0b013e31829d2549.

Obeyesekere, G. (1981). *Medusa's hair: An essay on personal symbols and religious experience*. Chicago: University of Chicago Press.

Patel, M., Phillips-Caesar, E., & Boutin-Foster, C. (2012). Barriers to lifestyle behavioral change in migrant south Asian populations. *Journal of Immigrant and Minority Health, 14*(5), 774–785. https://doi.org/10.1007/s10903-011-9550-x.

Patel, M., Phillips-Caesar, E., & Boutin-Foster, C. (2014). Attitudes and beliefs regarding cardiovascular risk factors among Bangladeshi immigrants in the US. *Journal of Immigrant and Minority Health, 16*(5), 994–1000. https://doi.org/10.1007/s10903-013-9868-7.

Patel, N. R., Chew-Graham, C., Bundy, C., Kennedy, A., Blickem, C., & Reeves, D. (2015). Illness beliefs and the sociocultural context of diabetes self-management in British South Asians: A mixed methods study. *BMC Family Practice, 16*, 58. https://doi.org/10.1186/s12875-015-0269-y.

Pool, R. (1987). Hot and cold as an explanatory model: The example of Bharuch district in Gujarat, India. *Social Science & Medicine, 25*(4), 389–399.

Rao, D. (2006). Choice of medicine and hierarchy of resort to different health alternatives among Asian Indian migrants in a metropolitan city in the USA. *Ethnicity & Health, 11*(2), 153–167. https://doi.org/10.1080/13557850500460306.

Rhodes, P. J., Small, N., Ismail, H., & Wright, J. P. (2008). The use of biomedicine, complementary and alternative medicine, and ethnomedicine for the treatment of epilepsy among people of south Asian origin in the UK. *BMC Complementary and Alternative Medicine, 8*, 7. https://doi.org/10.1186/1472-6882-8-7.

Saper, R. B., Phillips, R. S., Sehgal, A., Khouri, N., Davis, R. B., Paquin, J., et al. (2008). Lead, mercury, and arsenic in US- and Indian-manufactured Ayurvedic medicines sold via the internet. *JAMA, 300*(8), 915–923. https://doi.org/10.1001/jama.300.8.915.

Satow, Y. E., Kumar, P. D., Burke, A., & Inciardi, J. F. (2008). Exploring the prevalence of Ayurveda use among Asian Indians. *Journal of Alternative and Complementary Medicine, 14*(10), 1249–1253. https://doi.org/10.1089/acm.2008.0106.

Shah, M. (1966). *The general principles of Avincenna's "canon of medicine"*. Karachi: Naveed Clinic.

Shah, A. D., Vittinghoff, E., Kandula, N. R., Srivastava, S., & Kanaya, A. M. (2015). Correlates of prediabetes and type II diabetes in US south Asians: Findings from the mediators of atherosclerosis in south Asians living in America (MASALA) study. *Annals of Epidemiology, 25*(2), 77–83. https://doi.org/10.1016/j.annepidem.2014.10.013.

Shanbag, V. (1994). *A beginner's introduction to ayurvedic medicine*. New Canaan/Connecticut: Keats Publishing Inc.

Shweder, R., Much, N. C., Mahapatra, M., & Park, L. (1997). *The big three of morality (autonomy, community, divinity) and the big three explanations of suffering*. Morality and Health.

Tirodkar, M. A. (2005). *Adaptations of contemporary Ayurvedic medical practice in urban India*. Chicago: University of Chicago.

Tirodkar, M. A., Baker, D. W., Makoul, G. T., Khurana, N., Paracha, M. W., & Kandula, N. R. (2011). Explanatory models of health and disease among South Asian immigrants in Chicago. *Journal of Immigrant and Minority Health, 13*(2), 385–394. https://doi.org/10.1007/s10903-009-9304-1.

Trepanowski, J. F., & Bloomer, R. J. (2010). The impact of religious fasting on human health. [journal article]. *Nutrition Journal, 9*(1), 1–9. https://doi.org/10.1186/1475-2891-9-57.
Van Hollen, C. (2003). Birth on the threshold: A childbirth and modernity in South India. Berkeley: University of California Press.
Williams, E. D., Stamatakis, E., Chandola, T., & Hamer, M. (2011). Physical activity behaviour and coronary heart disease mortality among South Asian people in the UK: An observational longitudinal study. *Heart, 97*(8), 655–659. https://doi.org/10.1136/hrt.2010.201012.
Zhou, Q., Ye, M., Lu, Y., Zhang, H., Chen, Q., Huang, S., et al. (2015). Curcumin improves the Tumoricidal effect of Mitomycin C by suppressing ABCG2 expression in stem cell-like breast Cancer cells. *PLoS One, 10*(8), e0136694. https://doi.org/10.1371/journal.pone.0136694.

Chapter 5
Psychological Models of Health

Zunaira Jilani, Edward C. Chang, Jerin Lee, and Casey N.-H. Batterbee

Healthiness is indicative of both physical and mental well-being. In addition to investigating the biological models of health in the previous chapter, it is valuable to consider psychological factors that relate to health. Health psychology is the study of how beliefs, values, thoughts, feelings, attitudes, and other psychosocial factors impact health behaviors, and is a relatively new field (Taylor 1995). Not only has health psychology played an integral role in the mind-body relationship, but it has also elucidated that certain treatments and practices may be more successful in improving health outcomes for unique patient populations. Recent decades have seen rapid growth of the South Asian American population (e.g., Hoeffel et al. 2012) and dramatic increases in published psychological research on South Asian Americans. Yet, the study of South Asian American health remains in its formative stages and dwarfs in comparison to the extant literatures for other minority populations in the U.S. (e.g., African Americans; East Asian Americans). Applying existing health psychology models to the South Asian American population will improve understanding of the connection between health beliefs (i.e., convictions about health that influence behaviors) and health behaviors (i.e., decisions or actions related to health) for this growing ethnic minority. In turn, this knowledge could be useful in generating effective and culturally adaptive health-related interventions and treatment. A key issue in the application of psychological frameworks and interventions to any cultural population is the sociocultural context in which the psychological frameworks were developed (most frequently developed by European

Z. Jilani (✉)
Wayne State University, Detroit, MI, USA
e-mail: zunaira.jilani@wayne.edu

E. C. Chang · J. Lee · C. N.-H. Batterbee
University of Michigan, Ann Arbor, MI, USA
e-mail: changec@umich.edu; jerinlee@umich.edu; caseybat@umich.edu

M. J. Perera, E. C. Chang (eds.), *Biopsychosocial Approaches to Understanding Health in South Asian Americans*, Cross-Cultural Research in Health, Illness and Well-Being, https://doi.org/10.1007/978-3-319-91120-5_5

Americans in Western society). Throughout this chapter, we will explore this issue by first examining established psychological models of health and their application to South Asian Americans in Part I, and then discussing psychological processes and practices used in intervention that are unique and indigenous to this ethnic population in Part II.

5.1 Part I: Psychological Models of Health

Researchers over the past few decades have developed several models that seek to clarify the motivational factors underlying health beliefs and health behaviors (e.g., Social Cognitive Theory, Bandura 1986). The structure of each model can be applied to South Asian Americans to identify and assess predictors of health habits and behaviors in this population. Circumstantial and potentially malleable factors that are predictive of health beliefs and behaviors can be identified and used by researchers to develop interventions and services to elicit higher rates of behavioral compliance as well as address health outcomes specific to this group (e.g., heart disease; Enas and Senthilkumar 2005). Although an overall understudied area, there are differences in health beliefs, behaviors, and risks within Asian sub-groups (e.g., Chinese, Indian, Filipino; Ghosh 2003). For instance, Indian adults are twice as likely to be told they have heart disease than Korean adults, and twice as likely to have diabetes than Chinese and Japanese adults (Barnes et al. 2008). Thus, it is important to examine how psychological models of health apply specifically to South Asian Americans. This chapter begins with an overview of established health psychology models and discusses how these models have been (or have yet to be) applied to health problems in the South Asian American population.

5.1.1 The Health Belief Model

The Health Belief Model (HBM; Becker 1974; Rosenstock 1966) suggests that health behavior is explained by two variables: the patient's psychological state of readiness to take a specific action in regards to his/her own health (*perception of health threat*) and the extent to which the patient believes that the action will improve his/her health (*perceived threat reduction*). The psychological state of readiness refers to the patient's interest and concern about his/her health status and is comprised of *perceived susceptibility* (the subjective risks of experiencing a health condition) and *perceived seriousness* (the emotional arousal from either the thought of the health concern or its associated risks and difficulties). According to Rosenstock (1974), changes in health behavior depend on the patient's belief about the perceived benefits and effectiveness of a given treatment *and* if the result of the required change in the patient's behavior for the treatment is worth undergoing the treatment. For instance, a treatment program may seem like the most effective option, but if it involves a procedure or behavior that is deemed inconvenient, expensive, painful, disconcerting, or unsatisfactory in some regard, the patient may reconsider pursuing the treatment. Alternatively, an individual may perceive changing a health habit or pursuing a treatment to be a worthwhile decision. These factors all contribute to predicting the likelihood of health behavior change.

The HBM can be useful in assessment of beliefs and behaviors pertinent to health issues impacting South Asian Americans, and can identify potential modifiable health beliefs and behaviors that contribute to poor health outcomes. Past research has assessed for concepts discussed in the HBM (e.g., perceptions of health, perceptions on treatments) in various South Asian populations globally (e.g., Rodrigues et al. 2014). A cross-cultural study examining Pakistanis, British South Asians, and Westerners by Sheikh and Furnham (2000) found that culturally determined beliefs of the cause of mental health issues contributed to attitudes towards seeking professional help for psychological distress for both groups of South Asians. These findings indicate that South Asians have a conceptualization of mental distress that is different from Westerners' conceptualization and impacts help-seeking behavior.

A specific health condition that the HBM has been applied to in South Asian Americans is breast cancer (Sadler et al. 2001). Wu et al. (2006) applied the HBM to assess for cultural differences in beliefs related to cancer-screening practices (e.g., breast self-exam, clinical breast exam, mammography) among Asian American subgroups, including Filipino, Chinese, and Asian-Indian women. Across the three groups, Asian-Indian women reported the lowest levels of perceived susceptibility (i.e., do not perceive cancer to be a serious illness, do not perceive themselves as vulnerable to breast cancer) and were nine times less likely to be aware of where to receive a mammogram than Filipino and Chinese women. Furthermore, lower income Asian-Indian women perceived greater barriers to getting screened (e.g., waiting time is too long, do not need a mammogram if feeling OK) than higher income Asian-Indian women. Thus, it might be beneficial to both focus on increasing availability of preventative treatments, such as mammogram screenings for lower income South Asian Americans, as well as improving health literacy and providing psychoeducation on preventative screening practices for all South Asian American women to increase perceived threat reduction. These results also indicate a need to be conscientious of multi-intersectional identities, such as ethnicity and socioeconomic status, when developing health interventions for South Asian Americans.

Several researchers (e.g., Lim et al. 2009; Vadaparampil et al. 2004) have expressed that a major discrepancy of applying the HBM to differing ethnic and racial populations populations is its disregard for the role of culture in health beliefs and behaviors. It may be important to explore models of health that consider cultural/societal context. Further, the HBM focuses specifically on attitudes about health but it may be important to also focus on the behavioral outcome, thereby providing a holistic analysis of a health situation (e.g., Champion and Skinner 2008).

5.1.2 Theory of Planned Behavior

The Theory of Planned Behavior (TPB; Ajzen 1991; Ajzen and Madden 1986), a model originally evolved from the Theory of Reasoned Action (TRA; Ajzen and Fishbein 1980), states that a patient's behavioral intention is directly linked to health behavior, and it is composed of three key factors. The first factor, *attitudes,* addresses individual beliefs of a specific health behavior and consideration of the associated outcomes. The second factor, *subjective norms,* denotes the process by which one evaluates the normative actions to be taken and the motivation to follow norms. The last factor, *perceived behavioral control*, is the extent to which one believes they have the ability to complete the health behavior and achieve the desired outcome. These factors collectively generate a behavioral intention that propagates change in behavior. This psychological model of health is particularly useful in understanding how factors like health beliefs impact health behavior directly.

The TPB framework is distinct from the HBM because it considers that social context can play a significant role in a patient's health behavior and health outcome. It is crucial that researchers, practitioners, and health professionals recognize that models, therapeutic techniques, and psychoeducation are often based on European American values of individualism, a concept that may not be entirely applicable to populations of varying cultures. Western society tends to take on a more egocentric psychological view, where the focus lies on the individual, holding dominant views on individualism, autonomy, personal achievement, materialism, and preference for individual locus of control (Stairs 1992). Alternatively, Asian culture imposes a more sociocentric-self, with high value placed on collectivism, interdependence, cooperation, honor, filial piety, and familism (Kirmayer 2007). Many Western healthcare professionals unknowingly follow these socio-normative perceptions of the self and may be unaware of the potential ineffectiveness of their methods in minority populations with hybrid identities (e.g., Asian Americans). Increasing awareness on these psychological views of cultural populations that are related to health (e.g., beliefs, behaviors, perceptions of diseases) may play a crucial role in identifying solutions to health issues within different diverse populations.

In exploring differences between Western and non-Western patient responses to mental health issues, TPB models have been applied to South Asians in India to understand the public perception of controversial mental illnesses (e.g., schizophrenia; Saravanan et al. 2007). Likewise, in applying the TPB to South Asian Americans in order to understand differences in subjective and cultural norms, researchers have focused on identifying behavioral factors that may play a role in eliciting healthcare-seeking behavior. One study examining HIV/AIDS among South Asian Americans highlighted the importance of considering various contextual factors (e.g., societal, cultural, economic, environmental norms; Bhattacharya 2004) when developing treatment programs promoting changes in health behavior. Indeed, increased cognizance of diverse mentalities and how a population understands a health issue allows for better-informed and therefore better-received methods of intervention, and South Asian Americans may require adapted models of health that differ from other ethnicities (e.g., European Americans). For instance, although some South Asian Americans may be more acculturated to Western society and adopt Western societal norms (e.g., seeking healthcare, using Western biomedicine), others may hold stronger ties with Eastern societal norms (e.g., alternative medicine), resulting in an internal struggle of deciding which values, attributes, and perceptions to align with, an issue often encountered in those with hybrid identities. Alternatively, European Americans may not encounter such internal conflicts and their own cultural identity may already fit with the societal norms of the Western society in which they reside.

These concerns point toward the need for healthcare professionals using the TPB to adopt cultural awareness to effectively address health issues in diverse populations. Some researchers have challenged the model to be heavily geared towards Westerners, while others have argued the model's cross-cultural adaptability in over fifty countries through the use of a method referred to as elicitation (e.g., Fishbein 2000). Elicitation consists of conducting interviews to define relevant health related factors (beliefs, behaviors, environmental influences, potential barriers) from the population's perspective. While elicitation may provide some more insight on this group's subjective norms, it may be difficult to predict where these post-immigrant hybrid-identity individuals fall on the spectrum from South Asian to Western cultural norms. This discrepancy in applying the TPB to new diverse populations may potentially explain the limited existing studies examining the present model among South Asian Americans in particular.

5.1.3 *Health Locus of Control*

The Health Locus of Control model (HLC; Wallston et al. 1976), derived from Rotter's (1966) conceptualization of Internal-External Locus of Control, assesses how expectancies related to health are attributed either to oneself or to an external factor. Approximately a decade later, the HLC progressed into a more elaborate model known as the Multidimensional Health Locus of Control model (MHLC; Wallston et al. 1978). The MHLC assesses for specific sources that may exert control over health-related behaviors, including internal locus of control (the control one has over their own health), external locus of control (the control that others, such as health professionals, have in the situation), and control left to chance. Different from its previous iteration, the MHLC also assesses the extent to which one believes healthcare professionals have the knowledge, power, and ability to improve their health outcome. Patients who believe that they have high control over their own health are more likely to partake in behaviors to improve their health than individuals who believe that their health is left up to fate, or some external source of control.

Researchers have demonstrated ethnic differences in health locus of control (e.g., Cohen and Azaiza 2007; Lim et al. 2009). Interestingly, Wrightson and Wardle (1997) found that South Asian women scored higher on the *chance* (the notion that health is left up to fate), and *powerful others* (control wielded by others outside the self and fate) locus of control, compared to Caucasian and Afro-Caribbean women. Echoed by the results of other studies, these findings point towards the role of religiosity in both health locus of control and in the exploration of alternative treatment options. One possible explanation is that some followers of South Asian religions believe that bad health is a result of karma, a concept in which individuals own responsibility in the present and future for actions committed in the past or even in a past life. Some also believe that acts of a deity (or deities) may exert more control over their health than they do. Individuals from more sociocentrically driven (typically Eastern) cultures tend to have a stronger sense of external locus of control compared to individuals from more egocentrically driven (typically Western) cultures (Hamid 1994; Sastry and Ross 1998).

Interestingly, studies conducted on the health locus of control in European South Asians (e.g., Ismail et al. 2005a; Ismail et al. 2005b; Macaden and Clarke 2010) report that a major limitation was conflicting traditional vs. Western ideals among hybrid identity patients. More specifically, while some South Asians believe an external locus of control (e.g., powerful other, deity) is responsible for health issues, it may not prevent them from seeking Western healthcare in addition to engaging in prayer. Alternatively, while some do believe in an external power, they may still assume some internal responsibility for their ailments. These possibilities do not fit the mold of MHLC, and it remains important to be cognizant of the patient's and their family's beliefs and understanding of the health condition in both assessment and treatment. While it is reasonable to assume that similar limitations exist in applying the MHLC to South Asians in North America, further research is warranted.

5.1.4 Transtheoretical Model of Health Behavior Change

Another psychological model of health that arose shortly after these frameworks is the Transtheoretical Model of Health Behavior Change (TTM; Prochaska et al. 1994; Prochaska and Velicer 1997). This model originated from the Transtheoretical Model of Change, which is used in therapy settings (Prochaska and DiClemente 1982). The TTM is based on decision-making and highlights six specific stages involved in an individual's progress towards health-related behavioral change: precontemplation, contemplation, preparation, action, maintenance, and termination. Cognitive processes that influence the transition between stages are then applied to elicit higher rates of change in health behavior. Compared to aforementioned models, this theoretical framework defines distinct stages of behavior change, providing researchers and clinicians with a means to recognize problematic stages and develop stage-specific interventions.

Application of the TTM to various at-risk, ethnic/racial populations allows researchers to identify clear differences in change across stages, allowing for more effective health promotion. The TTM has been successfully used to develop interventions for South Asian Americans as it recognizes clearer distinctions between stages among different cultural groups. The TTM's conceptualization of behavioral change as a continuum from pre-contemplation, contemplation, preparation, action, maintenance, and termination, allows for easier identification of which stage to intervene in when addressing a health issue. For example, Ahmad et al. (2005) found that the stage-specific TTM was better suited in demonstrating specific explanatory components than the HBM model when tailoring interventions to promote breast cancer awareness among South Asian women in Canada because it targeted early stages, resulting in increased knowledge and reduced perceived barriers related to breast cancer screening.

The TTM was also applied to alcohol addiction recovery among South Asian and European American men, finding spirituality and religion played a more prominent role among South Asians than European Americans in recovery (Morjaria and Orford 2002). More specifically, researchers found that the lowest level defined as "needing help", was correlated with a "pre-existing low-level belief in God" and that the last step of recovery "abstinence/ controlled drinking" was correlated with "greater sense of connectedness with God" among South Asians. These findings highlight the need to account for such cultural values (e.g., religion) when developing interventions, supporting Orford's (2001) claim that the TTM is lacking significant elements involved in behavioral change: the social, spiritual, and moral. For instance, a key difference between the ethnic populations engaging in this recovery program was that Western participants were non-practicing members of a religion developing a sense of faith, while South Asian participants identified more as practicing believers strengthening their pre-existing faith. Considering the emphasis placed among these elements in South Asian culture/religions, this may be a major issue when applying the TTM to this particular population.

5.1.5 *Further Research*

This section offered a brief summary of major established psychological models of health and their relevance to South Asian Americans. Although some past literature has provided valuable insight, potential discrepancies (e.g., lack of a cultural component, the hybrid identity conflict, limited research on the population) exist when applying the models to South Asian Americans. For instance, several models have been used in studies and/or successfully applied to South Asians or (East) Asian Americans, while only a few studies have been conducted on specifically South Asian Americans, even though South Asian Americans may have different experiences than South Asians not residing in the Western hemisphere, and from other subgroups of Asian Americans (e.g., Chinese). Additionally, despite the several studies, there is no solid evidence that one model is stronger than the other (e.g., Noar and Zimmerman 2005; Weinstein and Rothman 2005), most likely due to most of the constructs across the models measuring the same concepts but with different names. However, it is also noteworthy that most studies examined the models using a majority Western population, thus it is unknown if perhaps there is indeed a model best fit for this particular population until further research is conducted. Given the recently increased value placed on the exploration of biopsychosocial factors of health, the growing population of South Asian Americans, and the limited research on this population, further studies must be conducted using South Asian American samples. It is important to research the relevance of existing models through a culturally informed psychological lens to encourage a more nuanced understanding of health behavior. Such knowledge may be useful in not only developing adapted or newer, better fitting models for this population, but also be in application of culturally sensitive interventions.

5.2 Part II: Psychological Processes and Interventions

Throughout this section, we will examine various existing relevant interventions that originated from South Asian culture and discuss their processes, associated health benefits, and practical reasons to increase the study of these practices and interventions. Not only will the exploration of psychological models and practices indigenous to Easterners benefit South Asian Americans, but there may also be advantages in examining their usefulness for other racial/ethnic minority groups in the U.S. In this section, South Asian cultural traditions, psychological processes emphasizing consciousness, and religious/spiritual practices will be considered as they pertain to current forms of treatment. The integration of such practices can provide rich and practical ways to address health concerns cross-culturally, again indicating the importance of further research in the development of culturally sensitive, meaningful, and sufficiently nuanced psychological models and interventions.

5.2.1 Mindfulness

The art of mindfulness dates back thousands of years to the Asian practices of Buddhism, where historically mindfulness was denoted as ‘the heart’ of Buddhist meditation (Thera 1962). Mindfulness is an intricate concept often entailing multiple meanings, but it is most commonly referred to as the quality of awareness or attention in a particular moment. A more complex understanding of mindfulness is that it is a mental process, a psychological trait, a specific meditative technique, a collection of techniques, or an outcome of the practice itself (Bishop et al. 2004). The Buddhist philosophies from which mindfulness stems are rooted deeply in the release of pain and suffering; notably, there is a significant distinction between releasing and suppressing suffering (Hanh 1975). In mindfulness meditation, one is trained to be aware of feelings and thoughts as they arise, accept the feelings and thoughts, and let the feelings and thoughts flow freely while maintaining focus on one’s breathing. Difficult thoughts and feelings are not ignored or pushed away but rather are accepted with openness and compassion to be released after they have been experienced.

Mindfulness meditation has been implemented in stress reduction programs through the usage of breathing techniques, experience of bodily sensations, and incorporation of a useful emotion regulation strategy known as cognitive reappraisal (Kabat-Zinn 1990). Practicing mindfulness meditation can also contribute to increased quality in sleeping patterns, improved mood, and the development of deeper concentration (e.g., Brown and Ryan 2003). Mindfulness entered the clinical setting and has been useful in many interventions aimed at the improvement of psychological and physiological health outcomes. However, it is important to be conscientious when using this practice in the West, as this setting may embody a different cultural paradigm in contrast to the cultural origin of mindfulness-based practices (Kabat-Zinn 2003).

Mindfulness-Based Stress Reduction (MBSR; Kabat-Zinn 1990) is an 8- or 10-week program geared towards the cultivation of mindfulness skills including the experience of bodily sensations, (Hatha) yoga postures, and meditation. Studies from recent decades have demonstrated that participants of this program have reported reduced levels of stress, reduced chronic pain, increased sense of control in their health and lives, higher levels of spirituality, and improvement in symptomology associated with both mental and physical health issues (e.g., Astin 1997; Carmody and Baer 2008; Kabat-Zinn 1982; Miller et al. 1995; Speca et al. 2000). Furthermore, numerous meta-analyses have found evidence for the successful use of mindfulness meditation programs not only for individuals suffering with psychological maladjustment (e.g., anxiety, depression; Hofmann et al. 2010) or chronic medical diseases (e.g., cancer; Bohlmeijer et al. 2010), but also for healthy people (e.g., Chiesa and Serretti 2009) and medical health professionals (e.g., Shapiro et al. 2005). Accordingly, Grossman et al. (2004) conducted a meta-analysis that found MBSR to be useful in alleviating distress associated with physical, psychosomatic, and psychiatric disorders.

Mindfulness has also been found to be useful for health issues through encouragement during mundane activities. One activity is eating, as applied through Mindfulness-Based Eating Awareness Training (MB-EAT; Kristeller and Wolever 2011). Studies have found mindful eating (e.g., increasing awareness of physical vs. psychological hunger, making conscious food choices, etc.) to be beneficial for both weight loss among obese patients and improved glycemic control among patients with type 2 diabetes (e.g., Mason et al. 2015; Miller et al. 2012). This is particularly important considering that South Asian Americans are not only prone to a greater risk for obesity and type 2 diabetes due to genetics, but also have an even higher susceptibility due to Western unhealthy environmental influences on eating behaviors (e.g., Chowdhury et al. 2014; Hall et al. 2010). Mindful eating as an intervention has yet to be studied as a treatment for South Asian American health issues.

Given its multifaceted nature, mindfulness has been broken down into several dimensions including compassion for others, loving-kindness, self-compassion, nonjudgmental attitudes, and equanimity. Several studies have shown support for the positive benefits of practicing mindfulness. Fredrickson et al. (2009) found that those who participated in loving-kindness mediation reported lower levels of stress, higher sense of purpose in life, greater perceived social support, reduced illness, decreased depressive symptoms, and increased life satisfaction as opposed to those who did not participate. Self-compassion, described as being vigilant of one's flaws in order to better oneself in a nonjudgmental way and learning to be content with and love oneself (Neff 2003), has been shown to play a significant role in the cultivation of positive health behaviors, including healthy diet, physical activity, adequate sleep, and stress management (Sirois et al. 2015). Additionally, high self-compassion and acceptance have also been found to help overcome maladaptive psychological processes common among South Asians (e.g., isolation, self-criticism, perfectionism; Neff et al. 2007; Slaney et al. 2000). Furthermore, overall increased levels of mindfulness have been linked to lower levels of psychological distress among Asian Americans (e.g., Masuda et al. 2010).

Despite the abundance of research on mindfulness and its attributes in relation to both psychological and physiological well-being, there are limited studies on the role of such aspects of mindfulness in health on the specific subgroup of South Asian Americans. In fact, few studies have even included South Asian Americans in the study sample (e.g., Davidson et al. 2003; Ostafin et al. 2006), let alone studied large samples of South Asian Americans. For instance, Masuda et al. (2014) conducted a study on an Asian American sample (25% South Asian American) and demonstrated that increased mindfulness was associated with lower levels of depression and anxiety. However, it is still unclear how these relationships varied between groups within the small Asian American sample (e.g., Chinese vs. Asian Indian). Similarly, while some studies have found that Asian ethnicity was not significantly interactive with dispositional trait mindfulness (mindfulness as a facet in one's personality) in comparison to other ethnicities in the U.S., sample sizes may have been too small and power too low to determine any noteworthy relationship (e.g., Creswell et al. 2007; Shapiro et al. 1998). This makes it difficult to generalize these results to Asian Americans, especially South Asian American populations. For these reasons, further research in this population is important, as it is unknown how successful such qualities of mindfulness (e.g., compassion, acceptance) may be among South Asian Americans when incorporated in various methods of treatment, such as acceptance and commitment therapy (e.g., Hayes et al. 2011) or cognitive behavioral therapies (e.g., Brown et al. 2011).

5.2.2 Yoga

Described as an ancient Indian way of life, yoga is a traditional South Asian philosophical practice that has been adapted in the West. Swami Satchidananda, a well-known translator of *The Yoga Sutras of Patanjali,* stated that the original purpose of yoga philosophy was to understand and master the mind, originating approximately 2,000 years ago. The term Raja Yoga (royal union, referring to the union of *Atman,* meaning self or soul, and *Brahman,* or universal consciousness of God) was first used for this purpose by Patanjali Maharishi in the *Yoga Sutras* (Satchidananda 1990) and was later expounded upon by Swami Vivekananda in his book *Raja Yoga* (1896/2016). Vivekananda discusses an array of concepts in the context of Patanjali's *Yoga Sutras,* or the eight limbs of yoga: *Yama* (universal ethics), *Niyama* (individual ethics), *Asana* (physical postures), *Pranayama* (breath control), *Pratyahara* (strengthening senses), *Dharana* (concentration), *Dhyana* (meditation), and *Samadhi* (self-realization). The emphasis on physical practice of yoga is a fairly new development utilized in the West (Satchidananda 1990). For instance, Hatha Yoga, the type of yoga most commonly practiced in the United States, is composed of mainly physical postures, breath control, and/or meditation.

There has been a large wave of empirical research supporting the positive health benefits associated with yoga practice. Brown and Gerbarg (2005) found Sudarshan Kriya Yoga (SKY), the use of rhythmic hyperventilation at different rates of breathing, to be a useful, low-risk and low-cost alternative and complementary treatment for stress, anxiety, depression, post-traumatic stress disorder (PTSD), substance abuse, and stress-related chronic diseases. Yoga has also been demonstrated to be beneficial for physiological health. Balaji et al. (2012) summarized several studies and noted a significant association between the practice of Hatha Yoga and lower cardiovascular risk factors (e.g., reduction in resting pulse rate, reduce blood pressure), lower risk of obesity (e.g., lower BMI, decreased cholesterol, better weight management), improvement in arthritis (e.g., less pain), improved balance, and even reduced DNA damage among cancer patients undergoing radiation. Additionally, Youngwanichsetha et al. (2014) found that pregnant Thai women with gestational diabetes mellitus who participated in yoga exercise consisting of deep-breathing during the repetition of yoga poses and movements showed improvement in glycemic control. More specifically, the movement of the yoga exercises increased blood circulation, improving insulin sensitivity and therefore, increasing utilization of glucose by muscle cells, thus reducing blood sugar among the diabetic pregnant women (Kuntsevich et al. 2010). Mamtani and Mamtani (2005) argue that yoga, when contextualized as part of Ayurvedic Medicine and Indian culture, benefited diabetics by reducing blood sugar levels and patients suffering from heart diseases and hypertension by reducing anxiety, promoting well-being, and improving overall quality of life. Thus, given that South Asian Americans have a higher prevalence of diabetes than other populations (e.g., Mohanty et al. 2005) and often suffer from higher cardiovascular risks including hypertension (Jonnalagadda and Diwan 2005), the practice of yoga may be especially useful in this population. Despite the origins of yoga in South Asian culture, research examining yogic treatments among South Asian Americans is limited.

Interestingly, much of the yogic practices in Western culture focus more on yogic postures, viewing yoga as more of a practice for bodily exercise, while Indian culture values the meditative aspects of yoga in combination with breathing techniques and regards it as a spiritual practice. For instance, yoga poses in Indian tradition are often accompanied with a verse style prayer called *Shloka.* While many yoga routines practiced in the West may have roots in ancient yoga practices, they are somewhat incongruent to the type of yoga valued in the East, further emphasizing the differences between these cultures. Feuerstein (2014) argued that yoga as it is conceptualized in Indian culture has a "distinct advantage over contemporary psychology when it comes to the issue of spiritual freedom and the path to freedom" (p. 235). This distinction underscores the significance of cultivating cultural awareness, but also points toward the need to differentiate indigenous and modified variations of such practices. Accordingly, models exported to the West are often misconstrued and can result in cultural appropriation of these practices. To avoid the potentially insincere adoption of indigenous models, it is important to provide culturally sensitive explanations of procedures that pay sincere homage to the traditional roots. Furthermore, it may be beneficial to compare and contrast the Indian-rooted vs. the Western-adapted elements of models in relation to health issues in South Asian Americans to measure the utility and effectiveness of the elements.

5.2.3 Transcendental Meditation

Another useful ancient Indian meditative practice that has been developed over the past century in the West is Transcendental Meditation (TM). Established by Maharishi Mahesh Yogi in the 1950s, TM is described as an internal control of attention and the act of cogitating a specific series of words, known as a *mantra* (a concept not inherent to the Transcendental Meditation movement, but inspired from ancient Indian practices of meditation). TM, found to be positively associated with high levels of energy, self-esteem, and happiness has been particularly useful in diminishing psychological stress by promoting relaxation, creativity, intelligence, learning ability, self-development, and a higher quality of life while reducing insomnia, anxiety, and depression (e.g., Roth 1987; Sedlmeier et al. 2012). Thus, considering that psychological stress has negative effects on various body mechanisms, including the autonomic nervous system, cardiovascular system, and immune system (McEwen 1998), it is not surprising that researchers and clinicians often turn to TM for research and treatment of several physiological aspects of health (e.g., blood pressure, cortisol levels, heart rate, breathing; Anderson et al. 2008; Dillbeck and Orme-Johnson 1987; MacLean et al. 1997; Wallace 1970). For instance, findings by Balaji et al. (2012) indicate that TM was effective in reducing a wide range of health risks including hypertension, obesity, heart failure, and stress, while improving cognition. Additionally, TM has been particularly successful in coronary artery disease risk reduction (e.g., Zamarra et al. 1996). Given that South Asian Americans are at high risk of coronary artery disease (e.g., Mooteri et al. 2004), TM might be especially useful in treating this population.

5.2.4 Prayer

Although the psychological practices mentioned thus far have attracted attention in research and been included in treatment options in Western medicine, it is still necessary to continue to explore understudied cultural and spiritual rituals that may be related to patients' perceptions of their health. As mentioned in Part I, religiosity and spirituality are highly valued in South Asian culture due to their significant role in shaping South Asian health beliefs and relevance as a form of comfort and/or stress relief when coping with adversity (e.g., experiencing a health issue). One unobserved and neglected practice crucial to a large South Asian American population is the practice of prayer.

While several studies have shown that practicing religious activities and high levels of spirituality are associated with positive psychological and physical well-being (e.g., Yonker et al. 2012), it is essential to note that most forms of spiritual and religious interventions in the health setting are often catered towards Christian populations. Considering the prevalence of religious beliefs like Hinduism, Islam, Buddhism etc., among South Asian Americans, one way to gain the trust and compliance of these individuals is to develop services that are more inclusive and cater to these religious populations. As avenues of expressing spirituality have been discussed in the context of Hinduism and Buddhism (in relation to yoga and meditation), it may also be valuable to explore expression of spirituality through the lens of Islam, a religion that is popularly followed among the South Asian American population. Muslim prayer, or *salat,* is an obligatory religious activity prescribed to be performed five times daily at specific times throughout the day. *Salat* involves yogic qualities through its different postures, which include standing, bowing, prostrating, and sitting, as well as meditative qualities (the *Shoklas* mentioned earlier), through the recitation of Quranic verses that accompany each posture. Doufesh et al. (2014) found that during the performance of *salat*, parasympathetic activity in the nervous system increased while sympathetic activity decreased, suggesting that this practice may be beneficial in inducing relaxation while reducing anxiety and cardiovascular risk. This recent study only provides promising preliminary evidence warranting further investigation of the role of prayer in health.

Although *salat* shares qualities of yoga and meditation, one aspect that might make this practice unique is its association with community. Not only is it important to form a relationship with God and generate inner spirituality through *salat,* but Islamic principles also endorse the strengthening of community, which is driven by the notion that joint-prayer is rewarded more highly than praying in solitude. This cultivation of community provides Muslims with a support system that may be beneficial to fostering spirituality/religiosity, psychological adjustment, and managing distress stemming from sociocultural factors like acculturation and discrimination. This is particularly relevant considering the recent negative depiction of the South Asian American Muslim community in Western social and political spheres (e.g., post 9/11, Islamophobia, negative portrayal in the media, stereotypes). Thus, it is necessary for researchers, clinicians, and health professionals to investigate, implement, and provide culturally sensitive resources and treatment for the health of this population.

5.2.5 Cognitive Behavioral Therapy

Several forms of intervention and therapy have emerged over the past few decades that have been useful in addressing health concerns cross-culturally, including cognitive-behavioral therapy (CBT; Beck 2011). CBT employs cognitive restructuring to alter a client's situation and to alleviate distress surrounding unsolvable issues. Cognitive restructuring is development of the ability to recognize dysfunctional thoughts and negative tendencies in order to facilitate change.

CBT is a flexible model of treatment that allows for modification of schemas in a culturally sensitive manner to best fit traditional values and nuances. According to Hays (2009), there are several steps to deliver culturally competent CBT. These steps include (1) the assessment of the client's needs based on a culturally respectful interaction between therapist and client (e.g., therapist awareness that cultures have different norms in relation to actions that are respectful or disrespectful, such as maintaining eye contact), (2) identification of culturally related strengths and supports (e.g., pride in one's cultural, religious, spiritual identity), and (3) an understanding of the client's external and internal aspects with attention to cultural influences (e.g., factors mentioned in Part 2). Therapists may also be advised not to challenge core cultural beliefs of clients, but rather to provide culturally sensitive methods of solutions.

In terms of treatment, researchers and clinicians have found that not only are Asian Americans less likely to have patience for ambiguous forms of therapy and would rather seek a more structured, practical, and immediate solution to their problems, but also that Eastern culture does not align with Western views of placing importance on autonomy and the individual (e.g., Chen and Davenport 2005; Leong 1986). Therefore, it might be beneficial to contextualize a patient's cognitive/affective experiences when conducting CBT (Hwang et al. 2006). CBT may be useful for South Asian Americans since this group includes individuals of varying degrees of cultural and religious identity and involves a mixture of both South Asian and Western influences. Studies have shown the usefulness of CBT in South Asian populations seeking treatment for substance abuse (Rastogi and Wadhwa 2006), depression (Tewary et al. 2012), and acculturation issues within the family (Dattilio and Bahadur 2005).

There has also been progress towards creating adaptive CBT frameworks for non-Western cultures, such as Pakistani culture. Naeem et al. (2009) found that key limitations of the original framework for this population was focusing on therapy factors and failing to emphasize factors related to health beliefs and the health system in Pakistan. Unlike the Western world, not only are there fewer qualified healthcare professionals and accessible facilities, but many Pakistanis simply do not have the knowledge, trust, money, ability, or other resources to seek appropriate treatment.

Thus, Naeem and colleagues (Naeem et al. 2009; Naeem et al. 2010) developed a framework that accounted for several aspects of variability due to culture (e.g., religion/spirituality, family, language), capacity and circumstances (e.g., gender, education level, capacity of the health system), and cognitions (e.g., beliefs about health, treatment, doctors, diseases) to address the barriers faced by this particular population. Overall, this team of researchers believe that the adaptation process of CBT includes awareness of relevant cultural issues (such as those previously mentioned), assessment (e.g., identifying if the client is from an individualistic or collectivist culture to assess the importance of focusing on involving family into therapy), engagement (e.g., therapist opening up to patients about their own family may make patients feel warmer and more comfortable towards the therapist), and implementing adjustments in therapy (e.g., patients may find it easier to read, write, and speak in their native language with the therapist; Naeem et al. 2015). Although specific to Pakistan, assessing the functionality of this model among South Asian Americans may be useful since this group may hold different religious and philosophical values than South Asian Hindu/Buddhist American groups (e.g., some Hindu and Buddhist Americans may prefer meditative and yoga practices over prayer). The development of this adaptation of CBT shows that not only is it possible to modify existing frameworks, but also that evidence exists for the utility of CBT in South Asian culture (Naeem et al. 2011). Additionally, this adaptation points to importance of consulting therapists' cultural expertise and increasing open communication between the client and therapist to avoid mistakes, like stereotyping and misinterpretation of patients' behaviors based on cultural assumptions (Naeem et al. 2010). To culturally adapt models within the Western hemisphere, therapists need to commit to recognition of their own cultural biases and seek to continually increase their cultural awareness for the betterment of their clients (Dobson 2009).

5.2.6 Further Research

While the psychological models discussed have opened a meaningful dialogue, the exploration of culturally sensitive psychological practices among South Asian Americans warrants further research. The aforementioned practices only begin to touch on a few significant methods in response to specific health issues. Indeed, there are several ways to encourage behavior change including exposure, cognitive change, self-management, relaxation, acceptance, or any combination of these. Combinations and overlap of ideologies in existing models also expand across several other interventions that have not yet been mentioned. For instance, acceptance and commitment therapy (ACT; Hayes et al. 2011) uses similar strategies to those found in mindfulness or meditation, such as observing the self, emotions, and thoughts from an external perspective (Baer 2003). Additionally, mindfulness-based cognitive therapy (MBCT; Teasdale et al. 1995) consists of methods from both mindfulness meditation and CBT. Moreover, transcendental meditation and mindfulness not only share roots in history, but have also been found to be significantly associated (Alexander et al. 1989). Furthermore, it has been argued that some mindfulness interventions like MBSR are not embedded in Western models of psychotherapy, and serve more as complementary methods of treatment outside of traditional interventions when contrasted with CBT. Indeed, the examination of such practices through a culturally sensitive lens opens up the pathway of "mutual enrichment" of both traditional Eastern and Western psychology (Walsh and Shapiro 2006). Though previous studies have shown the utility and effectiveness of such behavioral interventions and practices among certain populations, some uncertainty still remains in the ability to generalize results to South Asian Americans. In addition, there seems to be a gap in the literature regarding practices that may be more specific to South Asian American groups, such as meditation, yoga, and prayer. Considering that such indigenous practices among South Asians have shown success in treating diverse populations, it may be beneficial to research the usefulness of such methods among various populations with differing cultural backgrounds. Finally, further research on South Asian American health practices will provide researchers with more useful information to aid in the creation of improved psychological models of health.

5.3 Implications and Concluding Thoughts

Overall, this chapter supports that the biopsychsocial approach to health may be especially useful in improving the trajectory of South Asian American health research and well-being. Accordingly, as the field of health psychology continues to progress, researchers and clinicians must aim to become more culturally competent and increase health literacy (awareness of mental health risks, health beliefs, health behaviors, and useful interventions) among not only themselves, but also South Asian Americans. As noted by Inman et al. (2014) in a three-decade analysis on psychological research among this population, it is evident that previous literature regarding South Asian American psychological health is scarce. In addition, much of the existing literature assesses South Asian immigrants, which is problematic because the increasing population of South Asian Americans consists of post-immigrant generations. For these reasons, there is a greater need to study second and third generation individuals and examine the extent of acculturation as it relates to health.

By looking through the cultural lens of pertinent populations, researchers and clinicians are able to address ethnic differences by creating adaptive interventions and models of health. Given that studies reported higher compliance rates among patients treated by culturally competent health professionals (e.g., Anderson et al. 2003), current research must be broadened to explore treatment preferences of South Asian Americans and the effectiveness of treatments discussed earlier among this population. For example, it is crucial for health professionals to be aware of the Westernization of meditative practices (Walsh and Shapiro 2006) when considering their application to non-Western patient populations. On one hand, some South

Asian Americans may appreciate a mixture between Western and Eastern practice, as some individuals identify with both cultures and mentalities, such as yoga exercises. On the other hand, some may prefer more traditional meditative treatments, such as TM or prayer, because of their cultural, spiritual, and religious familiarity. As evident in the discussion of the present chapter, aside from understanding which types of treatment would be most fitting for minority populations, it is imperative to improve the methods by which health issues among diverse populations are assessed by researchers through existing, and perhaps insufficient, models of health.

Thus, it is important to continue exploring and adapting the models discussed earlier in this chapter since key elements relevant to understanding South Asian American health may still be missing, such as perceptions of the psychological self. According to Markus and Kitayama (2010), the *self* is composed of both biological and sociocultural psychological realities (Markus and Kitayama 1991), and functions as a basis for self-regulatory schemas (the notion that conscious and unconscious processes regulate individual attention, perception, cognition, emotion, motivation, etc.) and tacitly extends to several psychological processes involved in health behavior. Indeed, past self-report surveys, experimental research, and field studies have indicated evidence of cross-cultural variations of the self (e.g., Kapoor et al. 2003; Morling and Lamoreaux 2008). Many of the explanatory models of health discussed thus far are built on functional influences of behavior that can discount differences prevailing in the psychological self. Understanding key cultural differences in the psychological self may be useful in identifying how culture plays a role in explaining how self-focused processes are involved in acting on health issues. For instance, one distinction to draw upon from the psychological health behaviors of South Asian Americans compared to other ethnic populations is that of coping. A recent study by Perera and Chang (2015) examining ethnic differences in coping strategies, found that South Asian Americans facing a stressful event reported the highest use of avoidant emotional coping strategies. This strategy type was also more strongly associated with depression in South Asian Americans, as compared to European Americans. Not only do these findings suggest that this population may be at higher risk of turning to maladaptive coping strategies (in that they have a positive, robust association with psychological maladjustment), but they acknowledge that there may be sociocultural influences in how South Asian Americans cope. Health beliefs may also be influenced by an individual's family (e.g., familial behavior, familial expectations, traditions, teachings) and the development of health perceptions through socialization. Influential factors of health like bicultural/hybrid identity, collectivism, familial influence etc., will be discussed in the following chapter on sociocultural models of health.

References

Ahmad, F., Cameron, J. I., & Stewart, D. E. (2005). A tailored intervention to promote breast cancer screening among South Asian immigrant women. *Social Science & Medicine, 60*, 575–586.

Alexander, C. N., Langer, E. J., Newman, R. I., Chandler, H. M., & Davies, J. L. (1989). Transcendental meditation, mindfulness, and longevity: An experimental study with the elderly. *Journal of Personality and Social Psychology, 57*, 950–964.

Anderson, L. M., Scrimshaw, S. C., Fullilove, M. T., Fielding, J. E., Normand, J., & Task Force on Community Preventive Services. (2003). Culturally competent healthcare systems: A systematic review. *American Journal of Preventive Medicine, 24*, 68–79.

Anderson, J. W., Liu, C., & Kryscio, R. J. (2008). Blood pressure response to transcendental meditation: A meta-analysis. *American Journal of Hypertension, 21*, 310–316.

Ajzen, I. (1991). The theory of planned behavior. *Organizational Behavior and Human Decision processes, 50*, 179–211.

Ajzen, I., & Fishbein, M. (1980). *Understanding attitudes and predicting social behavior.* Englewood Cliffs: Prentice-Hall.

Ajzen, I., & Madden, T. J. (1986). Prediction of goal-directed behavior: Attitudes, intentions, and perceived behavioral control. *Journal of Experimental Social Psychology, 22*, 453–474.

Astin, J. A. (1997). Stress reduction through mindfulness meditation. *Psychotherapy and Psychosomatics, 66*, 97–106.

Baer, R. A. (2003). Mindfulness training as a clinical intervention: A conceptual and empirical review. *Clinical Psychology: Science and Practice, 10*, 125–143.

Balaji, P. A., Varne, S. R., & Ali, S. S. (2012). Physiological effects of yogic practices and transcendental meditation in health and disease. *North American Journal of Medical Sciences, 4*, 442–448.

Bandura, A. (1986). *Social foundations of thought and action: A social cognitive theory.* Englewood Cliffs: Prentice-Hall.

Barnes, P. M., Adams, P. F., & Powell-Griner, E. (2008). *Health characteristics of the Asian adult population: United States, 2004–2006. Advance data from vital and health statistics no. 394.* Hyattsville: National Center for Health Statistics.

Beck, J. S. (2011). *Cognitive behavior therapy: Basics and beyond.* New York: Guilford Press.

Becker, M. H. (1974). The health belief model and personal health behavior. *Health Education Monographs, 2*, 324–508.

Bhattacharya, G. (2004). Health care seeking for HIV/AIDS among South Asians in the United States. *Health & Social Work, 29*, 106–115.

Bishop, S. R., Lau, M., Shapiro, S., Carlson, L., Anderson, N. D., Carmody, J., et al. (2004). Mindfulness: A proposed operational definition. *Clinical Psychology: Science and Practice, 11*, 230–241.

Bohlmeijer, E., Prenger, R., Taal, E., & Cuijpers, P. (2010). The effects of mindfulness-based stress reduction therapy on mental health of adults with a chronic medical disease: A meta-analysis. *Journal of Psychosomatic Research, 68*, 539–544.

Brown, L. A., Gaudiano, B. A., & Miller, I. W. (2011). Investigating the similarities and differences between practitioners of second- and third-wave Cognitive-Behavioral Therapies. *Behavior Modification, 35*, 187–200.

Brown, R. P., & Gerbarg, P. L. (2005). Sudarshan kriya yogic breathing in the treatment of stress, anxiety, and depression: Part II-clinical applications and guidelines. *Journal of Alternative & Complementary Medicine, 11*, 711–717.

Brown, K. W., & Ryan, R. M. (2003). The benefits of being present: mindfulness and its role in psychological well-being. *Journal of Personality and Social Psychology, 84*, 822–848.

Carmody, J., & Baer, R. A. (2008). Relationships between mindfulness practice and levels of mindfulness, medical and psychological symptoms and well-being in a mindfulness-based stress reduction program. *Journal of Behavioral Medicine, 31*, 23–33.

Champion, V. L., & Skinner, C. S. (2008). The health belief model. *Health behavior and health education: Theory, research, and practice, 4*, 45–65.

Chen, S. W. H., & Davenport, D. S. (2005). Cognitive-behavioral therapy with Chinese American clients: Cautions and modifications. *Psychotherapy: Theory, Research, Practice, Training, 42*, 101–110.

Chiesa, A., & Serretti, A. (2009). Mindfulness-based stress reduction for stress management in healthy people: A review and meta-analysis. *The Journal of Alternative and Complementary Medicine, 15*, 593–600.

Chowdhury, R., M Venkat Narayan, K., Zabetian, A., Raj, S., & Tabassum, R. (2014). Genetic studies of type 2 diabetes in South Asians: a systematic overview. *Current Diabetes Reviews, 10*, 258–274.

Cohen, M., & Azaiza, F. (2007). Health-promoting behaviors and health locus of control from a multicultural perspective. *Ethnicity and Disease, 17*, 636.

Creswell, J. D., Way, B. M., Eisenberger, N. I., & Lieberman, M. D. (2007). Neural correlates of dispositional mindfulness during affect labeling. *Psychosomatic Medicine, 69*, 560–565.

Dattilio, F. M., & Bahadur, M. (2005). Cognitive-behavioral therapy with an East Indian family. *Contemporary Family Therapy, 27*, 367–382.

Davidson, R. J., Kabat-Zinn, J., Schumacher, J., Rosenkranz, M., Muller, D., Santorelli, S. F., et al. (2003). Alterations in brain and immune function produced by mindfulness meditation. *Psychosomatic Medicine, 65*, 564–570.

Dillbeck, M. C., & Orme-Johnson, D. W. (1987). Physiological differences between transcendental meditation and rest. *American Psychologist, 42*, 879–881.

Dobson, K. S. (Ed.). (2009). *Handbook of cognitive-behavioral therapies*. New York: Guilford Press.

Doufesh, H., Ibrahim, F., Ismail, N. A., & Wan Ahmad, W. A. (2014). Effect of Muslim prayer (salat) on α electroencephalography and its relationship with autonomic nervous system activity. *The Journal of Alternative and Complementary Medicine, 20*, 558–562.

Enas, E. A., & Senthilkumar, A. (2005). Coronary artery disease in Asian Indians: An update and review. *Coronary Artery Disease, 3*, 21–57.

Feuerstein, G. (2014). *The psychology of yoga: Integrating Eastern and Western approaches for understanding the mind*. Boston: Shambhala Publications.

Fishbein, M. (2000). The role of theory in HIV prevention. *AIDS care, 12*, 273–278.

Fredrickson, B. L., Cohn, M. A., Coffey, K. A., Pek, J., & Finkel, S. M. (2009). Open hearts build lives: Positive emotions, induced through loving-kindness meditation, build consequential personal resources. *Journal of Personality and Social Psychology, 95*, 1045–1062.

Ghosh, C. (2003). Healthy People 2010 and Asian Americans/Pacific Islanders: Defining a baseline of information. *American Journal of Public Health, 93*, 2093–2098.

Grossman, P., Niemann, L., Schmidt, S., & Walach, H. (2004). Mindfulness-based stress reduction and health benefits: A meta-analysis. *Journal of Psychosomatic Research, 57*, 35–43.

Hall, L. M., Moran, C. N., Milne, G. R., Wilson, J., MacFarlane, N. G., Forouhi, N. G., et al. (2010). Fat oxidation, fitness and skeletal muscle expression of oxidative/lipid metabolism genes in South Asians: implications for insulin resistance? *PLoS One, 5*, e14197.

Hamid, P. N. (1994). Self-monitoring, locus of control, and social encounters of Chinese and New Zealand students. *Journal of Cross-Cultural Psychology, 25*, 353–368.

Hanh, T. N. (1975). *The miracle of mindfulness: An introduction to the practice of meditation* (trans: Ho, M.). Boston: Beacon Press.

Hays, P. A. (2009). Integrating evidence-based practice, cognitive–behavior therapy, and multicultural therapy: Ten steps for culturally competent practice. *Professional Psychology: Research and Practice, 40*, 354–360.

Hayes, S. C., Strosahl, K. D., & Wilson, K. G. (2011). *Acceptance and commitment therapy: The process and practice of mindful change*. New York: Guilford Press.

Hoeffel, E. M., Rastogi, S., Kim, M. O., & Shahid, H. (2012). *The Asian Population: 2010. 2010 Census Briefs*. Washington, DC: U.S. Census Bureau.

Hofmann, S. G., Sawyer, A. T., Witt, A. A., & Oh, D. (2010). The effect of mindfulness-based therapy on anxiety and depression: A meta-analytic review. *Journal of Consulting and Clinical Psychology, 78*, 169–183.

Hwang, W. C., Wood, J. J., Lin, K. M., & Cheung, F. (2006). Cognitive-behavioral therapy with Chinese Americans: Research, theory, and clinical practice. *Cognitive and Behavioral Practice, 13*, 293–303.

Inman, A. G., Devdas, L., Spektor, V., & Pendse, A. (2014). Psychological research on South Asian Americans: A three-decade content analysis. *Asian American Journal of Psychology, 5*, 364–372.

Ismail, H., Wright, J., Rhodes, P., & Small, N. (2005a). Religious beliefs about causes and treatment of epilepsy. *British Journal of General Practice, 55*, 26–31.

Ismail, H., Wright, J., Rhodes, P., Small, N., & Jacoby, A. (2005b). South Asians and epilepsy: Exploring health experiences, needs and beliefs of communities in the north of England. *Seizure, 14*, 497–503.

Jonnalagadda, S. S., & Diwan, S. (2005). Health behaviors, chronic disease prevalence and self-rated health of older Asian Indian immigrants in the US. *Journal of Immigrant Health, 7*, 75–83.

Kabat-Zinn, J. (1982). An outpatient program in behavioral medicine for chronic pain patients based on the practice of mindfulness meditation: Theoretical considerations and preliminary results. *General Hospital Psychiatry, 4*, 33–47.

Kabat-Zinn, J. (1990). *Full catastrophe living: Using the wisdom of your body and mind to face stress, pain and illness*. New York: Delacorte.

Kabat-Zinn, J. (2003). Mindfulness-based interventions in context: Past, present, and future. *Clinical Psychology: Science and Practice, 10*, 144–156.

Kapoor, S., Hughes, P. C., Baldwin, J. R., & Blue, J. (2003). The relationship of individualism–collectivism and self-construals to communication styles in India and the United States. *International Journal of Intercultural Relations, 27*, 683–700.

Kirmayer, L. J. (2007). Psychotherapy and the cultural concept of the person. *Transcultural Psychiatry, 44*, 232–257.

Kristeller, J. L., & Wolever, R. Q. (2011). Mindfulness-based eating awareness training for treating binge eating disorder: The conceptual foundation. *Eating Disorders, 19*, 49–61.

Kuntsevich, V., Bushell, W. C., & Theise, N. D. (2010). Mechanisms of yogic practices in health, aging, and disease. *Mount Sinai Journal of Medicine: A Journal of Translational and Personalized Medicine, 77*, 559–569.

Leong, F. T. (1986). Counseling and psychotherapy with Asian-Americans: Review of the literature. *Journal of Counseling Psychology, 33*, 196–206.

Lim, J. W., Gonzalez, P., Wang-Letzkus, M. F., & Ashing-Giwa, K. T. (2009). Understanding the cultural health belief model influencing health behaviors and health-related quality of life between Latina and Asian-American breast cancer survivors. *Supportive Care in Cancer, 17*, 1137–1147.

Macaden, L., & Clarke, C. L. (2010). The influence of locus of control on risk perception in older South Asian people with type 2 diabetes in the UK. *Journal of Nursing and Healthcare of Chronic Illness, 2*, 144–152.

MacLean, C. R., Walton, K. G., Wenneberg, S. R., Levitsky, D. K., Mandarino, J. P., Waziri, R., et al. (1997). Effects of the transcendental meditation program on adaptive mechanisms: Changes in hormone levels and responses to stress after 4 months of practice. *Psychoneuroendocrinology, 22*, 277–295.

Mamtani, R., & Mamtani, R. (2005). Ayurveda and yoga in cardiovascular diseases. *Cardiology in Review, 13*, 155–162.

Markus, H. R., & Kitayama, S. (1991). Culture and the self: Implications for cognition, emotion, and motivation. *Psychological Review, 98*, 224–253.

Markus, H. R., & Kitayama, S. (2010). Cultures and selves: A cycle of mutual constitution. *Perspectives on Psychological Science, 5*, 420–430.

Mason, A. E., Epel, E. S., Kristeller, J., Moran, P. J., Dallman, M., Lustig, R. H., et al. (2015). Effects of a mindfulness-based intervention on mindful eating, sweets consumption, and fast-

ing glucose levels in obese adults: data from the SHINE randomized controlled trial. *Journal of Behavioral Medicine*, 1–13.
Masuda, A., Mandavia, A., & Tully, E. C. (2014). The role of psychological inflexibility and mindfulness in somatization, depression, and anxiety among Asian Americans in the United States. *Asian American Journal of Psychology, 5*, 230.
Masuda, A., Wendell, J. W., Chou, Y. Y., & Feinstein, A. B. (2010). Relationships among self-concealment, mindfulness and negative psychological outcomes in Asian American and European American college students. *International Journal for the Advancement of Counselling, 32*, 165–177.
McEwen, B. S. (1998). Stress, adaptation, and disease: Allostasis and allostatic load. *Annals of the New York Academy of Sciences, 840*, 33–44.
Miller, J. J., Fletcher, K., & Kabat-Zinn, J. (1995). Three-year follow-up and clinical implications of a mindfulness meditation-based stress reduction intervention in the treatment of anxiety disorders. *General Hospital Psychiatry, 17*, 192–200.
Miller, C. K., Kristeller, J. L., Headings, A., Nagaraja, H., & Miser, W. F. (2012). Comparative effectiveness of a mindful eating intervention to a diabetes self-management intervention among adults with type 2 diabetes: A pilot study. *Journal of the Academy of Nutrition and Dietetics, 112*, 1835–1842.
Mohanty, S. A., Woolhandler, S., Himmelstein, D. U., & Bor, D. H. (2005). Diabetes and cardiovascular disease among Asian Indians in the United States. *Journal of General Internal Medicine, 20*, 474–478.
Mooteri, S. N., Petersen, F., Dagubati, R., & Pai, R. G. (2004). Duration of residence in the United States as a new risk factor for coronary artery disease (The Konkani heart study). *The American Journal of Cardiology, 93*, 359–361.
Morjaria, A., & Orford, J. (2002). The role of religion and spirituality in recovery from drink problems: A qualititative study of Alcoholics Anonymous members and South Asian men. *Addiction Research & Theory, 10*, 225–256.
Morling, B., & Lamoreaux, M. (2008). Measuring culture outside the head: A meta-analysis of individualism–collectivism in cultural products. *Personality and Social Psychology Review, 12*, 199–221.
Naeem, F., Ayub, M., Gobbi, M., & Kingdon, D. (2009). Development of Southampton Adaptation Framework for CBT (SAF-CBT): A framework for adaptation of CBT in non-western culture. *Journal of Pakistan Psychiatric Society, 6*, 79–84.
Naeem, F., Phiri, P., Munshi, T., Rathod, S., Ayub, M., Gobbi, M., & Kingdon, D. (2015). Using cognitive behaviour therapy with South Asian Muslims: Findings from the culturally sensitive CBT project. *International Review of Psychiatry, 27*, 233–246.
Naeem, F., Phiri, P., Rathod, S., & Kingdon, D. (2010). Using CBT with diverse patients: Working with South Asian Muslims. In M. Mueller, H. Kennerley, F. McManus, & D. Westbrook (Eds.), *Oxford Guide to Surviving as a CBT Therapist* (pp. 41–55). Oxford: Oxford University Press.
Naeem, F., Waheed, W., Gobbi, M., Ayub, M., & Kingdon, D. (2011). Preliminary evaluation of culturally sensitive CBT for depression in Pakistan: Findings from Developing Culturally-sensitive CBT Project (DCCP). *Behavioural and Cognitive Psychotherapy, 39*, 165–173.
Neff, K. (2003). Self-compassion: An alternative conceptualization of a healthy attitude toward oneself. *Self and Identity, 2*, 85–101.
Neff, K. D., Kirkpatrick, K. L., & Rude, S. S. (2007). Self-compassion and adaptive psychological functioning. *Journal of Research in Personality, 41*, 139–154.
Noar, S. M., & Zimmerman, R. S. (2005). Health Behavior Theory and cumulative knowledge regarding health behaviors: are we moving in the right direction? *Health Education Research, 20*, 275–290.
Orford, J. (2001). *Excessive appetites: A psychological view of addictions*. John Wiley & Sons Ltd.
Ostafin, B. D., Chawla, N., Bowen, S., Dillworth, T. M., Witkiewitz, K., & Marlatt, G. A. (2006). Intensive mindfulness training and the reduction of psychological distress: A preliminary study. *Cognitive and Behavioral Practice, 13*, 191–197.

Perera, M. J., & Chang, E. C. (2015). Depressive symptoms in South Asian, East Asian, and European Americans: Evidence for ethnic differences in coping with academic versus interpersonal stress? *Asian American Journal of Psychology, 6*, 350–358.

Prochaska, J. O., & DiClemente, C. C. (1982). Transtheoretical therapy: Toward a more integrative model of change. *Psychotherapy: Theory, Research & Practice, 19*, 276–288.

Prochaska, J. O., & Velicer, W. F. (1997). The transtheoretical model of health behavior change. *American Journal of Health Promotion, 12*, 38–48.

Prochaska, J. O., Velicer, W. F., Rossi, J. S., Goldstein, M. G., Marcus, B. H., Rakowski, W., et al. (1994). Stages of change and decisional balance for 12 problem behaviors. *Health Psychology, 13*, 39–46.

Rastogi, M., & Wadhwa, S. (2006). Substance abuse among Asian Indians in the United States: A consideration of cultural factors in etiology and treatment. *Substance Use & Misuse, 41*, 1239–1249.

Rodrigues, G., Jongbloed, L., Li, Z., & Dean, E. (2014). Ischaemic heart disease-related knowledge, behaviours, and beliefs of Indo-Canadians and Euro-Canadians: Implications for physical therapists. *Physiotherapy Canada, 66*, 208–217.

Rosenstock, I. M. (1966). Why people use health services. *The Milbank Memorial Fund Quarterly, 44*, 94–127.

Rosenstock, I. M. (1974). The health belief model and preventive health behavior. *Health Education Monographs, 2*, 354–386.

Roth, R. (1987). *Transcendental meditation*. New York: Donald I. Fine.

Rotter, J. B. (1966). Generalized expectancies for internal versus external control of reinforcement. *Psychological Monographs: General and Applied, 80*, 1–28.

Sadler, G. R., Dhanjal, S. K., Shah, N. B., Shah, R. B., Ko, C., Anghel, M., & Harshburger, R. (2001). Asian Indian women: Knowledge, attitudes and behaviors toward breast cancer early detection. *Public Health Nursing, 18*, 357–363.

Saravanan, B., Jacob, K. S., Johnson, S., Prince, M., Bhugra, D., & David, A. S. (2007). Belief models in first episode schizophrenia in South India. *Social Psychiatry and Psychiatric Epidemiology, 42*, 446–451.

Sastry, J., & Ross, C. E. (1998). Asian ethnicity and the sense of personal control. *Social Psychology Quarterly*, 101–120.

Satchidananda, S. (1990). *The Yoga Sutras of Patanjali*. Yogaville: Integral Yoga Publications.

Sedlmeier, P., Eberth, J., Schwarz, M., Zimmermann, D., Haarig, F., Jaeger, S., & Kunze, S. (2012). The psychological effects of meditation: A meta-analysis. *Psychological Bulletin, 138*, 1139–1171.

Shapiro, S. L., Astin, J. A., Bishop, S. R., & Cordova, M. (2005). Mindfulness-based stress reduction for health care professionals: Results from a randomized trial. *International Journal of Stress Management, 12*, 164–176.

Shapiro, S. L., Schwartz, G. E., & Bonner, G. (1998). Effects of mindfulness-based stress reduction on medical and premedical students. *Journal of Behavioral Medicine, 21*, 581–599.

Sheikh, S., & Furnham, A. (2000). A cross-cultural study of mental health beliefs and attitudes towards seeking professional help. *Social Psychiatry and Psychiatric Epidemiology, 35*, 326–334.

Sirois, F. M., Kitner, R., & Hirsch, J. K. (2015). Self-compassion, affect, and health-promoting behaviors. *Health Psychology, 34*(6), 661–669.

Slaney, R. B., Chadha, N., Mobley, M., & Kennedy, S. (2000). Perfectionism in Asian Indians exploring the meaning of the construct in India. *The Counseling Psychologist, 28*, 10–31.

Speca, M., Carlson, L. E., Goodey, E., & Angen, M. (2000). A randomized, wait-list controlled clinical trial: The effect of a mindfulness meditation-based stress reduction program on mood and symptoms of stress in cancer outpatients. *Psychosomatic Medicine, 62*, 613–622.

Stairs, A. (1992). Self-image, world-image: Speculations on identity from experiences with Inuit. *Ethos, 20*, 116–126.

Taylor, S. E. (1995). *Health psychology* (3rd ed.). New York: McGraw-Hill.

Teasdale, J. D., Segal, Z. V., & Williams, J. M. G. (1995). How does cognitive therapy prevent depressive relapse and why should attentional control (mindfulness) training help? *An information processing analysis. Behaviour Research & Therapy, 33*, 25–39.

Tewary, S., Jani, N., & Anstadt, S. P. (2012). Cognitive behavior therapy: A potential treatment for depression among Asian Indian immigrant women in the United States. *Journal of Human Behavior in the Social Environment, 22*, 463–478.

Thera, N. (1962). *The heart of Buddhist meditation: A handbook of mental training on the Buddha's way of mindfulness*. London: Rider.

Vadaparampil, S. T., Champion, V. L., Miller, T. K., Menon, U., & Skinner, C. S. (2004). Using the Health Belief Model to examine differences in adherence to mammography among African-American and Caucasian women. *Journal of Psychosocial Oncology, 21*, 59–79.

Vivekananda, S. (2016). *Raja yoga: Conquering the internal nature*. Advaita Ashrama. (Original work published in 1896).

Wallace, R. K. (1970). Physiological effects of transcendental meditation. *Science, 167*, 1751–1754.

Wallston, K. A., Wallston, B. S., & DeVellis, R. (1978). Development of the Multidimensional Health Locus of Control (MHLC) Scales. *Health Education & Behavior, 6*, 160–170.

Wallston, B. S., Wallston, K. A., Kaplan, G. D., & Maides, S. A. (1976). Development and validation of the Health Locus of Control (HLC) Scale. *Journal of Consulting and Clinical Psychology, 44*, 580–585.

Walsh, R., & Shapiro, S. L. (2006). The meeting of meditative disciplines and Western psychology: A mutually enriching dialogue. *American Psychologist, 61*, 227–239.

Weinstein, N. D., & Rothman, A. J. (2005). Commentary: Revitalizing research on health behavior theories. *Health Education Research, 20*, 294–297.

Wrightson, K. J., & Wardle, J. (1997). Cultural variation in health locus of control. *Ethnicity &Health, 2*, 13–20.

Wu, T. Y., West, B., Chen, Y. W., & Hergert, C. (2006). Health beliefs and practices related to breast cancer screening in Filipino, Chinese and Asian-Indian women. *Cancer Detection and Prevention, 30*, 58–66.

Yonker, J. E., Schnabelrauch, C. A., & DeHaan, L. G. (2012). The relationship between spirituality and religiosity on psychological outcomes in adolescents and emerging adults: A meta-analytic review. *Journal of Adolescence, 35*, 299–314.

Youngwanichsetha, S., Phumdoung, S., & Ingkathawornwong, T. (2014). The effects of mindfulness eating and yoga exercise on blood sugar levels of pregnant women with gestational diabetes mellitus. *Applied Nursing Research, 27*, 227–230.

Zamarra, J. W., Schneider, R. H., Besseghini, I., Robinson, D. K., & Salerno, J. W. (1996). Usefulness of the transcendental meditation program in the treatment of patients with coronary artery disease. *The American Journal of Cardiology, 77*, 867–870.

Zunaira Jilani is a graduate student in the Social Psychology PhD program at Wayne State University, Detroit. She received her M.S. in Clinical Psychology and B.A. with a double major in Psychology (with honors) and International Studies of Global Health from the University of Michigan. Ms. Jilani has conducted, presented, and published research on a wide range of topics, ranging from hope, spirituality/religiosity, sexual assault, and personality factors, to trauma, eating disturbances, negative affective conditions, and suicide risk. Currently, Ms. Jilani is interested in understanding the role of biopsychosocial factors in predicting health beliefs and behaviors in different racial/ethnic groups. Corresponding author: zunaira.jilani@wayne.edu

Edward C. Chang is Professor of Psychology and Social Work in the Department of Psychology and the School of Social Work at the University of Michigan. His interests involve optimism/pessimism, perfectionism, coping, and cultural influences on behavior.

Jerin Lee is an undergraduate student at the University of Michigan majoring in Psychology and minoring in Applied Statistics. Her research is focused on cross-cultural influences on motivation, coping, psychological and physical adjustment, positive psychological processes in diverse groups, and decision-making processes in adults. After college, she hopes to further her education in Psychology and pursue a PhD.

Casey N.-H. Batterbee is an undergraduate student in the Department of Psychology at the University of Michigan. His research is focused on psychological and physical adjustment in marginalized groups, the role of culture on health, and the role of positive psychological processes, including spirituality and religiosity.

Chapter 6
South Asian American Health: Perspectives and Recommendations on Sociocultural Influences

Riddhi Sandil and Ranjana Srinivasan

As outlined in earlier in this text, Asian Americans are one of the fastest growing ethnic groups in the United States, comprised of 19.4 million individuals (5.1% of the total U.S. population (U.S. Census 2012). This number reflects a 46% increase in population from 2008 when Asian Americans constituted close to 12% of the total population (11.9 million individuals). Historically, the term "Asian American" referenced individuals from East Asia, namely China, Japan, Korea, and the Philippines (Khandelwal 1988). This conceptualization of Asian Americans was somewhat accurate prior to the 1970s when 96% of Asians in the United States were of Chinese, Japanese, or Filipino heritage (Pew Research Center 2012a). However, the face of Asian Americans has since changed. Specifically, South Asian Americans (individuals who identify their ethnic origins to Bangladesh, Bhutan, India, the Maldives, Nepal, Pakistan, and Sri Lanka) are one of the fastest growing Asian American subgroups, with a population growth of 81% between 2000 and 2010 (1.9 million individuals to 3.4 million individuals) (U.S. Census 2012). Amongst the South Asian Americans, Asian Indians comprise the third largest group of Asian Americans in the United States at a population of 3.18 million, preceded only by Chinese Americans (3.79 million) and Filipino Americans (3.41 million). When combined with Pakistani and Bangladeshi Americans, the population of South Asian Americans surpasses that of Filipino Americans, thus becoming the second largest Asian American minority currently residing in in the United States (U.S. Census 2012).

Although South Asian Americans are rapidly becoming majority of the Asian American population in the United States, they are underrepresented in health research (Hussain-Gambles et al. 2004). Often grouped with other Asian Americans, unique concerns shared by South Asian Americans are often diluted or

R. Sandil (✉) · R. Srinivasan
Teachers College, Columbia University, New York, NY, USA
e-mail: sandil@tc.columbia.edu; rs3359@tc.columbia.edu

M. J. Perera, E. C. Chang (eds.), *Biopsychosocial Approaches to Understanding Health in South Asian Americans*, Cross-Cultural Research in Health, Illness and Well-Being, https://doi.org/10.1007/978-3-319-91120-5_6

underrepresented in research (Chen 2005). Studies suggest that South Asian Americans experience unique health disparities when compared to their Caucasian and East Asian American peers. Enas et al. (1996) reported that Asian Indians show higher incidence of coronary heart disease, diabetes, and hypertriglyceridemia when compared to White Americans. Similarly, Hsu et al. (2015) found that when compared to other Asian Americans, South Asian Americans had higher incidence of diabetes and associated complications. Misra and Vikram (2004) further suggest that along with the aforementioned health conditions, South Asian Americans might also be more likely to central obesity which can make this population particularly vulnerable to cardiovascular disease. Health disparities experienced by South Asians are also well documented in studies done in other Western countries (Bhopal et al. 1999; Williams et al. 2010; Whitty et al. 1999). Similar to South Asian Americans, South Asians in the United Kingdom and Canada also report higher incidences of coronary heart disease and diabetes when compared to other ethnic minorities in the United Kingdom and Canada (Williams et al. 2010).

Along with susceptibility to the aforementioned health conditions, South Asian Americans might not be oriented toward preventative health care (Bottorff et al. 1998). For example, physical activity has been shown to reduce the risk of contracting cardiovascular diseases and diabetes (Nelson et al. 2007). However, only 40% of South Asian Indian Americans reported engaging in regular physical activity (Misra et al. 2000). In their meta-analysis of physical activity in Asian Indians, Daniel and Wilbur (2011) found similar results with at least 40% of the examined studies indicating low physical activity in this population.

Asian Americans share distinct cultural values that can be linked to their ethnic and racial identity (Kim et al. 2001). Namely collectivism, family honor, and adherence to religious and moral expectations are Asian American cultural values that are endorsed by South Asian American individuals (Ibrahim et al. 1997). There is agreement that given their distinct ethnic and cultural heritage, South Asian Americans exhibit unique variances of these shared Asian cultural values and these, subsequently, may impact the health of South Asian Americans.

Firstly, this chapter will substantiate on the impact of common South Asian American cultural values including religiosity, collectivism, morality, and adherence to traditional gender roles on the health of South Asian Americans. Secondly, experiences that are salient in this population, including acculturation and racial discrimination, will be expanded upon, particularly as they relate to the physical well-being of this unique population. Lastly, recommendations for culturally-sensitive practice will be provided as existing research indicates that the specific needs of South Asian Americans are commonly overlooked in the current health care system (Ahmed and Lemkau 2000).

6.1 South Asian Cultural Values

Given the complexity and diversity of South Asian cultures, there are significant differences in cultural practices of South Asian populations. For example, India is composed of 29 states, each with its own cultural practices and traditions. Hence, individuals from different parts of the country might exhibit unique cultural characteristics. Religion, collectivism, morality, and gender can have a significant influence on these varied South Asian populations, which in turn could impact health practices of this population. These cultural values and their subsequent influence on South Asian health are expanded on below.

6.1.1 Religion and Religious Identity

According to the Religious Landscape Study conducted by the Pew Research Center (2015), the most prominent religious identities for Asian Americans include Hindu, Buddhist, Muslim, Catholic, and non-religious. Although religious identity by South Asian subgroup was not examined, data on religious affiliation for Indian Americans show 51% identifying as Hindu, 10% as Muslim, 18% as Christian, 5% as Sikh, 2% as Jain, and 10% as unaffiliated (Pew Research Center 2012b). Hannay (1980) explored the relationship between active versus passive religious allegiance and its association with symptom frequencies, and found that the further people are from their cultural base, the more important religious activity becomes in order to find a sense of stability. This phenomenon seems to be true for South Asian Americans with research suggesting that South Asian immigrants are often more religious after immigrating than they were in their host country, and that religious activities help South Asian Americans feel more connected to their ethnicity and heritage, and allow them to bequeath cultural practices with future generations (Dasgupta 1998; Williams 1988). With regard to religiosity and health beliefs, Bhattacharya (2004) suggests that South Asians may have a sense that certain experiences, including health concerns, are unavoidable. Therefore, instead of seeking health care in a timely manner to alleviate their symptoms, this population might view their situation as a destiny they must accept.

Frequent correlations have also been noticed between an individual's level of religiosity and quality of physical health (Clements and Ermakova 2012). Actively practicing a religion has been shown to reduce involvement in harmful health behaviors such as unhealthy diet and the practice of unsafe sex (Jones 2004). In addition, as discussed in the prior chapter, many religious practices such as meditation and centering prayer elicit a sort of "relaxation response" that contributes a reduction in sympathetic nervous system activity, reduced muscle tension, reduced activity of the anterior pituitary/adrenocortical axis, lower blood pressure, and lower heart rate (Benson 1996). People involved in religious institutions are also provided with a support system, which can play a positive role in maintaining healthy mental and physical behaviors. Jones also noted that people who identify as religious are more attentive and compliant to treatment plans given by their medical providers, and have increased optimism towards their treatment (2004). Indeed, optimism mediates the relationship between religion and health in the face of serious illness, such as coping with cancer (Sherman and Simonton 2001).

Specific studies have examined South Asian religious practices and its ability to lead to improved health. For example, Sudsuang et al. (1991) conducted a study with Thai college students to understand the relationship between Buddhist meditation and serum cortisol levels, serum protein levels, and blood pressure. The subjects spent two months within a monastery, meditating between two to four hours a day. Measurements were taken before the program began, three weeks into the program, and six weeks into the program. The results showed that for the experimental group there were reductions in blood pressure, pulse rate, and serum cortisol level. Asian religious practices such as meditation may serve as protective factors among practicing South Asian Americans.

Similarly, Hsiao et al. (2006) studied the relationship between complementary and alternative medicine practice in a sample of 9187 Asian Americans living in California. Nearly 75% of the sample population had engaged in alternative medicine treatments such as using an Ayurvedic practitioner, chiropractor, massage therapist, and acupuncturist. Asian Americans who reported a high level of spirituality were more likely to engage in alternative medicine practices. Hsiao et al. (2006) suggest that the Asian Americans might be more likely to consolidate Eastern and Western perspectives of healing when managing their health care needs. The correlation between the increased use of alternative medicinal practices and religiosity suggests that these techniques may provide South Asians' additional spiritual support beyond traditional Western health practices.

6.1.2 Collectivism

The common hierarchical structure of South Asian American families creates an environment in which each person has a specific role they must adhere to for the family to adequately function. These given roles are often interdependent and dictated by traditional Asian values (Sue and Sue 1993). Within a typical family unit, fathers are considered to be the head of the household and the decision makers of the family (Matthews 2000). Mothers are frequently seen as caretakers of the husband, the children, and the extended family members. Sons often have immense pressure to achieve at a high level in order to carry on the family name, and are also viewed as additional providers for the family. Daughters are to perform domestic duties and to be subservient to the family as a whole (Kim et al. 2001). For all family members, there is an obligation to the larger group that is put before individual needs, thereby suggesting that collectivism might be a salient concept for South Asian Americans (Ballard 1982).

For the South Asian American population, the concept of "family" often extends beyond the immediate bloodline, as family friends are called "aunties" and "uncles," and cousins are considered as close as brothers and sisters (Das and Kemp 1997). Family roles and responsibilities are shared amongst the larger community and family members greatly lean on one another, which at times involves having shared living spaces amongst multiple families (Das and Kemp 1997).

Due to the collectivistic nature of the community, personal decision-making and problem solving are also considered to be a family matter. Kitano and Matsushima (1981) noted that Asian Americans often turn to authority figures in the community for assistance with problems due to their increased expertise and vast experience in life. The term "*filial piety*" has been used to describe how traditional Asian cultures put an immense importance on showing respect and compliance to elders and parental figures (Zhan and Montgomery 2003). This can specifically manifest itself with younger South Asian American generations. They are typically expected to show reverence and admiration to elders, which in turn could increase the hesitation in discussing sensitive topics with older individuals (Chung et al. 2005).

Within the Asian American community, individuals are thought to be a representation of their larger household (Kim et al. 2001). This requires much time and energy to be directed towards upholding the family name and keeping the family unit intact. Within this community, individual achievements and successes are directed not only towards the individual, but to the family as a whole. This expectation to serve as family representatives is also seen in protecting the family from adverse societal judgments. It reflects negatively on the family, and in turn, brings shame to the whole community (Sue and Sue 1993). Due to the collectivistic atmosphere of South Asian culture, individuals may feel a strong sense of attachment to their cultural group, and a requirement to bring esteem to their family.

Family honor also manifests itself within South Asian health due to the pride and avoidance of accepting one's health issues and the impact that the health issues might have on the family as a whole. Frey and Roysircar (2006) posited three underlying reasons that Asian Americans do not utilize health services: (1) lack of trust in helping professionals and their services, (2) lack of knowledge about the availability of services and (3) stigma associated with formal help seeking. Within the culture, it is thought to be taboo to speak about individual problems or difficulties because it will stigmatize not only the person who needs help, but also the entire family (Das and Kemp 1997). This perspective affects the utilization of health and mental health treatment for the South Asian American community because bringing attention to one's own health problems creates a "me" identity instead of a "we" identity. In addressing personal health concerns, South Asian Americans may feel the stigma that is associated with various diagnoses such as human immunodeficiency virus infection and acquired immune deficiency syndrome (HIV/AIDS), and feel that they are a poor reflection on their families. Along with this, South Asian Americans have great pride and honor in their culture, and often make it a priority to continue cultural traditions within the acculturation process.

Collectivism could also have a unique impact on compliance of health care intervention within South Asian populations. In their study on South Asians living in

Canada, Bannerji et al. (2010) found that South Asians participants were more likely to complete a cardiac rehabilitation program if the program had community member endorsement. Similarly, Ahmed et al. (2004) found South Asian Canadian women to be more likely to seek health care information from community members and social networks.

Collectivism can also influence what is or is not shared with health care providers. At times, uncomfortable topics, including stigmatized mental and physical health conditions, may be left out of conversation to preserve the family harmony (Gudykunst 2001). The collectivistic nature of addressing concerns and problems causes South Asian individuals to be less forthcoming in speaking about health-related issues. Understandably, this discretion could have serious ramifications on the well-being of South Asian Americans.

6.1.3 Morality

Similar to religious values, South Asian Americans may have cultural moral values that can be linked to well-being (Saran 1985). For example, chastity and virginity are highly valued in Asian Indian culture, and dating is frequently only acceptable within the context of a possible marriage (Dhruvarajan 1993; Saran 1985). An Asian Indian woman's sexuality may be viewed as a threat to her family and community, and engaging in sexual relationships before marriage can be interpreted as betrayal of one's family (Dasgupta and Dasgupta 1996; Inman et al. 2001). These cultural moral values can be challenged when South Asians, and particularly Asian Indian women, assimilate to the United States where dating and sexual relationships are regarded as an important part of self-development. This contrasting and new American environment (that is more accepting of premarital romantic relationships) might invoke feelings of confusion, envy, and conflict in South Asian Americans. Discussing or acknowledging these feelings could be construed as a betrayal of family and cultural values, and South Asian American women might be less likely to discuss these issues with family and friends (Sweta 2005). Further, the control of the immigrant South Asian American women's sexuality can be disguised under the notion of cultural preservation (Madan-Bahel 2008). Thus, South Asian American women might be reticent to seek sexual health care given the cultural values of morality and chastity.

Similarly, along with revering chastity and virginity, identification as lesbian, gay, bisexual, transgender, and/or queer (LGBTQ) is also highly discouraged within the community (Bhattacharya 2004). For some, being gay is viewed as a deviant and unacceptable behavior that brings dishonor and shame to one's family (Szymanski and Sung 2013). The purpose of sexual behavior is thought to be strictly for procreation, therefore these identities go against this ideal and are socially not accepted.

Sandil et al. (2015) applied the Minority Stress Theory and the Feminist Multicultural Theory to the experiences of South Asian lesbian gay, bisexual, and queer (LGBQ) individuals to examine incidents of discrimination due to multiple marginalized identities, and effects on mental health. The results indicated that South Asian LGBQ participants who have experienced heterosexist discrimination and have higher levels of internalized heterosexism also report higher levels of psychological stress. Additionally, it shows that the collectivistic nature of South Asian culture can intensify the psychological stress experienced by this population. South Asian sexual minorities often have difficulty in identifying as gay, lesbian, and bisexual because of the negative conceptualizations of LGBQ identities in the community. These individuals often engage in heterosexual relationships in order to avoid the discriminatory stress (Choudhury et al. 2009).

These beliefs around dating and sexuality often prevent South Asian American individuals from engaging in health care treatments related to their sexual activity or sexuality. An individual may choose not to be tested for HIV/AIDS or disclose a positive result due to the shame that could be put on their family and community (Bhattacharya 2004). There is also a lack of sex education within the population, and many are not aware of contraceptive options. Unsafe abortions contribute to deaths of South Asian Americans from hemorrhage and sepsis due to the pressures of purity on women (Fikree and Pasha 2004). For South Asian women, there is also importance placed on maintaining one's dignity and practicing modesty, and this also applies within a health care setting. According to Bottorff et al. (1998), within breast cancer research, many South Asian women reported feeling shy about having male physicians examine their breasts, and had an overall hesitancy to be touched by a male physician or to undress for examinations. Along with this, many women said that they were uncomfortable doing a self-breast examination due to the possibility of it being misconstrued as being inappropriate.

6.1.4 Gender Role

Gender is a socio-cultural construction that outlines specific characteristics and behavior expectations based on one's biological sex (Abraham 1995). Children are socialized from infancy to adhere to strict gender norms as outlined by their culture (Bem 1983). Das and Kemp (1997) suggest that first generation South Asian immigrant families have well-defined hierarchical gender roles which impact family roles and dynamics. Typically, women hold the subordinate position within the family structure, thereby, taking on the role of caregivers whereas men hold the responsibility for earning an income and financially supporting the family. These familial expectations also extend to other gender-defined roles. In accordance with other Asian beliefs, there are primary roles ascribed for women: daughter, wife, and mother (Ibrahim et al. 1997; Ibrahim 1994). Conversely, men are seen as protectors and expected to assume a dominant role within the family structure. As expected, these role expectations can have consequences on the well-being of South Asian Americans.

South Asian gender roles expect that women carry the primary responsibility of taking care of the home, preparing meals, and child care (Dasgupta 1998; Choudhry

2001). These gender role expectations also have an impact of physical well-being of South Asian women. When asked about physical exercise, South Asian women often report that they do not have time for exercise given their household duties and expectations (Sriskantharajah and Kai 2007). When asked about barriers to physical exercise, using a sample of South Asian women with coronary heart disease and diabetes, Sriskantharajah and Kai (2007) found that participants reported that reserving time in the day for exercise was a selfish activity, one that hindered a woman's ability to attend to other duties such as care-giving and cooking. Participants acknowledged the importance of physical activity but only when it contributed toward their other duties and expectations. For example, being active around the home was regarded as an acceptable way of engaging in physical exercise as this activity also led to caretaking of family members.

Similarly, Choudhry (2001) suggests that South Asian immigrant women may not prioritize their own health care and well-being since their primary concern is the health of their family. Thus, often, preventative programs failed to meet the needs of South Asian immigrant women as they had not been socialized to think about their health and thus might not participate in prevention programs (Choudhry 2001). This socialization was also evident in a study by Weerasinghe and Numer (2011) where South Asian Canadian immigrant, widowed women stated that they were not allowed to participate in physical activity as children and young adults as this was not acceptable given their gender. This lack of agency was also noted in later life, where women reported that even after retirement, they could not engage in health-promoting leisure activities as they felt responsible for caretaking of their children and grandchildren. Thus, gender role socialization has a long-term impact on the ability of and likelihood of South Asian populations engaging in health promotion and maintenance activities.

6.2 Unique Experiences of South Asian Populations and Impact on Health

Along with having unique cultural characteristics, South Asian American populations also share experiences that are specific and related to cultural heritage and identity. Literature suggests that intimate partner violence, acculturation/acculturative stress, and racism not only contribute to poorer psychological well-being but also can impact physical health of South Asian populations (Gee and Ponce 2010; Kalra et al. 2004; Raj et al. 2005). The following section expands on the aforementioned experiences and their unique influence on South Asian health.

6.2.1 Intimate Partner Violence

The World Health Organization (WHO) estimates that 15–71% of women worldwide will experience violence through an intimate partner (WHO 2008). Intimate partner violence is any behavior of one intimate partner that causes physical, sexual or emotional harm to the other partner in the relationship (WHO 2002; Ahmed et al. 2013). 25–40% of South Asian women in the United States have experienced physical violence through an intimate partner (Ayyub 2000; Dasgupta 2000; Raj and Silverman 2002). These rates are much higher than those reported by other ethnic minorities in the United States (for example, 29% for African Americans and 23.4% for Hispanic Americans [Women of Color Network 2006]), and within the Asian American community at large (Raj and Silverman 2002). Even with these staggering prevalence rates, South Asian American communities are often overlooked when examining the etiology of domestic violence incidents (Midlarsky et al. 2006). Theorists posit that this occurs due to several factors: South Asian individuals are viewed as the model minority, there is a propensity to deny the existence of domestic violence in Asian American households, and there might be a different cultural understanding of what constitutes physical, sexual and emotional abuse (Midlarsky et al. 2006; Tjaden and Thoennes 2000).

South Asian cultural norms can dictate how abuse is perceived within the community. For example, sexual abuse defined as unwelcome touching and forced sexual activity is not always viewed as abuse in the context of South Asian marriages (Midlarsky et al. 2006). Cultural norms suggest that sexual activity within a marriage is the right of a husband and considered male privilege (Midlarsky et al. 2006). Similarly, verbal violence is only considered abuse when it is done in a public setting and includes derogation and insults (Midlarsky et al. 2006). This nuanced understanding of what constitutes abuse leads to lower reporting within South Asian communities and, as a result, lower help-seeking behaviors (Raj and Silverman 2002).

With regards to health, intimate partner violence (IPV), physical and sexual abuse, has an impact on women's reproductive health. Studies with White American women and Latinas have linked HIV risk with a history of abuse and lower relationship autonomy (Quina et al. 2000; Pulerwitz et al. 2002). Similarly, Beadnell et al. (2000) found that women who were in a relationship with active physical violence were less likely to engage in safe sex and HIV prevention interventions compared to women who were not in physically abusive relationships. IPV has also been linked to overall poorer reproductive health, with survivors reporting higher rates of menstrual abnormalities, unwanted pregnancies, termination of pregnancies and pelvic pain than women who have not been in a physically abusive relationship (Heise et al. 2002).

To understand the impact of IPV on the health of South Asian American women, Raj et al. (2005) sampled 208 South Asian heterosexual women living in the United States. The study found that when compared to South Asian American women who were not in violent relationships, victims of IPV were almost 3 times more likely to experience distressing health outcomes including burning during urination, discolored vaginal discharge, and unwanted pregnancies. There are significant health concerns for women in violent relationships.

To capture a more in-depth understanding of the experiences of South Asian victims of IPV, Raj et al. (2005) then conducted in-depth interviews with 23 survivors of IPV. Incident rates in this group were even higher, with almost 61% of the sample reporting burning during urination, 21% stated having discoloration in vaginal discharge, and 40% of the sample experienced an unwanted pregnancy. Additionally, approximately 11% of the sample had also undergone reproductive sterilization, with some of the participants reporting that they resorted to sterilization because of gynecological damage inflicted during sexual assault by their husbands. Along with the pervasive health consequences for South Asian American women in violent relationships, this study also highlighted the lack of preventative reproductive health practices in this population since approximately one third of the population in both samples admitted that they had not had a pap smear in the previous year. South Asian victims in the United States were found not only to be vulnerable to poorer health outcomes but also less likely to engage in preventative gynecological interventions (Raj et al. 2005).

Similar health consequences were reported by Hurwitz et al. (2006). With a sample of 208 South Asian women living in the United States, results showed that victims of IPV were four times more likely to report poor physical health (such as illness, injury, chronic pain, and stress headaches) in seven of the last 30 days, two times more likely to report sleep disturbances and three times more likely to report health inhibited daily activity for seven or more days in the last month (Hurwitz et al. 2006). In their qualitative study, Hurwitz et al. (2006) found that victims of IPV struggled with ongoing pain as result of physical violence in their relationships and this usually manifested itself in the form of headaches, backaches, and gastrointestinal concerns. Victims of IPV also reported that their injuries prevented them from normal life functioning including care-taking, spending time with family and work, thereby impacting overall life satisfaction. Lastly, sleep disturbances were also seen in this population. Victims attributed post-traumatic stress symptoms, such as anticipation of abuse and nightmares, to their disruptive sleep patterns (Hurwitz et al. 2006). Victims of IPV suffered significantly higher physical health ramifications when compared to South Asian women who had not been victimized, indicating that South Asian American female survivors of IPV are at greater risk for health problems.

6.2.2 Acculturation and Acculturative Stress

The earliest definition of acculturation was "those phenomena which result when groups of individuals having different cultures come into continuous, firsthand contact with subsequent changes in the original cultural patterns of either or both groups" (Redfield et al. 1936, p. 149). Thus, acculturation can influence both the immigrant and the host culture of a society. Throughout the acculturation process, many changes might take place at the individual level. These changes can be physical (moving to a new country, differences in physical environments), biological (exposure to different diseases, adapting to a new diet), cultural (exposure to different religions, new forms of government, novel languages and customs) and psychological (changes in mental health of an individual as they try to adapt to a new environment) (Berry and Kim 1988). These difficulties are often grouped together and referred to as *acculturative stress* (Berry and Annis 1974).

Research suggests that acculturative stress can have lasting negative impact on the health of immigrants (for example overall cancer rates, high blood pressure, nicotine use and adolescent pregnancy) in the United States (Vega and Amaro 1994). As immigrants integrate into the United States they are more vulnerable to experiencing discrimination and exclusion, which are linked to psychological stress, which is further connected with poorer mental and physical health outcomes such as increased blood pressure and anxiety (Vega and Amaro 1994; Kuo 1995). Studies have also tried to establish connection between acculturation and health outcomes in Asian immigrants, specifically vulnerability to health conditions such as cardiovascular disease and preventative healthy behaviors such as attitudes toward help seeking behavior and routine physicals (Atkinson and Gim 1989; Frisbie et al. 2001; Tang et al. 2000; Unger et al. 2000; Uppaluri et al. 2001). Frisbie et al. (2001) also found that length of stay in the United States had a detrimental impact on the health of migrants with their health declining with continued residence in the United States. It should be noted that health in this study was measured by participant self-assessment of health, activity limitation due to illness as number of days a participant was bedridden because of health concerns, and number of visits to a physician. This study also found that access and utilization of health care services amongst Asian immigrants was less than the national average, and newer immigrants (individuals who had been in the United States for less than 10 years) were three to four times more likely to report no regular contact with medical professionals.

With regards to South Asian Americans, most of the existing research has examined the link between acculturation and psychological well-being (Bhugra 2004; Mehta 1998; Samuel 2009). Studies that have examined the link between acculturation/acculturative stress and physical health correlates of South Asian Americans are sparse. Kalra et al. (2004) examined the relationship between perceptions of cardiovascular disease in 57 Asian Indians living in northern California. While the participants demonstrated knowledge about cardiovascular health risk factors, they were more likely to attribute cardiovascular health to genetic propensity and disposition. Interestingly, when discussing stress related risk factors, participants outlined acculturative stress as a concern that impacts their physical well-being. Specifically, participants highlighted loss of social support upon migration, occupational distress (particularly taking jobs for which immigrants were overqualified), supporting extended family in their host country and lastly, being worried that their children would not retain their South Asian cultural values as potential factors that impacted their stress and subsequently cardiovascular health (Kalra et al. 2004).

Similarly, Tirodkar et al. (2011) reported that South Asian immigrants living in Chicago adhered to a biopsychosocial perspective when conceptualizing their own health and risk for disease. Participants mentioned acculturative stress as one of the factors contributing to poorer health (in particular, diabetes and cardiovascular disease) and suggested that a lack of stress would logically result in a lack of sickness. Women in this study were more likely to highlight acculturative stress as it related to a loss of social support upon migration whereas men highlighted being under employed, overworked or having financial struggles as the manifestations of their migration related stress (Tirodkar et al. 2011). Thus, there is evidence to suggest that South Asian immigrants understand the impact of acculturation and migration related stress on their physical well-being.

6.2.3 Racism and Racial Discrimination

Clark et al. (1999) defined racism as "beliefs, attitudes, institutional arrangements or acts that tend to denigrate individuals or groups due to phenotypic characteristics or ethnic group affiliation" (p.805). Similar to other ethnic minorities, South Asian Americans have a long-standing history of experiencing systemic discrimination and racism in the United States (Sheth 1995). South Asians were denied land ownership and prevented from immigrating to the United States due to exclusionary institutional laws such as the Barred Zone Act in 1917 and the Asian Exclusion Act of 1924. Even post 1965, when immigration laws were relaxed in the United States, South Asian Americans continued to experience harassment and discrimination due to their ethnic identity (Sheth 1995). An example, post-September 11 terrorist attacks, South Asian Americans reported an increase in their experience of race based harassment or discrimination (Bhatia 2008; Inman et al. 2007).

Research has examined the role of racism on psychological well-being and it is evident that experiences of racism and race based trauma are linked to poorer psychological health for South Asian Americans (Lee 2003; Liang et al. 2004). Experiences of being perceived as a perpetual foreigner, treated with mistrust given one's accent and/or religion, and of being discriminated because of wearing a turban or hijab are some examples of race-based trauma experienced by South Asian Americans (Cheryan and Monin 2005; Devos and Banajee 2005). Dasgupta (2006) also adds that South Asian Americans tend to deny or diminish these experiences of racism thereby leading to an increase in psychological distress.

Recent literature has examined the link between racism and physical health correlates and found that race-based discrimination has a negative impact on the physical health (such as increased psychological stress, use of nicotine, an increased risk of cardiovascular disease) of ethnic minorities (Gee et al. 2007; Landrine et al. 2006; Utsey et al. 2000). Some studies have also linked racism to poorer cardiovascular health through psychological stress and cardiovascular health (Gee and

Walsemann 2009; Lewis et al. 2010; Troxel et al. 2003). Additionally, experiences of racism can also result in maladaptive coping behaviors such as substance use in Asian Americans (Chae et al. 2008). With regards to South Asian Americans, similar results have emerged. In their study on 423 Asian Indian Americans living in Michigan, Yoshihama et al. (2012) found that day-to-day discrimination negatively impacted psychological and physical health of the participants. In particular, men in this study reported that discrimination negatively impacted their general health and overall well-being.

In their study on racism and well-being with six Asian American ethnic groups, Gee and Ponce (2010) found interesting links between racial discrimination, self-reported health and activity limitation. Similar to other Asian Americans in this study, South Asian Americans limited their activity on days that they experienced racial discrimination. Additionally, racial discriminatory experiences were linked with experiences of ill-health for some Asian American subgroups. Interestingly, however, racial discrimination was not associated with increased reports of ill-health by South Asian Americans in this study (Gee and Ponce 2010).

Thus, there is evidence to suggest that persistent experiences of racial discrimination might be negatively impacting the health South Asian Americans. As with other ethnic groups in the United States, it is evident that racial discrimination can have a substantial impact on the psychological and physical well-being of South Asian Americans (Gee et al. 2009) and it's important to be mindful of experiences of discrimination when working with South Asian Americans.

6.3 Recommendations for Culturally Competent Care: Meeting the Needs of South Asian American Individuals

South Asians are particularly vulnerable to cardiovascular-related problems and diseases. For instance, South Asian Americans are two times more likely than their Euro-American peers to develop coronary artery disease (Nair and Prabhakaran 2012). Further, South Asian Americans may be at higher risk for such diseases due to multiple factors such as acculturation, ethnic identity, lack of awareness regarding healthful practices and inability of health care providers to provide culturally competent care. In addition, South Asian Americans do not appear to be as oriented toward preventative care as other Americans. This section will provide a list of recommendations and considerations for health care providers working with and treating this unique population.

6.3.1 Inclusion of Cultural Factors in Treatment Planning and Intervention.

As outlined earlier, South Asian Americans have unique cultural characteristics that impact treatment adherence and implementation. It is recommended that health care providers be aware of cultural characteristics such as religiosity, collectivism, family honor and morality when working with South Asian Americans. Regarding religion, it is important for health care providers to take into account that South Asian clients may have specific treatment needs due to their religious affiliation, and that certain religious practices may become prominent within their clients' lives during times of illness (Ahmed and Lemkau 2000). Religiosity has been positively related to overall wellness and health, and it could be beneficial to acknowledge the presence of religion in client's lives and incorporate their religious practices into treatment.

Cultural attitudes around pre-marital sexuality, LGBTQ identities, and the female body often prevent South Asian Americans from accessing and taking part in appropriate health care. Health care providers should be mindful around cultural values such as modesty and morality to address health concerns in a sensitive and multicultural manner. Family relationships are important in this population, and including family members in preventative care may be beneficial. It is important for health care professionals to be aware that the South Asian patient may choose to make health-related decisions in consultation with his/her family. When appropriate, medical professionals are encouraged to be open to the family unit as involved with the health related decision-making processes. An example, Walker et al. (2015), suggest that having grandchildren (as opposed to health care providers) explain the benefits of exercise and physical activity might be more salient for elderly South Asian Americans. Furthermore, it is also common for South Asian Americans, particularly women, to rely on family members when dealing with health concerns and patients often seek medical help after encouragement from family members (Grewal et al. 2005). It is important for medical professionals to recognize cultural factors that can impact prognosis and seeking of services among the South Asian American population.

Lastly, Srinivasan and Guillermo (2000) explains that there are several gaps within the knowledge of health care for minority specific needs. Currently the information for determining dosage levels for Asian Americans does not take into account the varied metabolisms, diets, heights, and weights of this population. The lack of recognition of their needs and the fear of being misunderstood or misdiagnosed by a health care provider who does not understand them may cause more resistance to engage in the health care system.

6.3.2 Recognizing the Unique Role of Gender and Gender Role Expectations in Treatment Planning and Health Care Interventions.

South Asian Americans often adhere to strict gender roles which can impact the success of health interventions. It may be important for health care providers to understand and respect the patient's gender and its possible impact on adherence to health interventions. For example, Astin et al. (2008) found that male South Asian family members, whether they were patients or not, were most influential with regards to dietary decisions and modifications. Even when female caregivers were willing to make dietary changes for male cardiac patients, they often did not do so as South Asian men were unwilling to follow through with dictary modifications. Furthermore, data suggested that dietary modifications were often made to accommodate the male patient's needs and not when the cardiac patient was a woman. When women were expected to make dietary modifications, they stated that they often had to make separate meals for themselves and given the extra time and effort this required, they would soon stop following their dietary regime. Thus, in this study it was clear that male members of families had higher influence when it came to the diet and food decisions even though the primary preparers of meals were women. Hence, it is important for health care providers to explore how gender might impact a patient's ability to conform to a treatment plan.

6.3.3 Being Mindful of Intimate Partner Violence When Working With South Asian American Women

Gender also has a salient impact on the health of South Asian American women. As highlighted earlier, South Asian women are more susceptible to intimate partner violence (IPV), which can have pervasive and permanent harmful effects on physical health. However, research suggests that South Asian women might not be able to distinguish between violent and culturally normative behavior. It is possible that a health care provider might be a victim's first point of contact and thus it is important that providers are equipped to screen for IPV when working with this population (Hurwitz et al. 2006). It is also suggested that health care providers be ready to educate a victim of the various manifestations of IPV such as emotional and financial control and connect the victim to culturally appropriate services such as legal aid and counseling (Hurwitz et al. 2006). Lastly, given the stigma and shame associated with IPV, it is important that a health care professional emphasize the importance of patient-provider confidentiality and assure women that their concerns would not be shared with family and/or community members (Grewal et al. 2005).

6.3.4 *Assessing Acculturation and Acculturative Stress during Patient Evaluations*

Acculturation and acculturative stress can negatively impact South Asian health (Tirodkar et al. 2011). Thus, it is important that health care professionals are mindful to these factors when working with South Asian Americans. Walker et al. (2015) suggest that when working with South Asian Americans, integrated family members (second or third generation South Asian Americans) could be involved in treatment planning and adherence, especially when explaining the health care interventions to less acculturated family members.

Annie (2014) further suggests that Asian immigrants might be particularly vulnerable to acculturative stress at two different points in their migration: one immediately following migration and manifested in the form of low social support, adjustment and language difficulties and the second occurring 15 years post migration when an individual becomes aware of systemic inequities and social barriers to complete inclusion in United States society. Thus, health care professionals should continually assess for migration related stress and provide a safe space for patients to talk about stress related to migration, assimilation and discrimination (Park et al. 2014).

6.3.5 *Assessing for Experiences of Racism and Discrimination during Patient Evaluations*

Given the stigma associated with discrimination, ethnic minorities typically tend to underreport their experiences of discrimination (Nancy et al. 2010). This underreporting may be particularly salient for South Asian Americans as they also burdened by upholding the desire to be viewed as the model minority and, perhaps, saving face in the community (Gee et al. 2009). Thus, health care providers should be sensitive to possible discrimination experienced by their South Asian American patients. Cinnamon et al. (2006) suggest that health care providers might present their patients with resources related to stress management and healthy coping of discrimination. It is also important that health care professionals undergo training in order to become more culturally competent when working with South Asian Americans.

6.4 Concluding Comments

South Asian Americans are one of the fastest growing minority populations in the United States, and are particularly vulnerable to serious health concerns including cardiovascular disease, diabetes mellitus, obesity and hypertriglyceridemia. It is essential that health care providers attend to the unique needs of this rapidly-growing population, and implementation of effective preventative and treatment interventions is crucial for this population. As health care in the United States moves toward cultural competence, it's important that health care providers are trained to work with, and for the needs of, South Asian Americans. Health care providers should be mindful of South Asian cultural values (such as collectivism, gender roles, family honor, morality) along with experiences of systemic inequities such as acculturative stress and race-based discrimination that might be particularly important when treating South Asian American patients.

References

Abraham, M. (1995). Ethnicity, gender and marital violence: South Asian women's organizations in the United States. *Gender & Society, 9*, 450–468. https://doi.org/10.1177/089124395009004004.

Ahmad, F., Shik, A., Vanza, R., Cheung, A., George, U., & Stewart, D. E. (2004). Popular health promotion strategies among Chinese and East Indian immigrant women. *Women & Health, 40*, 21–40. https://doi.org/10.1300/J013v40n01_02.

Ahmad, F., Rai, N., Petrovic, B., Erickson, P. E., & Stewart, D. E. (2013). Resilience and resources among south Asian immigrant women as survivors of partner violence. *Journal of Immigrant and Minority Health, 15*, 1057–1064. https://doi.org/10.1007/s10903-013-9836-2.

Ahmed, S. M., & Lemkau, J. P. (2000). Cultural issues in the primary care of south Asians. *Journal of Immigrant Health, 2*, 89–96. https://doi.org/10.1023/A:1009585918590.

Annie, R. (2014). The Longer You Stay, the Worse Your Health? A Critical Review of the Negative Acculturation Theory among Asian Immigrants. *International Journal of Environmental Research and Public Health, 11*(8), 8038–8057.

Astin, F., Atkin, K., & Darr, A. (2008). Causal attributions, lifestyle change, and coronary heart disease: Illness beliefs of patients of South Asian and European origin living in the United Kingdom. *Heart & Lung: The Journal of Acute and Critical Care, 37*, 91–104. https://doi.org/10.1016/j.hrtlng.2007.03.004.

Atkinson, D. R., & Gim, R. H. (1989). Asian-American cultural identity and attitudes toward mental health services. *Journal of Counseling Psychology, 36*, 209–212. https://doi.org/10.1037/0022-0167.36.2.209.

Ayyub, R. (2000). Domestic violence in the south Asian Muslim immigrant population in the United States. *Journal of Social Distress and the Homeless, 9*, 237–248. https://doi.org/10.1023/A:1009412119016.

Ballard, C. (1982). South Asian families. In R. N. Rapoport & M. P. Fogarty (Eds.), *Families in Britain*. London: Routledge and Kegan Paul.

Banerjee, A. T., Grace, S. L., Thomas, S. G., & Faulkner, G. (2010). Cultural factors facilitating cardiac rehabilitation participation among Canadian South Asians: A qualitative study. *Heart & Lung: The Journal of Acute and Critical Care, 39*(6), 494–503. https://doi.org/10.1016/j.hrtlng.2009.10.021.

Beadnell, B., Baker, S. A., Morrison, D. M., & Knox, K. (2000). HIV/STD risk factors for women with violent male partners. *Sex Roles, 42*, 661–689. https://doi.org/10.1023/A:1007003623810.

Bem, S. L. (1983). Gender schema theory and its implications for child development: Raising gender-aschematic children in a gender-schematic society. *Signs, 8*, 598–616.

Benson, H. (1996). *Timeless healing: The power and biology of belief.* New York: Fireside Books.

Berry, J. W., & Kim, U. (1988). Acculturation and mental health. In P. R. Dasen & J. W. Berry (Eds.), *Health and cross-cultural psychology: Toward applications* (pp. 207–236). Thousand Oaks: Sage Publications.

Berry, J. W., & Annis, R. C. (1974). Acculturative stress: The role of ecology, culture and differentiation. *Journal of Cross-Cultural Psychology, 5*, 382–406. https://doi.org/10.1177/002202217400500402.

Bhatia, S. (2008). 9/11 and the Indian diaspora: Narratives of race, place and immigrant identity. *Journal of Intercultural Studies, 29*, 21–39. https://doi.org/10.1080/07256860701759923.

Bhattacharya, G. (2004). Health care seeking for HIV/AIDS among South Asians in the United States. *Health & Social Work, 29*, 106–114 https://doiorgezproxy.cul.columbia.edu/10.1093/hsw/29.2.106.

Bhopal, R., Unwin, N., White, M., Yallop, J., Walker, L., Alberti, K. G. M. M., & Tavridou, A. (1999). Heterogeneity of coronary heart disease risk factors in Indian, Pakistani, Bangladeshi, and European origin populations: Cross sectional study. *British Medical Journal, 319*, 215–220. https://doi.org/10.1136/bmj.319.7204.215.

Bhugra, D. (2004). Migration and mental health. *Acta Psychiatrica Scandinavica, 109*, 243–258. https://doi.org/10.1046/j.0001-690X.2003.00246.x.

Bottorff, J. L., Johnson, J. L., Bhagat, R., Grewal, S., Balneaves, L. G., Clarke, H., & Hilton, B. A. (1998). Beliefs related to breast health practices: The perceptions of south Asian women living in Canada. *Social Science & Medicine, 47*, 2075–2085. https://doi.org/10.1016/S0277-9536(98)00346-3.

Chae, D. H., Takeuchi, D. T., Barbeau, E. M., Bennett, G. G., Lindsey, J. C., Stoddard, A. M., & Krieger, N. (2008). Alcohol disorders among Asian Americans: Associations with unfair treatment, racial/ethnic discrimination, and ethnic identification (the national Latino and Asian Americans study, 2002–2003). *Journal of Epidemiology and Community Health, 62*, 973–979. https://doi.org/10.2105/AJPH.2006.088401.

Chen, M. S. (2005). Cancer health disparities among Asian Americans. *Cancer, 104*, 2895–2902. https://doi.org/10.1002/cncr.21501.

Cheryan, S., & Monin, B. (2005). Where are you really from?: Asian Americans and identity denial. *Journal of Personality and Social Psychology, 89*, 717–730. https://doi.org/10.1037/0022-3514.89.5.717.

Choudhry, U. K. (2001). Uprooting and resettlement experiences of South Asian immigrant women. *Western Journal of Nursing Research, 23*, 376–393. https://doi.org/10.1177/019394590102300405.

Choudhury, P. P., Badhan, N. S., Chand, J., Chhugani, S., Choksey, R., Husainy, S., Lui, C., & Wat, E. C. (2009). Community alienation and its impact on help-seeking behavior among LGBTIQ South Asians in Southern California. *Journal of Gay & Lesbian Social Services, 21*, 247–266. https://doi.org/10.1080/10538720902772196.

Chung, P. J., Borneo, H., Kilpatrick, S. D., Lopez, D. M., Travis, R., Jr., Lui, C., Khandwala, S., & Schuster, M. A. (2005). Parent-adolescent communication about sex in Filipino American families: A demonstration of community-based participatory research. *Ambulatory Pediatrics, 5*, 50–55. https://doi.org/10.1367/A04-059R.1.

Cinnamon, S., Edith, C., & Gregory E., M. (2006). Written disclosure of experiences with racial discrimination and antibody response to an influenza vaccine. *International Journal of Behavioral Medicine, 13*(1), 60–68.

Clark, R., Anderson, N. B., Clark, V. R., & Williams, D. R. (1999). Racism as a stressor for African Americans: A biopsychosocial model. *American Psychologist, 54*(10), 805–816. https://doi.org/10.1037/0003-066X.54.10.805.

Clements, A. D., & Ermakova, A. V. (2012). Surrender to god and stress: A possible link between religiosity and health. *Psychology of Religion and Spirituality, 4*, 93–107. https://doi.org/10.1037/a0025109.

Daniel, M., & Wilbur, J. (2011). Physical activity among South Asian Indian immigrants: An integrative review. *Public Health Nursing, 28*, 389–401. https://doi.org/10.1111/j.1525-1446.2010.00932.x.

Das, A. K., & Kemp, S. F. (1997). Between two worlds: Counseling South Asian Americans. *Journal of Multicultural Counseling and Development, 25*, 23–33.

Dasgupta, S. D. (1998). *Sex Roles, 38*(11/12), 953–974.
Dasgupta, S. D. (2000). Charting the course: An overview of domestic violence in the South Asian community in the United States. *Journal of Social Distress and the Homeless, 9*, 173–185. https://doi.org/10.1023/A:1009403917198.
Das Gupta, M. (2006). *Unruly immigrants: Rights, activism, and transnational South Asian politics in the United States*. Durham, NC: Duke University Press.
Dasgupta, S. D., & Dasgupta, S. (1996). Women in exile: Gender relations in the Asian Indian community. In S. Maira & R. Srikanth (Eds.), *Contours of the Heart: South Asians Map North America* (pp. 381–481). New York, NY: Temple University Press.
Devos, T., & Banaji, M. R. (2005). American ?=White? *Journal of Personality and Social Psychology, 88*, 447–466. https://doi.org/10.1037/0022-3514.88.3.447.
Dhruvarajan, V. (1993). Ethnic cultural retention and transmission among first generation Hindu Asian Indians in a Canadian Prairie city. *Journal of Comparative Family Studies, 24*, 63–79.
Enas, E. A., Dhawan, J., & Petkar, S. (1996). Coronary artery disease in Asian Indians: Lessons learnt and the role of lipoprotein. *Indian Heart Journal, 49*, 25–34.
Fikree, F. F., & Pasha, O. (2004). Role of gender in health disparity: The South Asian context. *British Medical Journal, 328*, 823–826. https://doi.org/10.1136/bmj.328.7443.823.
Frey, L. L., & Roysircar, G. (2006). South Asian and East Asian international students' perceived prejudice, acculturation, and frequency of help resource utilization. *Journal of Multicultural counseling and development, 34*, 208–222. https://doi.org/10.1002/j.2161-1912.2006.tb00040.x.
Frisbie, W. P., Cho, Y., & Hummer, R. A. (2001). Immigration and the health of Asian and Pacific islander adults in the United States. *American Journal of Epidemiology, 153*, 372–380. https://doi.org/10.1093/aje/153.4.372.
Gee, G. C., & Ponce, N. (2010). Associations between racial discrimination, limited English proficiency, and health-related quality of life among 6 Asian ethnic groups in California. *American Journal of Public Health, 100*, 888–895. https://doi.org/10.2105/AJPH.2009.178012.
Gee, G., & Walsemann, K. (2009). Does health predict the reporting of racial discrimination or do reports of discrimination predict health? Findings from the National Longitudinal Study of youth. *Social Science & Medicine, 68*, 1676–1684. https://doi.org/10.1016/j.socscimed.2009.02.002.
Gee, G. C., Spencer, M. S., Chen, J., & Takeuchi, D. (2007). A nationwide study of discrimination and chronic health conditions among Asian Americans. *American Journal of Public Health, 97*, 1275–1282. https://doi.org/10.2105/AJPH.2006.091827.
Gee, G. C., Ro, A., Shariff-Marco, S., & Chae, D. (2009). Racial discrimination and health among Asian Americans: Evidence, assessment, and directions for future research. *Epidemiologic Reviews, 31*, 130–151. https://doi.org/10.1093/epirev/mxp009.
Grewal, S., Bottorff, J. L., & Hilton, B. A. (2005). The influence of family on immigrant South Asian women's health. *Journal of Family Nursing, 11*, 242–263. https://doi.org/10.1177/1074840705278622.
Gudykunst, W. B. (2001). *Asian American ethnicity and communication*. Thousand Oaks: Sage.
Hannay, D. R. (1980). Religion and health. *Social Science & Medicine. Part A: Medical Sociology, 14*, 683–685. https://doi.org/10.1016/S0271-7123(80)80079-4.
Heise, L., Ellsberg, M., & Gottmoeller, M. (2002). A global overview of gender-based violence. *International Journal of Gynecology & Obstetrics, 78*, S5–S14. https://doi.org/10.1016/S0020-7292(02)00038-3.
Hsiao, A. F., Wong, M. D., Goldstein, M. S., Becerra, L. S., Cheng, E. M., & Wenger, N. S. (2006). Complementary and alternative medicine use among Asian-American subgroups: Prevalence, predictors, and lack of relationship to acculturation and access to conventional health care. *Journal of Alternative and Complementary Medicine, 12*, 1003–1010. https://doi.org/10.1089/acm.2006.12.1003.

Hsu, W. C., Araneta, M. R. G., Kanaya, A. M., Chiang, J. L., & Fujimoto, W. (2015). BMI cut points to identify at-risk Asian Americans for type 2 diabetes screening. *Diabetes Care, 38*, 150–158. https://doi.org/10.2337/dc14-2391.

Hurwitz, E. J. H., Gupta, J., Liu, R., Silverman, J. G., & Raj, A. (2006). Intimate partner violence associated with poor health outcomes in U.S. south Asian women. *Journal of Immigrant and Minority Health, 8*, 251–261. https://doi.org/10.1007/s10903-006-9330-1.

Hussain-Gambles, M., Atkin, K., & Leese, B. (2004). Why ethnic minority groups are under-represented in clinical trials: A review of the literature. *Health & Social Care in the Community, 12*, 382–388. https://doi.org/10.1111/j.1365-2524.2004.00507.x.

Ibrahim, F. A. (1994). Suicidal behavior in Asian American women. In S. S. Canetto & D. Lester (Eds.), *Women and suicidal behavior*. New York: Springer.

Ibrahim, F. A., Ohnishi, H., & Sandhu, D. S. (1997). Asian American identity development: A culture specific model for South Asian Americans. *Journal of Multicultural Counseling and Development, 25*, 34–50. https://doi.org/10.1002/j.2161-1912.1997.tb00314.x.

Inman, A. G., Ladany, N., Constantine, M. G., & Morano, C. K. (2001). Development and preliminary validation of the cultural values conflict scale for South Asian women. *Journal of Counseling Psychology, 48*, 17–27. https://doi.org/10.1037/0022-0167.48.1.17.

Inman, A. G., Yeh, C. J., Madan-Bahel, A., & Nath, S. (2007). Bereavement and coping of South Asian families post 9/11. *Journal of Multicultural Counseling and Development, 35*, 101–115. https://doi.org/10.1002/j.2161-1912.2007.tb00053.x.

Jones, J. W. (2004). Religion, health, and the psychology of religion: How the research on religion and health helps us understand religion. *Journal of Religion and Health, 43*, 317–328. https://doi.org/10.1007/s10943-004-4299-3.

Kalra, P., Srinivasan, S., Ivey, S., & Greenlund, K. (2004). Knowledge and practice: The risk of cardiovascular disease among Asian Indians. Results from focus groups conducted in Asian Indian communities in Northern California. *Ethnicity & Disease, 14*, 497–504.

Khandelwal, M. (1988). In L. Hibayashi (Ed.), *Teaching Asian American: Diversity and the problem of community*. Boulder: Rowman & Littlefield Publishers.

Kim, B. S., Atkinson, D. R., & Umemoto, D. (2001). Asian cultural values and the counseling process current knowledge and directions for future research. *The Counseling Psychologist, 29*, 570–603. https://doi.org/10.1177/0011000001294006.

Kitano, H. H. L., & Matsushima, N. (1981). Counseling Asian Americans. In P. B. Pedersen, J. G. Draguns, W. J. Lonner, & J. E. Trimble (Eds.), *Counseling across cultures* (pp. 163–180). Honolulu: University of Hawaii Press.

Kuo, W. H. (1995). Coping with racial discrimination: The case of Asian Americans. *Ethnic and Racial Studies, 18*, 109–127. https://doi.org/10.1080/01419870.1995.9993856.

Landrine, H., Klonoff, E. A., Corral, I., Fernandez, S., & Roesch, S. (2006). Conceptualizing and measuring ethnic discrimination in health research. *Journal of Behavioral Medicine, 29*, 79–94. https://doi.org/10.1007/s10865-005-9029-0.

Lee, R. M. (2003). Do ethnic identity and other-group orientation protect against discrimination for Asian Americans? *Journal of Counseling Psychology, 50*, 133–141. https://doi.org/10.1037/0022-0167.50.2.133.

Lewis, T. T., Aiello, A. E., Leurgans, S., Kelly, J., & Barnes, L. L. (2010). Self-reported experiences of everyday discrimination are associated with elevated C-reactive protein levels in older African-American adults. *Brain, Behavior, and Immunity, 24*, 438–443.

Liang, C. T., Li, L. C., & Kim, B. S. (2004). The Asian American racism-related stress inventory: Development, factor analysis, reliability, and validity. *Journal of Counseling Psychology, 51*, 103–114. https://doi.org/10.1037/0022-0167.51.1.103.

Madan-Bahel, A. (2008). *Sexual health and bollywood films: A culturally based program for South Asian teenage girls*. Youngstown: Cambria Press.

Mathews, R. (2000). Cultural patterns of south Asian and southeast Asian Americans. *Intervention in School and Clinic, 36*, 101–104. https://doi.org/10.1177/105345120003600205.

Mehta, S. (1998). Relationship between acculturation and mental health for Asian Indian immigrants in the United States. *Genetic, Social, and General Psychology Monographs, 124*, 61–78.

Midlarsky, E., Venkatramani-Kothari, A., & Plante, M. (2006). Domestic violence in the Chinese and south Asian immigrant communities. *Annals of the New York Academy of Sciences, 1087*, 279–300. https://doi.org/10.1196/annals.1385.003.

Misra, A., & Vikram, N. K. (2004). Insulin resistance syndrome (metabolic syndrome) and obesity in Asian Indians: Evidence and implications. *Nutrition, 20*, 482–491. https://doi.org/10.1016/j.nut.2004.01.020.

Misra, R., Patel, T. G., Davies, D., & Russo, T. (2000). Health promotion behaviors of Gujarati Asian Indian immigrants in the United States. *Journal of Immigrant Health, 2*, 223–230. https://doi.org/10.1023/A:1009544414050.

Nair, M., & Prabhakaran, D. (2012). Why Do South Asians Have High Risk for CAD? *Global Heart, 7*(4), 307–314.

Nancy, K., Dana, C., Katie, L., Pamela D., W., Anna, K., & Mahzarin, B. (2010). Combining Explicit and Implicit Measures of Racial Discrimination in Health Research. *American Journal of Public Health, 100*(8), 1485–1492.

Nelson, M. E., Rejeski, W. J., Blair, S. N., Duncan, P. W., Judge, J. O., King, A. C., et al. (2007). Physical activity and public health in older adults: Recommendations from the American College of Sports Medicine and the American Heart Association. *Circulation, 116*, 1094–1105. https://doi.org/10.1161/CIRCULATIONAHA.107.185650.

Park, S. Y., Anastas, J., Shibusawa, T., & Nguyen, D. (2014). The impact of acculturation and acculturative stress on alcohol use across Asianimmigrant subgroups. *Substance Use & Misuse, 49*, 922–931. https://doi.org/10.3109/10826084.2013.855232.

Pew Research Center. (2012a). *Chapter 1: Portrait of Asian Americans*. Retrieved September 25, 2015, from http://www.pewsocialtrends.org/2012/06/19/chapter-1-portrait-of-asian-americans/?beta=true&utm_expid=53098246-2.Lly4CFSVQG2lphsg-KopIg.1&utm_referrer=https%3A%2F%2Fwww.google.com%2F.

Pew Research Center. (2012b). *Overview: Religious Affiliation*. Retrieved December 7, 2015, from http://www.pewforum.org/2012/07/19/asian-americans-a-mosaic-of-faiths-overview/.

Pew Research Center. (2015). *Appendix D: Detailed tables*. Retrieved December 7, 2015, from http://www.pewforum.org/religious-landscape-study/racial-and-ethnic-composition/.

Pulerwitz, J., Amaro, H., Jong, W. D., Gortmaker, S. L., & Rudd, R. (2002). Relationship power, condom use and HIV risk among women in the USA. *AIDS Care, 14*, 789–800. https://doi.org/10.1080/0954012021000031868.

Quina, K., Harlow, L. L., Morokoff, P. J., Burkholder, G., & Deiter, P. J. (2000). Sexual communication in relationships: When words speak louder than actions. *Sex Roles, 42*, 523–549. https://doi.org/10.1023/A:1007043205155.

Raj, A., & Silverman, J. (2002). Violence against immigrant women the roles of culture, context, and legal immigrant status on intimate partner violence. *Violence Against Women, 8*, 367–398. https://doi.org/10.1177/10778010222183107.

Raj, A., Liu, R., McCleary-Sills, J., & Silverman, J. G. (2005). South Asian victims of intimate partner violence more likely than non-victims to report sexual health concerns. *Journal of Immigrant Health, 7*, 85–91. https://doi.org/10.1007/s10903-005-2641-9.

Redfield, R., Linton, R., & Herskowitz, M. T. (1936). Memorandum for the study of acculturation. *American Anthropologist, 38*, 149–152.

Samuel, E. (2009). Acculturative stress: South Asian immigrant women's experiences in Canada's Atlantic provinces. *Journal of Immigrant & Refugee Studies, 7*(1), 16–34. https://doi.org/10.1080/15562940802687207.

Sandil, R., Robinson, M., Brewster, M. E., Wong, S., & Geiger, E. (2015). Negotiating multiple marginalizations: Experiences of South Asian LGBQ individuals. *Cultural Diversity and Ethnic Minority Psychology, 21*, 76–88. https://doi.org/10.1037/a0037070.

Saran, P. (1985). *The Asian Indian Experience in the United States*. Cambridge, MA: Schenkman Press.

Sheth, M. (1995). Asian Indian Americans. In P. G. Min (Ed.), *Asian American: Contemporary trends and issues* (pp. 1690–1198). Thousand Oaks: Sage.
Sherman, A., & Simonton, S. (2001). *Religious involvement among cancer patients* (pp. 167–194). Psychological Perspectives: Faith and Health. https://doi.org/10.1002/pon.523.
Srinivasan, S., & Guillermo, T. (2000). Toward improved health: Disaggregating Asian American and native Hawaiian/Pacific islander data. *American Journal of Public Health, 90*, 1731–1734.
Sriskantharajah, J., & Kai, J. (2007). Promoting physical activity among South Asian women with coronary heart disease and diabetes: What might help? *Family Practice, 24*, 71–76. https://doi.org/10.1093/fampra/cml066.
Sudsuang, R., Chentanez, V., & Veluvan, K. (1991). Effect of Buddhist meditation on serum cortisol and total protein levels, blood pressure, pulse rate, lung volume and reaction time. *Physiology & Behavior, 50*, 543–548. https://doi.org/10.1016/0031-9384(91)90543-W.
Sue, D., & Sue, D. W. (1993). Ethnic identity: Cultural factors in the psychological development of Asians in America. In D. R. Atkinson, G. Morten, & D. W. Sue (Eds.), *Counseling American minorities: A cross-cultural perspective* (pp. 199–210). Dubuque: W. C. Brown.
Sweta, T. (2005). Asian Indian Immigrant Women. *Journal of Human Behavior in the Social Environment, 11*(1), 1–22.
Szymanski, D. M., & Sung, M. R. (2013). Asian cultural values, internalized heterosexism, and sexual orientation disclosure among Asian American sexual minority persons. *Journal of LGBT Issues in Counseling, 7*, 257–273. https://doi.org/10.1080/15538605.2013.812930.
Tang, T. S., Solomon, L. J., & McCracken, L. M. (2000). Cultural barriers to mammography, clinical breast exam, and breast self-exam among Chinese-American women 60 and older. *Preventive Medicine, 31*, 575–583. https://doi.org/10.1006/pmed.2000.0753.
Tirodkar, M. A., Baker, D. W., Makoul, G. T., Khurana, N., Paracha, M. W., & Kandula, N. R. (2011). Explanatory models of health and disease among south Asian immigrants in Chicago. *Journal of Immigrant and Minority Health, 13*, 385–394. https://doi.org/10.1007/s10903-009-9304-1.
Tjaden, P., & Thoennes, N. (2000). Prevalence and consequences of male-to-female and female-to-male intimate partner violence as measured by the National Violence against Women Survey. *Violence Against Women, 6*, 142–161. https://doi.org/10.1177/10778010022181769.
Troxel, W. M., Matthews, K. A., Bromberger, J. T., & Sutton-Tyrrell, K. (2003). Chronic stress burden, discrimination, and subclinical carotid artery disease in African American and Caucasian women. *Health Psychology, 22*, 300–309. https://doi.org/10.1037/0278-6133.22.3.300.
Unger, J. B., Cruz, T. B., Rohrbach, L. A., Ribisl, K. M., Baezconde-Garbanti, L., Chen, X., & Johnson, C. A. (2000). English language use as a risk factor for smoking initiation among Hispanic and Asian American adolescents: Evidence for mediation by tobacco-related beliefs and social norms. *Health Psychology, 19*, 403–410. https://doi.org/10.1037/0278-6133.19.5.403.
Uppaluri, C. R., Schumm, L. P., & Lauderdale, D. S. (2001). Self-reports of stress in Asian immigrants: effects of ethnicity and acculturation. *Ethnicity & Disease, 11*, 107–114.
U.S. Census Bureau. (2012). *The Asian Population: 2010*. Retrieved August 25, 2015, from https://www.census.gov/prod/cen2010/briefs/c2010br-11.pdf.
Utsey, S. O., Ponterotto, J. G., Reynolds, A. L., & Cancelli, A. A. (2000). Racial discrimination, coping, life satisfaction, and self-esteem among African Americans. *Journal of Counseling & Development, 78*, 72–80. https://doi.org/10.1002/j.1556-6676.2000.tb02562.x.
Vega, W. A., & Amaro, H. (1994). Latino outlook: Good health, uncertain prognosis. *Annual Review of Public Health, 15*, 39–67.
Walker, G. J., Caperchione, C. M., Mummery, W. K., & Chau, S. (2015). Examining the role of acculturation in the leisure-time physical activity of South Asians living in Canada. *Journal of Science and Medicine in Sport, 18*, 156–160. https://doi.org/10.1016/j.jsams.2014.02.010.
Weerasinghe, S., & Numer, M. (2011). A life-course exploration of the social, emotional and physical health behaviours of widowed South Asian immigrant women in Canada: Implications for health and social programme planning. *International Journal of Migration, Health and Social Care, 6*, 42–56. https://doi.org/10.5042/ijmhsc.2011.0153.

Whitty, C., Brunner, E., Shipley, M., Hemingway, H., & Marmot, M. (1999). Differences in biologic risk factors for cardiovascular disease between three ethnic groups in the Whitehall II study. *Atherosclerosis, 142*, 279–286. https://doi.org/10.1016/S0021-9150(98)00239-1.

Williams, R. (1988). *Religions of immigrants from Indian and Pakistan*. New York: Cambridge University Press.

Williams, E. D., Nazroo, J. Y., Kooner, J. S., & Steptoe, A. (2010). Subgroup differences in psychosocial factors relating to coronary heart disease in the UK South Asian population. *Journal of Psychosomatic Research, 69*, 379–387. https://doi.org/10.1016/j.jpsychores.2010.03.015.

World Health Organization. (2002). *Understanding and addressing violence against women*. Retrieved from: http://apps.who.int/iris/bitstream/10665/77432/1/WHO_RHR_12.36_eng.pdf.

World Health Organization. (2008). *Preventing and addressing intimate partner violence against migrant and ethnic minority women: the role of the health sector*. Retrieved from: http://www.euro.who.int/__data/assets/pdf_file/0018/270180/21256-WHO-Intimate-Partner-Violence_low_V7.pdf

Yoshihama, M., Bybee, D., & Blazevski, J. (2012). Day-to-day discrimination and health among Asian Indians: A population-based study of Gujarati men and women in metropolitan Detroit. *Journal of Behavioral Medicine, 35*, 471–483. https://doi.org/10.1007/s10865-011-9375-z.

Zhan, H. J., & Montgomery, R. J. (2003). Gender and elder care in China: The influence of filial piety and structural constraints. *Gender & Society, 17*, 209–229. https://doi.org/10.1177/0891243202250734.

Part III
Major Health Conditions in South Asian Americans

Chapter 7
Type 2 Diabetes Mellitus in South Asian Americans

Suhaila Khan, Nilay Shah, Nisha Parikh, Divya Iyer, and Latha Palaniappan

7.1 Introduction

This chapter focuses on Type 2 Diabetes Mellitus (T2DM), since South Asian Americans suffer disproportionately higher from T2DM, and at lower levels of body weight compared to many other populations in the United States (U.S.).

South Asian Americans in the U.S. are primarily defined as individuals with origins in Bangladesh, Bhutan, India, the Maldives, Nepal, Pakistan, Sri Lanka, and sometimes Afghanistan (World Bank 2015). Increasing waves of South Asian immigration to the U.S. began upon the passage of the Immigration and Nationality Act of 1965, leading to an influx of professionals for high-skilled jobs (Kelkar 2011). Today, the South Asian American population is the fastest growing of all major ethnic groups in the U.S., with an 8s1% growth reported between 2000 and 2010. There are 3.4 million South Asian Americans in the U.S. Over 80% of South Asian

S. Khan (✉)
National Council of Asian Pacific Islander Physicians, San Francisco, CA, USA
e-mail: suhailak@shkglobalhealth.org

N. Shah
Stanford University Until Summer 2017, Stanford, CA, USA

Northwestern University Starting 2017, Chicago, IL, USA

N. Parikh
University of California, CA, San Francisco, USA
e-mail: Nisha.Parikh@ucsf.edu

D. Iyer
University of Connecticut School of Medicine, Farmington, CT, USA
e-mail: iyer@uchc.edu

L. Palaniappan
Stanford University, Stanford, CA, USA
e-mail: lathap@stanford.edu

M. J. Perera, E. C. Chang (eds.), *Biopsychosocial Approaches to Understanding Health in South Asian Americans*, Cross-Cultural Research in Health, Illness and Well-Being, https://doi.org/10.1007/978-3-319-91120-5_7

Americans identify as Asian Indians, who are the third largest Asian American subgroup in the U.S. South Asian Americans (particularly Asian Indians) tend to have high median annual household incomes, high levels of education, and are more likely to be foreign-born compared to the rest of the Asian American and the general population (Pew Research Center 2013).

7.1.1 South Asian Americans vs. South Asians

There are many similarities, especially cultural and linguistic, between South Asian Americans and South Asians. But there are many differences too, especially in terms of mortality and morbidity issues (see Table 7.1).

7.1.2 Leading Causes of Mortality in South Asian Americans

The top causes of death for adults in South Asia as of 2010 were (in descending order): 1. ischemic heart disease; 2. tuberculosis; 3. self-harm; 4. road injury; 5. HIV/AIDS; 6. chronic obstructive pulmonary disease; 7. diarrheal diseases; 8. cerebrovascular disease; 9. cirrhosis of the liver, and 10. fire/heat/hot substances (Lopez 2013). The South Asia region has seen decreased mortality and mortality burden from communicable, newborn, nutritional, and maternal causes since 1990, while non-communicable diseases (especially ischemic heart disease, stroke, diabetes, musculoskeletal disorders, and major depressive disorders) have increased substantially.

South Asian Americans show a different mortality profile than South Asians in South Asia. Most studies in the U.S. focus on Asian Indian populations (since Asian Indians are specifically disaggregated on U.S. death record data), while mortality studies on other South Asian American subgroups (from Afghanistan, Bangladesh, Bhutan, the Maldives, Nepal, Pakistan, and Sri Lanka) are largely lacking due to small sample sizes. An analysis of U.S. mortality records from 2003–2011 for Asians and non-Hispanic Whites (NHWs) in 36 states and the District of Columbia show that the leading causes of death for Asian Indians are heart diseases, cancers, cerebrovascular diseases, accidents, diabetes, respiratory tract diseases, renal diseases, and Alzheimer's (see Tables 7.2 and 7.3).

Asian Indians have lower mortality rates than non-Hispanic Whites (NHW), nearly by half (Hastings et al. 2015), as would be expected given the younger and largely healthy immigrant populations. New immigrants are regularly screened for tuberculosis, syphilis, mental illness and other medical conditions. Given that South Asian Americans are mostly comprised of new immigrants, lower relative mortality rates compared to NHWs should be expected among these groups due to self-selection into migration and the rigorous screening and selection process. Although

Table 7.1 Differences in mortality and morbidity in the USA, South Asian American, and South Asian populations

	USA	South Asian Americans	South Asia
Population	318 million (census)	4.0 million (census)	1.7 billion (WHO)
T2DM – Absolute #	21.9 million (CDC)	640,000–1.4 million (estimated using available prevalence rates)[a]	36 million (WHO)
T2DM – Prevalence rate	9.3% (CDC)	16%–35% (Venkataraman et al. 2004; Rajpathak et al. 2010)	5%–13.9% (Ramachandran et al. 2012)
Obesity	68.8% adults (CDC, NHANES/NHIS)	7%–20% adults in California (Wolstein et al. 2015; Jih et al. 2014)	10% adults (Ramachandran et al. Ramachandran and Snehalatha 2010)
Top 5 mortality causes	Heart disease, cancer, chronic lower respiratory diseases, stroke, unintentional injuries (Johnson et al. 2014)	Heart disease, cancer, stroke, diabetes, accidents/injuries (Hastings et al. 2015)	Ischemic heart disease, tuberculosis, self harm, road injury, HIV/AIDS (WHO)
		**For Asian Indians. Data not available for SAA	
Top 5 morbidity causes/ disease burden	Ischemic heart disease, lung cancer, stroke, chronic obstructive pulmonary disease, road injuries (Murray et al. 2013)	Data not available for SAA	Lower respiratory infections, preterm birth complications, diarrheal diseases, ischemic heart diseases, chronic obstructive pulmonary diseases (WHO)

[a]4 million x 16% = 640,000; 4 million x 35% = 1.4 million
[b]WHO = World Health Organization
[c]CDC = Centers for Disease Control

cancer is the leading cause of death for Asians as an aggregate group, the leading cause of death for Asian Indians was heart disease.

The proportion of death due to heart disease for Asian Indian males was nearly double that due to cancer (31% vs. 18%). This reflects trends that many studies conducted both in the U.S. (e.g. Enas et al. 1996) and abroad in the UK (Tillin et al. 2013; Balarajan 1991), Canada (Sheth et al. 1999; Anand et al. 2000), and South Asia (Xavier et al. 2008) have noted – South Asians are often at greater risk of heart disease than other racial/ethnic groups. Acute coronary syndrome (caused by a blockage in the blood vessels that supply blood and oxygen to the heart muscle) and overall cardiovascular mortality also occur approximately 7 to 11 years earlier, with increased severity in Asian Indians compared with other ethnic groups (Joshi et al. 2007; Rosengren et al. 2006). Asian Indians had greater proportionate mortality

Table 7.2 Mortality profile of Women in the U.S

Rank	Asian Indian women	Asian American women	NHW women
1	Diseases of the heart	Malignant neoplasms	Diseases of the heart
2	Malignant neoplasms	Diseases of the heart	Malignant neoplasms
3	Cerebrovascular diseases	Cerebrovascular diseases	Cerebrovascular diseases
4	Diabetes mellitus	Diabetes mellitus	Chronic lower respiratory diseases
5	Accidents – Unintentional injuries	Influenza and pneumonia	Alzheimer's disease
6	Influenza and pneumonia	Accidents – Unintentional injuries	Accidents – Unintentional injuries
7	Chronic lower respiratory diseases	Chronic lower respiratory diseases	Influenza and pneumonia
8	Renal diseases	Alzheimer's disease	Diabetes mellitus
9	Alzheimer's disease	Renal diseases	Renal diseases

Hastings et al. 2015
[a]NHW = Non-Hispanic White

Table 7.3 Mortality profile of Men in the U.S

Rank	Asian Indian men	Asian American men	NHW men
1	Diseases of the heart	Malignant neoplasms	Diseases of the heart
2	Malignant neoplasms	Diseases of the heart	Malignant neoplasms
3	Accidents – Unintentional injuries	Cerebrovascular diseases	Chronic lower respiratory diseases
4	Cerebrovascular diseases	Accidents – Unintentional injuries	Accidents – Unintentional injuries
5	Diabetes mellitus	Chronic lower respiratory diseases	Cerebrovascular diseases
6	Intentional self-harm	Diabetes mellitus	Diabetes mellitus
7	Influenza and pneumonia	Influenza and pneumonia	Intentional self-harm
8	Chronic lower respiratory diseases	Intentional self-harm	Influenza and pneumonia
9	Renal diseases	Renal diseases	Alzheimer's disease

Hastings et al. 2015
[a]NHW = Non-Hispanic White

burden from ischemic heart disease (caused by narrowing of the coronary arteries) than other racial/ethnic groups (1.12 for women, 1.43 for men). Asian Indians, like most other Asian subgroups, had higher proportionate mortality from hypertensive heart disease (overburdening of the heart and blood vessels by high blood pressures), (proportionate mortality 1.46 for women, 1.18 for men compared to NHWs) and hemorrhagic stroke than NHWs (proportionate mortality 1.78 for women, 1.45 for men) (Jose et al. 2014).

Jose et al. (2014) showed that temporal trends from 2003–2011 reflected increasing mortality from heart disease among Asian Indian women and stable mortality in Asian Indian men, although in the general population, the number of annual deaths from cardiovascular diseases (CVD) declined by 17% between 2000 and 2010 (Go et al. 2014). Temporal trends also showed increased mortality of cancer, diabetes, and stroke in Asian Indians. Among all Asian subgroups, Asian Indians had lowest cancer mortality rates, although rates are rising; average annual percent change for years 2003–2011 was 3.8% for women and 2.5% for men (Hastings et al. 2015). Exact reasons why cardiovascular mortality among Asian Indian women has increased, contrary to general trends, warrants further research. One recent analysis of California Health Interview Survey data (Bharmal et al. 2014) revealed that more recent South Asian immigrants (in the U.S. for <15 years) were more likely to be overweight/obese and have a sedentary lifestyle compared with South Asians who had lived in the U.S. for ≥15 years. However, there were no associations between length of residence in the U.S. and other CVD risk factors. Further research on changes in lifestyle due to acculturation and utilization of health services is needed in order to develop population-level prevention strategies.

Similarly, in another recent study (Qureshi et al. 2014) using U.S. multiple-cause-of-death and National Health and Interview Survey data, showed that annual incidence of stroke mortality in 2000 was lowest for Asian Indians (88 per 100,000) compared to Whites, African Americans, American Indian and Alaska Natives. However, the incidence of stroke mortality decreased in all race/ethnic categories by 2009 except in Asian Indians (average annual percentage increase of 13.5%). The lower rates of stroke are likely due to lower rates of hypertension, obesity, and cigarette smoking as reported in the analysis of the National Health Interview Survey. However, as in the case of heart disease, the reason for increase in stroke mortality among Asian Indians, contrary to trends in other race/ethnicity groups, remains unclear.

This section discussed the mortality patterns of South Asian Americans. The morbidity issues could not be discussed as such data are still not available on South Asian Americans.

7.2 Incidence and Prevalence of Type 2 Diabetes in South Asian Americans

Type 2 Diabetes Mellitus (T2DM) affects 9.3 million Americans (CDC 2014), with about 1.7 million new cases per year (7.8 per 1000 people). T2DM leads to complications such as heart and blood vessel disease, nerve damage, kidney damage, eye damage, foot damage, hearing impairment, skin conditions, and Alzheimer's (American Diabetes Association 2015). India has a higher number of people with diabetes than any other country in the world (32.7 million as of 2000), and Pakistan is among the top 10 world nations for high numbers of people with diabetes (Ghaffar et al. 2004). Diabetes is the 4th leading cause of death among Asian Indians in America (see Tables 7.2 and 7.3) (Hastings et al. 2015).

South Asian Americans carry the burden of T2DM much more than other racial/ethnic groups. Although national analyses of T2DM incidence and prevalence (McNeely and Boyko 2004) have traditionally grouped Asians and Pacific Islanders together, some studies of self-report data have disaggregated Asians by racial/ethnic subgroup. Analysis of National Health Interview Survey data from 1997–2005 (Oza-Frank et al. 2009) showed that Asian Indians were three times more likely to self-report having T2DM than non-Hispanic Whites (NHWs), even after adjustment for body mass index (BMI). Smaller regional studies in metropolitan areas like New York, Atlanta, and California also showed startlingly high self-reported T2DM rates in Asian Indians: 35% in New York (compared to 11% in NHWs) (Rajpathak et al. 2010), 18.3% in Atlanta (Venkataraman et al. 2004), and 29% in California (Kanaya et al. 2010).

Studies in large clinical populations (Karter et al. 2013; Wang et al. 2011; Choi et al. 2013) that did not depend on self-report show similar numbers. An analysis of 6768 South Asian adult members of Kaiser Permanente Northern California (Karter et al. 2013) showed that South Asians had 16% prevalence of T2DM and incidence of 17.2 per 1000 person-years. Another analysis of 5171 Asian Indians in a Northern California healthcare system (Wang et al. 2011) showed an age-and-BMI-standardized T2DM prevalence of 17% in women and 25% in men, odds that were 3.44 and 3.54 times higher relative to NHW women and men, respectively. When comparing South Asian Americans with four other racial/ethnic groups in the U.S. in two community-based cohorts, the Mediators of Atherosclerosis in South Asians Living in America (MASALA) study and the Multi-Ethnic Study of Atherosclerosis (MESA) (Kanaya et al. 2014), South Asians had significantly higher age-adjusted prevalence of diabetes (23%) than other ethnic groups (6% in whites, 18% in African Americans, 17% in Latinos, and 13% in Chinese Americans). Similar to South Asians, Filipino, Japanese and Native Hawaiian populations in the U.S., also tend to have high rates of diabetes (10–22%) (Araneta et al. 2010).

Prospective studies on incidence of T2DM in South Asians in the U.S. are largely lacking, but studies in Europe (Miller et al. 1989; Forouhi et al. 2006) have shown that the incidence of and mortality from CAD among Asian Indians are at least 2-fold higher than in whites, even when fully adjusted for the high rates of insulin resistance, and diabetes, as well as socioeconomic status.

T2DM remains a special burden on the South Asian population in the United States, and should remain a public health priority in minority health. Longitudinal studies and existing cohorts of South Asian populations will continue to provide important information on incidence and temporal trends.

7.3 Determinants of Type 2 Diabetes Mellitus in South Asian Americans

There are numerous determinants of T2DM. These include but are not limited to:

(a) Clinical risk factors such as body mass index (BMI), waist circumference, and body fat;
(b) Lifestyle risk factors such as diet, exercise, alcohol, and smoking;
(c) Social determinants such as race/ethnicity, insurance, language, nativity, and education.

7.3.1 Clinical Risk Factors: BMI, Waist Circumference, Body Fat

Among the known risk factors for the development of type 2 diabetes are body weight-related clinical measurements, which include body mass index (BMI) and waist circumference. It is well documented that the likelihood of developing diabetes increases with increasing weight and BMI (Narayan et al. 2007), and obesity has been identified as a major risk factor for type 2 diabetes (Sattar and Gill 2014). South Asians have a unique association between these measures of body fat and their risk for developing diabetes. Evidence suggests that individuals of South Asian background living in both the U.S. and Canada have higher risk for weight-related diseases, including diabetes, at lower BMI levels compared to their white counterparts (Chiu et al. 2011; Jih et al. 2014). While the standard definition of obesity (a BMI $\geq$ 30 kg/m^2) has been validated for white individuals, ethnic-specific BMI cutoff points have been proposed for Asian, and, in particular, South Asian, populations to better assess risk of diabetes and other chronic diseases given their elevated risk. The World Health Organization (2011) recommended potential BMI categories for people of Asian ancestry (underweight <18.5 kg/m^2, increasing but acceptable risk 18.5 to <23 kg/m^2, increased risk 23 to <27.5 kg/m^2, and high risk $\leq$27.5 kg/m^2), which have been validated to identify at-risk Asian Americans as a whole (Jih et al. 2014). While evidence validating these cutoff values is primarily available for Asian Indians living in India (Snehalatha et al. 2003), these lower body mass index values were also recently adopted by the American Diabetes Association, to identify Asian Americans who would benefit from glucose screening (Hsu et al. 2015).

Waist circumference has also been identified as a risk factor for diabetes in South Asians living in the United Kingdom and India (Bodicoat et al. 2014), and, similar to BMI, the risk for diabetes in South Asians may better be characterized at unique waist circumference cutoff points, rather than standard measurements. The International Diabetes Federation variably defines abdominal obesity based on an individual's ethnic group. For instance, obesity is defined as a waist circumference of $\geq$94 cm in men of European descent, versus a cutoff of $\geq$90 cm in men of South

Asian descent (obesity is defined as ≥80 cm in women of both ethnicities). Still other studies have indicated even more conservative measurements indicative of increased risk; in an analysis of over 10,000 Asian Indian adults in living in six Indian cities, waist circumference cutoff values of 85 cm in men, and 80 cm in women, optimized sensitivity and specificity of these measures for the risk of diabetes (Snehalatha et al. 2003).

Although the underlying reason for the trend of higher risk at lower BMI and waist circumference is not completely understood, studies in South Asian populations suggest that the characteristics of body fat in South Asian individuals may be a contributing factor. Central adiposity, indicative of abdominal obesity or visceral fat, has been implicated in the pathogenesis of atherosclerosis and glucose intolerance (Westphal 2008). South Asian individuals are known to carry body fat predominantly in the central/visceral abdominal region (Prasad et al. 2011) and therefore this type of fat may contribute to the differentially elevated risk in South Asians. Prior studies have demonstrated that large fat cell, or adipocyte, size may contribute to insulin resistance. Subcutaneous abdominal adipocytes are larger in South Asian men compared to white men (Chandalia et al. 2007) and have been identified as a potential mechanism for increased risk of diabetes and the metabolic syndrome.

Large studies have suggested that waist circumference (and a related measure, waist-hip ratio), primarily a measure of central adiposity, may better estimate the degree of risk for cardiovascular diseases and diabetes than BMI, an overall measure of a person's weight relative to his or her height (Yusuf et al. 2005). Notably, in a comparison between South Asians and other ethnic groups in multiple international studies in the U.S., United Kingdom, India, and Australia, it was found that South Asians have increased abdominal fat and greater levels of insulin resistance at similar BMI levels, supporting the evidence that BMI alone may not reliably indicate risk level in South Asians (Gupta and Brister 2006; Gupta et al. 2006; McKeigue et al. 1991; Hodge et al. 1996; Banerji et al. 1999). Regardless of the measurement used, it is overall clear that body weight and obesity contribute to the elevated risk for type 2 diabetes in South Asians.

There are many genetic locus variants that are proposed to result in a differential increased predisposition to type 2 diabetes, obesity, and the metabolic syndrome in South Asians – such as the FTO gene (Li et al. 2012) and the PC-1 gene (Abate et al. 2003), which both have been found to confer increased risk in South Asians – however research into the underlying role of genetic variation in South Asian body fat patterning and the predisposition to cardiovascular disease is ongoing.

7.3.2 *Lifestyle Factors: Diet, Exercise, Alcohol, and Smoking*

7.3.2.1 Diet / Exercise

In a 24-hour dietary recall study of food group intake and the dietary quality of middle-aged and older urban-dwelling Gujarati Asian Indian immigrants (45 years or older) in the U.S., participant diets were adequate in grain and vegetable intake but low in fruits and meats and too high in fat (according to guidelines of the U.S. Food Guide Pyramid) (Jonnalagadda et al. 2005). Another study reported that Asian Indian men reported eating less fruits and vegetables as compared to Caucasian men (Ghai et al. 2012). South Asian Americans also tend to consume more festival foods, which are high in refined grain, sugar, and fat (Azar et al. 2013). Vegetarian diet has been associated with less insulin resistance and relatively lower high density lipoprotein (or "good") cholesterol levels (Gadgil et al. 2014).

South Asians tend to have higher sedentary behavior than other ethnic groups (Ghai et al. 2012; Ye et al. 2009). Asian Indians were less likely to report moderate/vigorous physical activity ≥3.5 hours/week than Non-Hispanic White men. Among Asian immigrants in the United States, specific cultural barriers to engaging in Western exercise habits include existing health problems, risk of injury, and for women in particular, a desire to engage in women-only group exercise (Kalavar et al. 2005; Jayprakash et al. 2016).

7.3.3 *Alcohol Consumption*

Alcohol has a U-shaped relationship with diabetes onset such that those with moderate consumption are relatively protected from diabetes whereas those who consume alcohol in relatively small or large quantities have higher risks of incident diabetes (Baliunas et al. 2009). South Asian Americans, as compared to other Asian subgroups (including Japanese, Chinese, Korean and Filipino Americans), had the lowest self-reported rates of both moderate and binge drinking. South Asians may be less likely to receive the protective benefits of low to moderate alcohol consumption on diabetes risk but may be as a group, less likely to suffer from increased diabetes incidence on the basis of binge drinking.

7.3.4 *Tobacco Use*

The CDC reports that smokers have a 30–40% increased risk of developing diabetes than non-smokers. Also, people with diabetes who smoke are more likely than non-smokers to have trouble with insulin dosing and with controlling their disease (CDC 2014).

Modes of tobacco consumption vary among South Asians and include cigarettes and cigars along with bidis (hand rolled tobacco flakes wrapped in leaves that are smoked), hookah (water pipe), and betel quid (tobacco wrapped in the Piper betel leaves along with areca nut, spices and slaked lime which is chewed) (Gupta and Ray 2003; Mukherjea et al. 2012). Studies vary in their report of South Asian tobacco in diaspora communities (Ghai et al. 2012; Ivey et al. 2006; Jonnalagadda et al. 2005; Ye et al. 2009) but use of tobacco in the general South Asian population is reported to be lower than in Non-Hispanic Whites and other Asian subgroups (Ivey et al. 2006). South Asian men and women in the United States reported current tobacco use at 7.9%, which was less than a third of the rate of Non-Hispanic Whites. Among 51,000 middle-aged male members of Kaiser Permanente Health Plan in California, 6.5% of South Asian men in the normal weight category reported current smoking whereas 11% of normal weight White men reported current smoking. Among men who were overweight or obese, rates of prevalent smoking were similar between both South Asian and White men at 9.8% and 9.9% respectively (Ghai et al. 2012). Whereas smoking rates in the general population have reportedly been lower among South Asians, cigarette smoking remains an important risk factor among those with prevalent coronary artery disease. A recent report from 279,256 patients undergoing percutaneous coronary intervention for acute coronary syndromes from 2004 to 2011 from the British Cardiovascular Intervention Society national database (with n = 19,938 South Asian individuals) suggested higher rates of cigarette smoking among South Asian (28.8%) as compared to Caucasian (23.5%) men and women.

7.3.5 Social Determinants of Diabetes: Race/Ethnicity, Insurance, Language, Nativity, Education

Along with clinical and lifestyle risk factors there are also social determinants that affect access to and quality of care, and show great disparities in health and healthcare of Asian Americans, including South Asian Americans. These social determinants are: race/ethnicity, insurance, limited English proficiency (LEP), nativity status, education, and socio-economic status. South Asian Americans have some of the worst rates and the rates are worse at state, county and city levels compared to national levels. National data are average or aggregate data; information gets masked by aggregate data (e.g. 25 states may have high access to care and 25 states may have low access to care; national data will show only an average of these numbers). The rates at state, county, and city levels are disaggregated and represent smaller subpopulations and give more accurate representation.

Several studies have reported that South Asian Americans have a higher prevalence of T2DM compared to non-Hispanic White Americans, as reported in detail earlier in this chapter. However, only a few studies have investigated insurance,

LEP, nativity status, education, and socio-economic status in relation to T2DM in South Asian Americans.

Data from the New York Health and Nutrition Examination Survey showed that the prevalence of diabetes mellitus is higher for foreign-born South Asian Americans (34.5%) compared to Asian Americans (16.1%) or Whites (10.8%) (Rajpathak et al. 2010). Cultural factors (e.g., having traditional Indian beliefs) and clinical and lifestyle risk factors (e.g., higher obesity levels and lower physical activity levels) were associated with higher prevalence of T2DM (Kanaya et al. 2010). Potential reasons for the variation in prevalence could also be education and income rather than race/ethnicity. However, the prevalence rates of T2DM for South Asian Americans increased after controlling for education and income (Kanaya et al. 2014).

Other studies have shown that the risk of T2DM is higher in foreign-born Asians compared to US-born Asians (Jackson et al. 2015) and foreign-born Hispanics compared to US-born Hispanics (Oza-Frank et al. 2013). However, Jackson et al. (2015) did not report disaggregated data for any Asian subgroups. Oza-Frank et al. (2013) analyzed disaggregated data (i.e. the categories were Hispanic, Chinese, White, and Black), and the results were not significant for Chinese, White, or Black population. This indicates the necessity of analyzing disaggregated data and including more ethnic groups such as SAAs.

The lack of data on social determinants affecting T2DM is surprising given that these factors show great disparities at national and worse at state, county, and city levels. The following paragraphs illustrate these disparities with the 2013 American Community Survey data (Khan et al. 2015).

For example, having health insurance allows greater access to the U.S. healthcare system, which leads to greater likelihood of diagnosis and treatment of T2DM. Of the top 10 highest ***uninsured*** subgroups in the U.S., two are South Asian Americans (Pakistani 20.9%, Bangladeshi 18.2%). Uninsurance is 41.8% for Pakistanis in Harris County, Texas. The uninsurance rate for Asian Indians is 10.4%; while the rate is relatively low, this represents nearly 360,000 uninsured people. Possible explanations of why Pakistani and Bangladeshi Americans are the highest uninsured groups may be: high rates of foreign-born individuals who tend to be first generation immigrants (they are not used to having health insurance in their native countries and thus do not seek health insurance); high rates of LEP individuals in these communities and limited resources in South Asian languages; and a five-year waiting period for legal immigrants for any U.S. government health programs.

Language is another significant barrier to accessing the healthcare system in the U.S. There are high numbers of LEP residents in the U.S. and there is limited availability of translated resources in hospitals, clinics, and other healthcare facilities across the nation. Of the top 10 highest LEP groups, eight are Asian American ethnic groups and Bangladeshis are the second highest (Vietnamese 47.9%, Bangladeshi 42.8%, Hmong 40.5%, Chinese 40.1%, Taiwanese 38.3%, Cambodian 37.4%, Other 36%, Korean 35.8%, Laotian 34.7%). The LEP rate for Asian Indians is 19.7% in the U.S. This rate is higher at city and county levels (e.g., in Cook County, IL, Asian Indian LEP is 25.7%) (Khan et al. 2015). The national data are aggregated and mask the magnitude of the problem seen at city and county levels.

Nativity status affects the likelihood of benefiting from government programs, having health insurance, and accessing quality care, as foreign-born individuals may be undocumented, non-U.S. citizens, or LEP. Of the top 10 highest ***foreign-born*** groups, three are South Asian Americans (Bangladeshi 70.9%, Asian Indian 67.8%, and Pakistani 62.6%). Of the top 10 highest ***less than high school educated*** groups, six are Asian American and one is South Asian American (Other 39.8%, Hispanic 35.3%, Cambodian 34%, Hmong 30.2%, Laotian 30.1%, Vietnamese 26.7%, Bangladeshi 17.8%, American Indian/Alaskan Native 17.3%, Chinese 17.3%, Black 16.2%) (Khan et al. 2015). These demographics stress the importance of investigating the disaggregated social determinants of diabetes in order to avoid overlooking the inequalities that the different South Asian American ethnic groups can face.

7.4 Detection, Treatment, and Management of T2DM in South Asian Americans

While management of type 2 diabetes in South Asian populations has been previously studied, recommendations for diabetes care in South Asian Americans must often be extrapolated from studies in international South Asian communities due to the relative lack of data specifically from the U.S. Studies suggest that Canadian South Asians are frequently diagnosed with diabetes after the development of major complications such as retinopathy or nephropathy, indicating the need for improved screening efforts for identifying the presence of diabetes earlier in the disease course (Sohal 2008; Egede and Dagogo-Jack 2005; Misra and Vikram 2004). There remains a need for effective screening programs for this high-risk group in all regions. One study explored an outpatient screening strategy that aimed to detect impaired glucose tolerance and undiagnosed T2DM in South Asians living in the United Kingdom. A stepwise approach that started initially with a screening health questionnaire, followed by anthropometric measurements (including waist and hip circumference, sagittal diameter, and percentage body fat) and a clinical oral glucose tolerance test (OGTT) in those individuals who screened to be at moderate to high risk, was able to identify and diagnose 50% of the diabetes in the screened population (Hanif et al. 2008). These results suggest that the basic questions of a patient's medical history that were included in the screening questionnaire, including query of family history of diabetes, history of gestational diabetes, and history of ischemic heart disease or hypertension, could assist in determining who to further test for the presence of diabetes.

Laboratory screening tests, including OGTT and hemoglobin A1c, identify South Asians at increased risk using standard diagnostic cutoff values (generally, normal less than 5.7%, pre-diabetes 5.7–6.4%, diabetes 6.5% or higher). An investigation of the use of these tests in a population of South Asians in the Netherlands showed that individuals identified as being diabetic or pre-diabetic via either OGTT or hemoglobin A1c were all at increased metabolic risk. Notably, however, an assessment of test characteristics of using hemoglobin A1c to diagnose type 2 diabetes (as identified by OGTT as the gold standard) showed that hemoglobin A1c had a sensitivity of 46% and a specificity of 98%. The low sensitivity suggests that hemoglobin A1c may be inadequate as a screening test in this population, especially for identifying pre-diabetes (Vlaar et al. 2013). While low sensitivity of hemoglobin A1c in South Asians is not well understood, similar findings have been found in other ethnic groups (Vlaar et al. 2013), and these test characteristics support the World Health Organization's recommendation to not use hemoglobin A1c to diagnose pre-diabetes (WHO 2011).

Gestational diabetes represents a particular challenge in South Asian women, who are at higher risk for developing this pregnancy-related condition. The prevalence of gestational diabetes in South Asian American (Indian, Sri Lankan, Pakistani, and Fijian Indian) women was found to be higher than that in South-East Asian American and East Asian American women (Savitz et al. 2008). The adjusted relative risk in South Asian American women was as high as 7.1 (95% confidence interval 6.8 to 7.3) times as high compared to other ethnicities in this study. In a Canadian study of women with gestational diabetes, infants of South Asian mothers had a higher risk (nearly 60%) of adverse neonatal and maternal outcomes compared to infants of mothers from the general population (about 56%) (Mukerji et al. 2003). It is unclear how much health literacy, cultural factors, and physiologic factors play in this differential risk of adverse outcomes. At this time, there are no specific screening, diagnosis, or treatment differences for South Asian women, although evidence suggests that women from different ethnic groups require variable insulin therapy for gestational diabetes (Yuen and Wong 2015), and cultural customs such as diet must be accounted for in the recommendations provided for medical nutritional therapy in the management of gestational diabetes.

Treatment and management of diabetes in South Asians Americans follows the same lifestyle and pharmacotherapy recommendations as for other populations. As of yet, there are no specific guidelines for management of type 2 diabetes in South Asians Americans, or South Asians in any other international setting. Results from the Indian Diabetes Prevention Program demonstrated that the combination of metformin and lifestyle changes significantly reduced the incidence of diabetes in Asian Indians (Singh et al. 2012; Ramachandran et al. 2006). While certain studies have shown that South Asian patients can achieve similar levels of glycemic control in comparison to white Europeans (Close et al. 1995), there is some evidence suggesting that South Asians have less response to diabetes medications compared to other ethnic groups (James et al. 2012; Holland et al. 2013). In a study conducted in London of individuals with poorly controlled diabetes, 63% of whom were South Asian, the South Asians had less improvement in hemoglobin A1c after two years of follow-up compared to other ethnic groups. This finding was consistent across treatment types, including use of metformin alone, combined oral hypoglycemic treatment, or use of insulin (James et al. 2012). The reason for this lag in improvement in South Asians is unclear, and could represent inefficacy of the treatments, or could be related to cultural or social factors that preclude adherence to diabetes medication regimens in this population, such as a desire to avoid taking medications or beliefs about the inadequate efficacy of medications.

In addition to pharmacotherapy, the cultural nuances specific to South Asians must be considered in any management and risk reduction program. Lifestyle factors in South Asians also contribute to increased risk, and providing culturally-sensitive information that incorporates religious and linguistic differences may improve self-efficacy and promote self-management for lifestyle modification in these patients (Hill 2007). Successful, culturally appropriate lifestyle interventions for international South Asian communities have involved family members in creating diabetes management plans (Singh et al. 2012), and provided nutritional recommendations based on traditional South Asian diets such as alternatives for carbohydrate-rich South Asian foods including rice and chapati (Gupta et al. 2010), and involved patients in practical healthful cooking demonstrations incorporating South Asian dishes (Snowdon 1999). Clinical trials of lifestyle interventions for diabetes management in South Asians are ongoing, including in the United States, and there remains a need for an understanding of optimal management strategies that combine lifestyle approaches with pharmacologic treatment specifically for this high-risk group.

Diabetes may be diagnosed at later stages associated with secondary complications in South Asian individuals (Chowdhury and Lasker 2002). The reasons for this are not fully elucidated however, they could possibly be due to the fact that South Asians are likely to develop diabetes at lower average BMI's than individuals in Caucasian and other Asian ethnic subgroups (Ntuk et al. 2014) and thus may not be screened at early enough time points. A diabetes risk score, which has been validated among South Asians, suggests that waist circumference rather than BMI may be a more robust predictor of incident diabetes among South Asians (Mohan and Anbalagan 2013). Evidence from British Columbia, Canada suggest low adherence rates to both oral hypoglycemic and well as insulin among South Asian men and women with diabetes as compared to Caucasian individuals (Chong et al. 2014).

7.4.1 Barriers to Detection, Treatment, and Management

Early detection, treatment and self-management of T2DM reduces the risk of developing complications, and improves quality of life and health outcomes. However, there are several barriers that lead to poor prevention and treatment of T2DM in Asian Americans, including South Asian Americans.

Patient barriers may include lack of understanding of the relationship between diet and lifestyle in the risk for T2DM, or poor health literacy. Provider barriers may include the lack of use of multiple clinical assessments (e.g., body mass index, adipose tissue - visceral and subcutaneous, waist size/central obesity, glucose levels - HbA1c, oral glucose tolerance, impaired fasting glucose, insulin resistance), poor understanding of different physiological responses to drugs, and the use of multiple guidelines of varying accuracy (e.g., not using a lower BMI cut-off) to detect

T2DM. Such patient and provider barriers can also be enhanced by foreign-born status, uninsurance, low educational attainment, and lack of access to culturally and linguistically appropriate resources and care.

For example, there is a lack of in-language resources related to the Affordable Care Act (ACA) for LEP, uninsured, and immigrant South Asian American communities. "In-language" refers to the languages spoken by South Asian Americans (e.g. Hindi, Urdu, Bengali, Gujarati, Telegu, etc.). California has the highest number of Asian Indians in the U.S., of whom 21.9% are LEP. Yet, Covered California, the state marketplace for California, did not have any translated materials in any South Asian languages. Similarly, the Center for Medicare and Medicaid Services and Healthcare.gov (the federal marketplace for the ACA) also did not have any translated materials in any South Asian Languages (Khan et al. 2015). Lack of such in-language resources prevented many South Asian Americans from enrolling into a health insurance program through the ACA.

Lack of language support is associated with more emergency room visits, more lab tests, less follow-up from health providers, low health literacy among patients, and less overall satisfaction with health services (Ramakrishnan and Ahmad 2014). Patients who do not speak the same language as their physicians have difficulty communicating with their doctors, are less likely to report positive patient-physician interactions, and receive lower quality of care (AAPCHO 2005). Yet, specific data for South Asian Americans are not available.

Racial/ethnic disparities in T2DM awareness, access, and quality of healthcare have been well documented (Kim et al. 2012; Saxena et al. 2007; Harris 2001; Laiteerapong et al. 2015). Racial/ethnic minorities tend to visit the doctor less (Fiscella et al. 2002), adhere less to medications (Traylor et al. 2010), and are less aware of how to manage their disease (Thackeray et al. 2004; Osborn et al. 2011).

Attitudes, cultural differences, and religious and social beliefs affect prevention and management of diabetes in South Asians (Misra and Khurana 2011). Specific barriers in management include: delayed diagnosis, insufficient clinical evaluation and advice, and lack of access to affordable and specialized health care (Wilkinson et al. 1996). Studies on Bangladeshis in the United Kingdom indicated that poor diabetes knowledge, health care utilization barriers, lack of acculturation, lack of physical activity, changing diets, and language barriers exacerbated diabetes in this population (Choudhury et al. 2009).

A qualitative study of South Asian Americans found that most participants could identify, but only minimally or partially adhered to, practices such as self-care behaviors that were important to appropriately manage diabetes, e.g. regular exercise, self-monitoring of glucose levels, appointments with primary care physicians, consuming balanced meals, and taking prescription medications on time (Imran et al. 2015).

7.5 Relation with Cardiovascular Diseases

T2DM is an established risk factor for the development of cardiovascular disease (Grundy et al. 1999). It has been established that South Asian Americans have an increased burden of cardiovascular disease, specifically, a high risk of developing coronary heart disease (CHD; Enas et al. 1996; Palaniappan et al. 2010b), and a high proportionate mortality due to CHD and stroke (Jose et al. 2014).

Evidence suggests that this increased burden of cardiovascular disease in South Asian Americans is related to the high prevalence of T2DM and insulin resistance in this population (Gholap et al. 2011). Studies examining CVD in the South Asian diaspora have found that South Asians with diabetes have a two to three fold increased risk of cardiovascular death (Fernando et al. 2015; Yusuf et al. 2004).

South Asians often present with a cluster of health abnormalities referred to as metabolic syndrome; this syndrome confers an increased risk for coronary artery disease and other cardiovascular disease (Flowers et al. 2010). Impaired glucose tolerance and insulin resistance are two abnormalities included in the metabolic syndrome, along with central obesity, dyslipidemia, and hypertension (Flowers et al. 2013; Kalhan et al. 2001). Patients with metabolic syndrome have two times the risk of developing CVD in 5 to 10 years compared to patients without the syndrome (Alberti et al. 2009). The prevalence of metabolic syndrome is increasing among South Asians on the Indian subcontinent, and in South Asian migrant communities, and it is estimated that 20–25% of South Asians have already developed metabolic syndrome (Eapen et al. 2009). It has been hypothesized that excess body fat and adverse body fat patterning, found in South Asians even when they have a normal BMI, may contribute to the high prevalence of insulin resistance, which may underlie the tendency to develop both diabetes mellitus and early atherosclerosis (Misra and Vikram 2004).

To further understand the relationship between T2DM and cardiovascular disease, a parallel can be drawn between South Asian Americans and South Asians living in Europe. One European study demonstrated that South Asians admitted to hospitals after heart attacks have a 50% higher 6-month mortality compared to whites, a difference largely attributed to the higher prevalence of diabetes in the South Asian patients (Wilkinson et al. 1996). In another European analysis, the presence of heart disease as identified by electrocardiogram was strongly associated with glucose intolerance and hyperinsulinemia in young South Asians (McKeigue et al. 1993). Although these data are primarily in South Asian European populations, they strongly suggest that mitigating the risk for cardiovascular diseases in South Asians communities requires treating diabetes in those who have already developed the disease, and preventing the development of diabetes in those who have risk factors.

The impact of diabetes as a risk factor for CVD should be viewed within the larger context of other risk factors unique to South Asian Americans. South Asians Americans are at a higher risk for cardiovascular diseases compared to other Asian subgroups and non-Hispanic whites (Gupta et al. 2006). South Asians develop cardiovascular risk factors at a younger age than individuals of other ethnicities (Palaniappan et al. 2004) and a study from 2016 found that South Asians in Western countries display accelerated cardiac aging (Shantsila et al. 2016). The mean age at which South Asians suffer heart attacks, or acute myocardial infarction, is lower in South Asian countries than in other countries (Joshi et al. 2007). One of the harmful factors that contribute to this lower age at first heart attack is the higher prevalence of diabetes in South Asians and South Asian Americans compared to other groups (Bellary et al. 2010; Gupta and Brister 2006). The mean age at which South Asians Americans are diagnosed with diabetes is 44.9 years, compared with 55.4 years in non-Hispanic white Americans (Becerra and Becerra 2015). Both conditions manifest earlier on in the life of South Asian American patients, further supporting the association between T2DM and the development of cardiovascular disease.

The pathophysiologic changes that underlie the development of diabetes likely also lead to increased risk for cardiovascular disease. South Asians in the U.S. have a high prevalence of dyslipidemia; a lipid profile characterized by high plasma triglycerides, total cholesterol, LDL-C and low HDL-C, that increases the risk of developing CVD (Frank et al. 2014). In South Asian Americans, this atherogenic profile may be explained by an alarmingly high prevalence of insulin resistance (Chu et al. 2003; Reaven et al. 1993). Furthermore, studies have found that South Asians in the U.K. display a unique phenotype of impaired glucose tolerance associated with low HDL-C, and that this may be related to the high prevalence and risk of cardiovascular disease in this population (Hughes et al. 1989; McKeigue et al. 1989, 1991).

For South Asians in their native countries and abroad, theories regarding the pathogenesis of diabetes include the influence of evolution, genetics, and diet. For instance, the "thrifty gene" hypothesis suggests that the energy-producing efficiency of mitochondria enhanced the successful adaptation of South Asians to climactic (e.g., warm temperature) and nutritional exposures (e.g., periods of starvation). Consequently, South Asians' mitochondria are proposed to be more likely to produce and store energy, an adaptation that would be disadvantageous in a lifestyle of low physical activity and high caloric diet as is frequently found in American and increasingly found in South Asian settings (Sellayah et al. 2014).

Environmental influences, including high intake of total fat, saturated fatty acids, trans fatty acids, and carbohydrates, combined with low intake of monounsaturated fatty acids and certain micronutrients (e.g., magnesium, calcium, and vitamin D) that characterizes the traditional South Asian diet, have also been found to promote insulin resistance (Bakker et al. 2013). Further explanations of the pathogenesis of insulin resistance and diabetes in South Asians, including the roles of various types of fat and fat cells, inflammation, and muscular composition remain the subject of ongoing research. The American Heart Association calls for increased research in these areas, with special attention to disaggregating data in the heterogeneous Asian American subgroups (Palaniappan et al. 2010a).

7.6 Relation with Obesity and Weight Related Conditions

In a meta-analysis of several studies among all Asian ethnic subgroups in the United States, South Asians had the lowest rates of obesity (> 30 kg/m2) and overweight (BMI > =25 but <30 kg/m2), yet the highest rates of diabetes (Staimez et al. 2013). Indeed, South Asians have been recognized to develop insulin resistance at a lower BMI than individuals of other ethnicities. The World Health Organization has consequently recommended lower thresholds to define overweight (23–27 kg/m^2) and obesity (>27.5 kg/m^2) among South Asians specifically (Razak et al. 2007). The percent of persons who are currently misclassified as normal weight using standard overweight metrics (of 25–29 kg/m^2) is 12.6% and for obese ($\geq$ 30 kg/m^2) is 9.9% (Rao et al. 2015). A study of Midwestern-dwelling South Asian individuals in the U.S. demonstrated that overweight and obese South Asians tend to underestimate their weight and did not associate being overweight with the presence of their concomitant weight-related chronic diseases; 40% of overweight participants and 19% of obese participants perceived themselves as normal weight or underweight (Tang et al. 2012).

7.7 Economic Burden of Diabetes

One study estimated that diabetes costs Americans $245 billion annually, and that $175 billion is from direct medical costs and $69 billion from loss of productivity. This represents a $7888 per capita expenditure (Yang et al. 2013a, b). The study estimated the costs by state, and race/ethnicity for White, Black, Hispanic, and Other population. 70% of the costs are due to direct medical costs and a 30% of the costs are due to loss of productivity/indirect costs, whether at state level or by any specific race/ethnicity.

However, data are not currently available for Asian Americans, let alone for South Asian Americans. Yet South Asian Americans are one of the fastest growing populations and they already suffer from a greater burden of diabetes compared to other ethnic minority groups. This implies a greater number of diabetes cases in the future, and potentially increasing economic burden, with higher costs for patients, communities, and providers.

7.8 Systemic and Policy Issues

Systemic and policy issues contribute to and exacerbate the disparities in T2DM for South Asian Americans.

Only recently (2015) the American Diabetes Association recommended a lower BMI cut point (at 23 kg/m2) to better diagnose diabetes for Asian Americans (ADA

2015). These racial/ethnic specific cut points and guidelines have not yet been adopted by any federal (e.g., CDC, CMS, or United States Preventive Services Task Force) or private agencies (e.g., American Hospital Association). Health plans will not reimburse health providers unless such guidelines are officially adopted by federal and/or state agencies.

This is further complicated by the fact that data on most subgroups of the South Asian American community are not available - as data are not collected or reported (due to small sample sizes). Lack of disaggregated data at national, state, and local levels makes it challenging to effectively address diabetes disparities in small communities of color such as South Asian Americans.

Systemic and policy changes at local, state, and national levels are necessary to raise awareness, address quality of care and access to service, and prevent future cases and complications of diabetes in South Asian Americans. All these efforts need to include the South Asian American community, the health service providers, funders, and policymakers.

7.9 Conclusion

South Asian Americans suffer disproportionately higher from Type 2 Diabetes Mellitus compared to many other communities of color in the U.S. Early detection, treatment, and self-management of T2DM reduces the risk of developing complications, and improves quality of life and health outcomes. However, patients and providers have to deal with many barriers in preventing, diagnosing and appropriately treating T2DM in South Asian Americans.

A high percentage of foreign-born immigrants, lack of health insurance, and lack of access to culturally and linguistically appropriate resources and care perpetuate these disparities in diabetes. There is a need to collect and report disaggregated data of South Asian American subgroups as some groups (e.g., Bangladeshi, Pakistani) appear to be at higher risk than others (Asian Indian).

Systemic and policy changes are necessary at local, state, and national levels to raise awareness, increase screening, improve access to services, and prevent future cases of diabetes in South Asian Americans.

More research and policy efforts are necessary to better understand the prevalence and prevention strategies affecting the health outcomes and economic costs of Type 2 Diabetes Mellitus in this rapidly growing minority group in the U.S.

References

Abate, N., Carulli, L., Cabo-Chan, A., Chandalia, M., Snell, P., et al. (2003). Genetic polymorphism PC-1 K121Q and ethnic susceptibility to insulin resistance. *Journal of Clinical Endocrinology & Metabolism, 88*(12), 5927–5934.

Ahmad, F. Z. (2014). *State of Asian Americans and Pacific Islanders Series: A multifaceted portrait of a growing population.* Center for American Progress.

Alberti, K. G., Eckel, R. H., Grundy, S. M., Zimmet, P. Z., Cleeman, J. I., & Donato, K. A. (2009). Harmonizing the metabolic syndrome: A joint interim statement of the international diabetes federation task force on epidemiology and prevention; National heart, lung, and blood institute; American heart association; World heart federation; International atherosclerosis society; And international association for the study of obesity. *Circulation, 120*(16), 1640–1645. https://doi.org/10.1161/CIRCULATIONAHA.109.192644.

American Diabetes Association. (2015a). Standards of medical care in diabetes – 2015. *Diabetes Care, 38*(Suppl1).

American Diabetes Association. (2015b). *Living with diabetes: Complications* [Online]. American Diabetes Association. Retrieved from http://www.diabetes.org/living-with-diabetes/complications/

Anand, S., Yusuf, S., Vuksan, V., Devanesen, S., Teo, K., et al. (2000). Differences in risk factors, atherosclerosis, and cardiovascular disease between ethnic groups in Canada: The study of health assessment and risk in ethnic groups (SHARE). *Lancet, 356*(9226), 279–284.

Araneta, M., Grandinetti, A., & Chang, H. (2010). A1C and diabetes diagnosis among Filipino Americans, Japanese Americans, and Native Hawaiians. *Diabetes Care, 33*(12), 2626–2628.

Association of Asian Pacific Community Health Organizations. (2005). *AAPI limited English proficiency.* Association of Asian Pacific Community Health Organizations.

Azar, K., Chen, E., Holland, A., & Palaniappan, L. (2013). Festival foods in the immigrant diet. *Journal of Immigrant and Minority Health, 15*(5), 953–960.

Bakker, L. E., Sleddering, M. A., Schoones, J. W., Meinders, A. E., & Jazet, I. M. (2013). Pathogenesis of type 2 diabetes in South Asians. *European Journal of Endocrinology, 169*(5), R99–R114.

Balarajan, R. (1991). Ethnic differences in mortality from Ischaemic heart disease and cerebrovascular disease in England and Wales. *BMJ: British Medical Journal, 302*(6776), 560–564.

Baliunas, D., Taylor, B., Irving, H., Roerecke, M., Patra, J., et al. (2009). Alcohol as a risk factor for type 2 diabetes: A systematic review and meta-analysis. *Diabetes Care, 32*(11), 2123–2132.

Banerji, M., Faridi, N., Atluri, R., Chaiken, R., & Lebovitz, H. (1999). Body composition, visceral fat, leptin, and insulin resistance in Asian Indian men. *Journal of Clinical Endocrinology and Metabolism, 84*(1), 137–144.

Barnett, A., Dixon, A., Bellary, S., Hanif, M., O'Hare, J., et al. (2006). Type 2 diabetes and cardiovascular risk in the UK South Asian community. *Diabetologia, 49*(10), 2234–2246.

Becerra, M. B. & Becerra, B. J. (2015). Disparities in age at diabetes diagnosis among Asian Americans: Implications for early preventive measures. Brief. Centers for Disease Control and Prevention. *Preventing Chronic Disease, 12*, E46.

Bellary, S., O'Hare, J. P., Raymond, N. T., Mughal, S., Hanif, W. M., Jones, A., et al. (2010). Premature cardiovascular events and mortality in South Asians with type 2 diabetes in the United Kingdom Asian diabetes study - effect of ethnicity on risk. *Current Medical Research and Opinion, 26*(8), 1873–1879. https://doi.org/10.1185/03007995.2010.490468.

Bharmal, N., Kaplan, R., Shapiro, M., Mangione, C., Kagawa-Singer, M., et al. (2014). The association of duration of residence in the United States with cardiovascular disease risk factors among South Asian immigrants. *Journal of Immigrant and Minority Health, 17*(3), 781–790.

Bhopal, R., Unwin, N., White, M., Yallop, J., Walker, L., et al. (1999). Heterogeneity of coronary heart disease risk factors in Indian, Pakistani, Bangladeshi, and European origin populations: Cross sectional study. *BMJ: British Medical Journal, 319*(7204), 215–220.

Bodicoat, D., Gray, L., Henson, J., Webb, D., Guru, A., et al. (2014). Body mass index and waist circumference cut-points in multi-ethnic populations from the UK and India: The ADDITION-Leicester, Jaipur heart watch and New Delhi cross-sectional studies: T90813. *PLoS One, 9*(3).
Centers for Disease Control and Prevention. (2014a). *National diabetes statistics report: Estimates of diabetes and its burden in the United States*. Centers for Disease Control and Prevention.
Centers for Disease Control and Prevention. (2014b). *Smoking and diabetes*. Centers for Disease Control and Prevention. Retrieved from http://www.cdc.gov/tobacco/campaign/tips/diseases/diabetes.html
Chandalia, M., Lin, P., Seenivasan, T., Livingston, E. H., Snell, P. G., et al. (2007). Insulin resistance and body fat distribution in South Asian men compared to Caucasian men. *PLoS One, 2*(8), e812.
Choi, S., Liu, M., Palaniappan, L., Wang, E., & Wong, N. (2013). Gender and ethnic differences in the prevalence of type 2 diabetes among Asian subgroups in California. *Journal of Diabetes and its Complications, 27*(5), 429–435.
Chiu, M., Austin, P., Manuel, D., Shah, B., & Tu, J. (2011). Deriving ethnic-specific bmi cutoff points for assessing diabetes risk. *Diabetes Care, 34*(8), 1741–1748.
Chong, E., Wang, H., King-Shier, K., Quan, H., Rabi, D., et al. (2014). Prescribing patterns and adherence to medication among South Asian, Chinese and White people with type 2 diabetes mellitus: A population-based cohort study. *Diabetic Medicine, 31*(12), 1586–1593.
Chowdhury, T., & Lasker, S. (2002). Complications and cardiovascular risk factors in South Asians and Europeans with early-onset type 2 diabetes. *QJM-an International Journal of Medicine, 95*(4), 241–246.
Choudhury, S., Brophy, S., & Williams, R. (2009a). Understanding and beliefs of diabetes in the UK Bangladeshi population. *Diabetic Medicine, 26*(6), 636–640.
Choudhury, S., Brophy, S., Fareedi, M., Zaman, B., Ahmed, P., et al. (2009b). Examining the effectiveness of a peer-led education programme for type 2 diabetes and cardiovascular disease in a Bangladeshi population. *Diabetic Medicine, 26*(1), 40–44.
Chu, J. W., Abbasi, F., Kulkarni, K. R., Lamendola, C., McLaughlin, T. L., Scalisi, J. N., & Reaven, G. M. (2003). Multiple lipoprotein abnormalities associated with insulin resistance in healthy volunteers are identified by the vertical auto profile-II methodology. *Clinical Chemistry, 49*(6 Pt 1), 1014–1017 Retrieved from http://www.ncbi.nlm.nih.gov/pubmed/12766017.
Close, C., Lewis, P., Holder, R., Wright, A., & Nattrass, M. (1995). Diabetes care in South Asian and white European patients with type 2 diabetes. *Diabetic Medicine, 12*(7), 619–621.
Corazon, B. (2004). Appropriate body-mass index for Asian populations and its implications for policy and intervention strategies. *Lancet, 363*(9403), 157–163.
Dave, S. S., Craft, L. L., Mehta, P., Naval, S., Kumar, S., & Kandula, N. R. (2015). Life stage influences on U.S. South Asian women's physical activity. *American Journal of Health Promotion, 29*(3), e100–e108.
Eapen, D., Kalra, G. L., Merchant, N., Arora, A., & Khan, B. V. (2009). Metabolic syndrome and cardiovascular disease in South Asians. *Vascular Health and Risk Management, 5*, 731–743 Retrieved from http://www.ncbi.nlm.nih.gov/pubmed/19756165.
Enas, E. A., Garg, A., Davidson, M. A., Nair, V. M., Huet, B. A., & Yusuf, S. (1996). Coronary heart disease and its risk factors in first-generation immigrant Asian Indians to the United States of America. *Indian Heart Journal, 48*(4), 343–353 Retrieved from https://www.ncbi.nlm.nih.gov/pubmed/8908818.
Egede, L. E., & Dagogo-Jack, S. (2005). Epidemiology of type 2 diabetes: Focus on ethnic minorities. *Medical Clinics of North America, 89*(5), 949–975.
Fernando, E., Razak, F., Lear, S. A., & Anand, S. S. (2015). Cardiovascular disease in South Asian migrants. *Canadian Journal of Cardiology, 31*(9), 1139–1150. https://doi.org/10.1016/j.cjca.2015.06.008.
Fiscella, K., Frank, P., Doescher, M. P., & Saver, B. G. (2002). Disparities in health care by race, ethnicity, and language among the insured: Findings from a national sample. *Medical Care, 40*, 52–59.

Flowers, E., Molina, C., Mathur, A., Prasad, M., Abrams, L., Sathe, A., et al. (2010). Prevalence of metabolic syndrome in South Asians residing in the United States. *Metabolic Syndrome and Related Disorders, 8*(5), 417–423. https://doi.org/10.1089/met.2009.0097.

Flowers, E., Molina, C., Mathur, A., & Reaven, G. M. (2013). Adiposity and cardiovascular risk clustering in South Asians. *Metabolic Syndrome and Related Disorders, 11*(6), 434–440. https://doi.org/10.1089/met.2013.0081.

Forouhi, N., Sattar, N., Tillin, T., McKeigue, P., & Chaturvedi, N. (2006). Do known risk factors explain the higher coronary heart disease mortality in South Asian compared with European men? Prospective follow-up of the Southall and Brent studies, UK. *Diabetologia, 49*(11), 2580–2588.

Frank, A. T., Zhao, B., Jose, P. O., Azar, K. M., Fortmann, S. P., & Palaniappan, L. P. (2014). Racial/ethnic differences in dyslipidemia patterns. *Circulation, 129*(5), 570–579. https://doi.org/10.1161/CIRCULATIONAHA.113.005757.

Gadgil, M., Anderson, C., Kandula, N., & Kanaya, A. (2014). Dietary patterns in Asian Indians in the United States: An analysis of the metabolic syndrome and atherosclerosis in South Asians living in America study. *Journal of the Academy of Nutrition and Dietetics, 114*(2), 238–243.

Ghaffar, A., Reddy, K., & Singhi, M. (2004). Burden of non-communicable diseases in South Asia. *BMJ: British Medical Journal, 328*(7443), 807–810.

Ghai, N., Jacobsen, S., Van Den Eeden, S., Ahmed, A., Haque, R., Rhoads, G. G., & Quinn, V. P. (2012). A comparison of lifestyle and behavioral cardiovascular disease risk factors between Asian Indian and White non-Hispanic men. *Ethnicity & Disease, 22*(2), 168–174.

Gholap, N., Davies, M., Patel, K., Sattar, N., & Khunti, K. (2011). Type 2 diabetes and cardiovascular disease in South Asians. *Primary Care Diabetes, 5*(1), 45–56.

Go, A., Mozaffarian, D., Roger, V., Benjamin, E., Berry, J., et al. (2014). Heart disease and stroke statistics-2014 update a report from the American heart association. *Circulation, 129*(3), E28–E292.

Grundy, S., Benjamin, I., Burke, G., Chait, A., Eckel, R., et al. (1999). Diabetes and cardiovascular disease – A statement for healthcare professionals from the American Heart Association. *Circulation, 100*(10), 1134–1146.

Gupta, M., & Brister, S. (2006). Is South Asian ethnicity an independent cardiovascular risk factor? *Canadian Journal of Cardiology, 22*(3), 193–197.

Gupta, M., Singh, N., & Verma, S. (2006). South Asians and cardiovascular risk - what clinicians should know. *Circulation, 113*(25), E924–E929.

Gupta, N., Shah, P., Goel, K., Misra, A., Rastogi, K., et al. (2010). Imbalanced dietary profile, anthropometry, and lipids in urban Asian Indian adolescents and young adults. *Journal of the American College of Nutrition, 29*(2), 81–91.

Gupta, P., & Ray, C. (2003). Smokeless tobacco and health in India and South Asia. *Respirology, 8*(4), 419–431.

Hanif, M., Valsamakis, G., Dixon, A., Boutsiadis, A., Jones, A., et al. (2008). Detection of impaired glucose tolerance and undiagnosed type 2 diabetes in UK South Asians: An effective screening strategy. *Diabetes, Obesity and Metabolism, 10*(9), 755–762.

Harris, M. I. (2001). Racial and ethnic differences in health care access and health outcomes for adults with type 2 diabetes. *Diabetes Care, 24*, 454–459.

Hastings, K., Jose, P., Kapphahn, K., Frank, A., Goldstein, B., et al. (2015). Leading causes of death among Asian American subgroups (2003–2011). *PLoS One, 10*(4), E0124341.

Hill, J. (2007). Management of diabetes in South Asian communities in the UK. *Primary Health Care, 17*(3), 49.

Hodge, A., Dowse, G., Collins, V., Alberti, K., Gareeboo, H., et al. (1996). Abdominal fat distribution and insulin levels only partially explain adverse cardiovascular risk profile in Asian Indians. *Journal of Cardiovascular Risk, 3*(3), 263–270.

Holland, A., Zhao, B., Wong, E., Choi, S., Wong, N., et al. (2013). Racial/ethnic differences in control of cardiovascular risk factors among type 2 diabetes patients in an insured, ambulatory care population. *Journal of Diabetes and its Complications, 27*(1), 34–40.

Hsu, W., Araneta, M., Kanaya, A., Chiang, J., & Fujimoto, W. (2015). BMI cut points to identify at-risk Asian Americans for type 2 diabetes screening. *Diabetes Care, 38*(1), 150–158.

Hughes, L., Cruickshank, J., Wright, J., & Raftery, E. (1989). Disturbances of insulin in British Asian and white men surviving myocardial infarction. *BMJ: British Medical Journal, 299*(6698), 537–541.

Imran, T., Jauhari, S., & Chaudhry, N. (2015). Living diabetes: How disease perceptions and cultural factors influence self-care behaviors in South Asians in America. *Journal of Nature and Science, 1*(5), 98.

Ivey, S., Mehta, K., Fyr, C., & Kanaya, A. (2006). Prevalence and correlates of cardiovascular risk factors in South Asians: Population-based data from two California surveys. *Ethnicity and Disease, 16*(4), 886–893.

Jackson, H., Su, D., Wang, M., & Huang, T. (2015). Risk of type 2 diabetes among US and foreign born non-Hispanic Asians: Evidence from NHANES 2011-12. *Journal of Diabetes and Obesity, 2*(1), 1–4.

James, G., Baker, P., Badrick, E., Mathur, R., Hull, S., et al. (2012). Type 2 diabetes: A cohort study of treatment, ethnic and social group influences on glycated haemoglobin. *BMJ Open, 2*(5).

Jayprakash, M., Puri-Taneja, A., Kandula, N. R., Bharucha, H., Kumar, S., et al. (2016). Qualitative process evaluation of a community-based culturally tailored lifestyle intervention for underserved South Asians. *Health Promotion Practice, 17*(6), 802–813 1524839916650165.

Jih, J., Mukherjea, A., Vittinghoff, E., Nguyen, T., Tsoh, J., et al. (2014). Using appropriate body mass index cut points for overweight and obesity among Asian Americans. *Preventive Medicine, 65*, 1–6.

Johnson, N., Hayes, L., Brown, K., Hoo, E., & Ethier, K. (2014). CDC national health report: Leading causes of morbidity and mortality and associated behavioral risk and protective factors--United States, 2005–2013. *MMWR Supplements, 63*(4), 3–27.

Jonnalagadda, S., Diwan, S., & Cohen, D. (2005). US food guide pyramid food group intake by Asian Indian immigrants in the US. *Journal of Nutrition Health & Aging, 9*(4), 226–231.

Jose, P., Frank, A., Kapphahn, K., Goldstein, B., Eggleston, K., et al. (2014). Cardiovascular disease mortality in Asian Americans. *Journal of the American College of Cardiology, 64*(23), 2486–2494.

Joshi, P., Islam, S., Pais, P., Reddy, S., Dorairaj, P., et al. (2007). Risk factors for early myocardial infarction in South Asians compared with individuals in other countries. *JAMA, 297*(3), 286–294.

Kalavar, J. M., Kolt, G. S., Giles, L. C., & Driver, R. P. (2005). Physical activity in older Asian Indians living in the United States. *Activities, Adaptation and Aging, 29*, 47–67.

Kalhan, R., Puthawala, K., Agarwal, S., Amini, S. B., & Kalhan, S. C. (2001). Altered lipid profile, leptin, insulin, and anthropometry in offspring of South Asian immigrants in the United States. *Metabolism, 50*(10), 1197–1202. https://doi.org/10.1053/meta.2001.26704.

Kanaya, A., Herrington, D., Vittinghoff, E., Ewing, S., Liu, K., et al. (2014). Understanding the high prevalence of diabetes in US South Asians compared with four racial/ethnic groups: The MASALA and MESA studies. *Diabetes Care, 37*(6), 1621–1628.

Kanaya, A., Wassel, C., Mathur, D., Stewart, A., Herrington, D., et al. (2010). Prevalence and correlates of diabetes in South Asian Indians in the United States: Findings from the metabolic syndrome and atherosclerosis in South Asians living in America study and the multi-ethnic study of atherosclerosis. *Metabolic Syndrome and Related Disorders, 8*(2), 157–163.

Karter, A., Schillinger, D., Adams, A., Moffet, H., Liu, J., et al. (2013). Elevated rates of diabetes in Pacific Islanders and Asian subgroups the diabetes study of northern California (DISTANCE). *Diabetes Care, 36*(3), 574–579.

Kelkar, M. (2011). South Asian immigration in the United States: A gendered perspective. *Asian American Policy Review, 22*, 55–60.

Khan, S., Cha, L., Chi, L., Kantaria, T., Le, T., et al. (2015). *The impact of the Affordable Care Act on Asian Indian, Chinese, Filipino, Korean, Pakistani, and Vietnamese Americans*. Full report. National Council of Asian Pacific Islander Physicians.

Kim, G., Ford, K. L., Chiriboga, D. A., & Sorkin, D. H. (2012). Racial and ethnic disparities in healthcare use, delayed care, and management of diabetes mellitus in older adults in California. *Journal of the American Geriatrics Society, 60*, 2319–2325.

Laiteerapong, N., Fairchild, P. C., Chou, C. H., Chin, M. H., & Huang, E. S. (2015). Revisiting disparities in quality of care among US adults with diabetes in the era of individualized care, NHANES 2007–2010. *Medical Care, 53*, 25.

Lee, S. Y., Martins, S. S., & Lee, H. B. (2015). Mental disorders and mental health service use across Asian American subethnic groups in the United States. *Community Mental Health Journal, 51*(2), 153–160.

Li, H., Kilpelainen, T. O., Liu, Y., Hu, C., Yang, Z., et al. (2012). Association of genetic variation in FTO with risk of obesity and type 2 diabetes with data from 96,551 East and South Asians. *Diabetologia, 55*(4), 981–995.

Lopez, A. (2013). *Trends in death and disability in Asia and the pacific: Key findings from the Global Burden of Disease 2010 Study*. Regional World Health Summit: Asia. Singapore.

Martyn-Nemeth, P., Quinn, L., Menon, U., Shrestha, S., Patel, C., et al. (2016). Dietary profiles of first-generation South Asian Indian adolescents in the United States. *Journal of Immigrant and Minority Health.*

McKeigue, P. M., Ferrie, J. E., Pierpoint, T., & Marmot, M. G. (1993). Association of earlyonset coronary heart disease in South Asian men with glucose intolerance and Hyperinsulinemia. *Circulation, 87*(1), 152–161. https://doi.org/10.1161/01.CIR.87.1.152.

McKeigue, P. M., Miller, G. J., & Marmot, M. G. (1989). Coronary heart disease in South Asians overseas: A review. *Journal of Clinical Epidemiology, 42*(7), 597–609 Retrieved from https://www.ncbi.nlm.nih.gov/pubmed/2668448.

McKeigue, P., Shah, B., & Marmot, M. (1991). Relation of central obesity and insulin resistance with high diabetes prevalence and cardiovascular risk in South Asians. *Lancet, 337*(8738), 382–386.

McNeely, M., & Boyko, E. (2004). Type 2 diabetes prevalence in Asian Americans: Results of a national health survey. *Diabetes Care, 27*(1), 66–69.

Mehrotra, N., Gaur, S., & Petrova, A. (2012). Health care practices of the foreign born Asian Indians in the United States. A community based survey. *Journal of Community Health, 37*, 328–334.

Miller, G., Beckles, G., Maude, G., Carson, D., Alexis, S., et al. (1989). Ethnicity and other characteristics predictive of coronary heart disease in a developing community: Principal results of the St James survey, Trinidad. *International Journal of Epidemiology, 18*(4), 808–817.

Misra, A., & Khurana, L. (2011). Obesity related non-communicable diseases: South Asians vs White Caucasians. *International Journal Obesity (Lond), 35*(2), 167–187.

Misra, A., & Vikram, N. K. (2004). Insulin resistance syndrome (metabolic syndrome) and obesity in Asian Indians: Evidence and implications. *Nutrition, 20*(5), 482–491.

Mohan, V., & Anbalagan, V. (2013). Expanding role of the Madras Diabetes Research Foundation–Indian diabetes risk score in clinical practice. *Indian Journal of Endocrinology and Metabolism, 17*, 31–36.

Mukerji, G., Chiu, M., & Shah, B. R. (2003). Gestational diabetes mellitus and pregnancy outcomes among Chinese and South Asian women in Canada. *The Journal of Maternal-Fetal & Neonatal Medicine, 26*(3), 279–284.

Mukherjea, A., Morgan, P., Snowden, L., Ling, P., & Ivey, S. (2012). Social and cultural influences on tobaccorelated health disparities among South Asians in the USA. *Tobacco Control, 21*(4), 422–428.

Murray, C., Atkinson, C., Bhalla, K., Birbeck, G., Burstein, R., et al. (2013). The state of US health, 1990–2010: Burden of diseases, injuries, and risk factors. *JAMA, 310*(6), 591–608.

Narayan, K., Boyle, J., Thompson, T., Gregg, E., & Williamson, D. (2007). Effect of BMI on lifetime risk for diabetes in the U.S. *Diabetes Care, 30*(6), 1562–1566.

National Council of Asian Pacific Islander Physicians. (2012). *State of the sciences conference 2011. Diabetes in Asian Americans, Native Hawaiians, and Pacific Islanders. A call to action*. National Council of Asian Pacific Islander Physicians.

Ntuk, U., Gill, J., MacKay, D., Sattar, N., & Pell, J. (2014). Ethnic-specific obesity cutoffs for diabetes risk: Crosssectional study of 490,288 UK biobank participants. *Diabetes Care, 37*(9), 2500–2507.

Osborn, C. Y., Cavanaugh, K., Wallston, K. A., Kripalani, S., Elasy, T. A., et al. (2011). Health literacy explains racial disparities in diabetes medication adherence. *Journal of Health Communication, 16*, 268–278.

Oza-Frank, R., Ali, M., Vaccarino, V., & Narayan, K. (2009). Asian Americans: Diabetes prevalence across U.S. and World Health Organization weight classifications. *Diabetes Care, 32*(9), 1644–1646.

Oza-Frank, R., Chan, C., Liu, K., Burke, G., & Kanaya, A. (2013). Incidence of type 2 diabetes by place of birth in the multi-ethnic study of atherosclerosis (MESA). *Journal of Immigrant and Minority Health, 15*(5), 918–924.

Palaniappan, L. P., Araneta, M. R., Assimes, T. L., Barrett-Connor, E. L., Carnethon, M. R., Criqui, M. H., et al. Council on Cardiovascular, N. (2010a). Call to action: Cardiovascular disease in Asian Americans: A science advisory from the American Heart Association. *Circulation, 122*(12), 1242–1252. https://doi.org/10.1161/CIR.0b013e3181f22af4.

Palaniappan, L., Mukherjea, A., Holland, A., & Ivey, S. L. (2010b). Leading causes of mortality of Asian Indians in California. *Ethnicity & Disease, 20*(1), 53–57 Retrieved from https://www.ncbi.nlm.nih.gov/pubmed/20178183.

Palaniappan, L., Wang, Y., & Fortmann, S. P. (2004). Coronary heart disease mortality for six ethnic groups in California, 1990–2000. *Annals of Epidemiology, 14*(7), 499–506. https://doi.org/10.1016/j.annepidem.2003.12.001.

Pew Research Center. (2013). *Demographics of Asian Americans, social and demographic trends*. Pew Research Center.

Prasad, D., Kabir, Z., Dash, A., & Das, B. (2011). Abdominal obesity, an independent cardiovascular risk factor in Indian subcontinent: A clinico epidemiological evidence summary. *Journal of Cardiovascular Disease Research, 2*(4), 199–205.

Qureshi, A., Adil, M., Rahim, B., Khan, S., Khan, N., et al. (2014). Paradoxical increase in stroke mortality among Asian Indians in the United States. *Journal of Vascular and Interventional Neurology, 7*(1), 1.

Rajpathak, S., Gupta, L., Waddell, E., Upadhyay, U., Wildman, R., et al. (2010). Elevated risk of type 2 diabetes and metabolic syndrome among Asians and South Asians: Results from the 2004 New York City HANES. *Ethnicity & Disease, 20*(3), 225–230.

Ramachandran, A., Snehalatha, C., Mary, S., Mukesh, B., Bhaskar, A., et al. (2006). The Indian diabetes prevention programme shows that lifestyle modification and metformin prevent type 2 diabetes in asian indian subjects with impaired glucose tolerance (idpp-1). *Diabetologia, 49*(2), 289–297.

Ramachandran, A., & Snehalatha, C. (2010). Rising burden of obesity in Asia. *Journal of Obesity, 2010*, 1–8.

Rao, G., Powell-Wiley, T., Ancheta, I., Hairston, K., Kirley, K., et al. (2015). Identification of obesity and cardiovascular risk in ethnically and racially diverse populations a scientific statement from the American Heart Association. *Circulation, 132*(5), 457–472.

Razak, F., Anand, S., Shannon, H., Vuksan, V., Davis, B., et al. (2007). Defining obesity cut points in a multiethnic population. *Circulation, 115*(16), 2111–2118.

Reaven, G. M., Chen, Y. D., Jeppesen, J., Maheux, P., & Krauss, R. M. (1993). Insulin resistance and hyperinsulinemia in individuals with small, dense low density lipoprotein particles. *The Journal of Clinical Investigation, 92*(1), 141–146. https://doi.org/10.1172/JCI116541.

Rosengren, A., Wallentin, L., Simoons, M., Gitt, A., Behar, S., et al. (2006). Age, clinical presentation, and outcome of acute coronary syndromes in the euroheart acute coronary syndrome survey. *European Heart Journal, 27*(7), 789–795.

SAALT and AAF. (2012). *A demographic snapshot of South Asians in the United States*. South Asian Americans Leading Together (SAALT) and Asian American Federation (AAF).
Sattar, N., & Gill, J. (2014). Type 2 diabetes as a disease of ectopic fat? *BMC Medicine, 12*(1), 123.
Savitz, D. A., Jenevic, T. M., Engel, S. M., Kaufmann, J. S., & Herring, A. H. (2008). Ethnicity and gestational diabetes in New York City, 1995–2003. *BJOG, 115*(8), 969–978.
Saxena, S., Misra, T., Car, J., Netuveli, G., Smith, R., et al. (2007). Systematic review of primary healthcare interventions to improve diabetes outcomes in minority ethnic groups. *Journal of Ambulatory Care Management, 30*, 218–230.
Sellayah, D., Cagampang, F. R., & Cox, R. D. (2014). On the evolutionary origins of obesity: A new hypothesis. *Endocrinology, 155*(5), 1573–1588. https://doi.org/10.1210/en.2013-2103.
Shantsila, E., Shantsila, A., Gill, P. S., & Lip, G. Y. (2016). Premature cardiac aging in South Asian compared to Afro-Caribbean subjects in a community-based screening study. *Journal of the American Heart Association, 5*(11). https://doi.org/10.1161/JAHA.116.004110.
Sheth, T., Nair, C., Nargundkar, M., Anand, S., & Yusuf, S. (1999). Cardiovascular and cancer mortality among Canadians of European, South Asian and Chinese origin from 1979 to 1993: An analysis of 1.2 million deaths. *Canadian Medical Association Journal, 161*(2), 132–138.
Singh, H., Cinnirella, M., & Bradley, C. (2012). Support systems for and barriers to diabetes management in South Asians and whites in the UK: Qualitative study of patients' perspectives. *BMJ Open, 2*(6).
Snehalatha, C., Viswanathan, V., & Ramachandran, A. (2003). Cutoff values for normal anthropometric variables in Asian Indian adults. *Diabetes Care, 26*(5), 1380–1384.
Snowdon, W. (1999). Asian cookery clubs: A community health promotion intervention. *International Journal of Health Promotion and Education, 37*, 135–136.
Sohal, P. (2008). Prevention and management of diabetes in South Asians. *Canadian Journal of Diabetes, 32*(3), 206–210.
Staimez, L., Weber, M., Narayan, K., & Oza-Frank, R. (2013). A systematic review of overweight, obesity, and type 2 diabetes among Asian American subgroups. *Current Diabetes Reviews, 9*(4), 312–331.
Tang, J., Mason, M., Kushner, R., Tirodkar, M., Khurana, N., et al. (2012). South Asian American perspectives on overweight, obesity, and the relationship between weight and health. *Preventing Chronic Disease, 9*, E107–E108.
Thackeray, R., Merrill, R. M., & Neiger, B. L. (2004). Disparities in diabetes management practice between racial and ethnic groups in the United States. *The Diabetes Educator, 30*, 665–675.
Tillin, T., Hughes, A., Mayet, J., Whincup, P., Sattar, N., et al. (2013). The relationship between metabolic risk factors and incident cardiovascular disease in Europeans, South Asians, and African Caribbeans SABRE (Southall and Brent Revisited) - a prospective population-based study. *Journal of the American College of Cardiology, 61*(17), 1777–1786.
Traylor, A. H., Schmittdiel, J. A., Uratsu, C. S., Mangione, C. M., & Subramanian, U. (2010). Adherence to cardiovascular disease medications: Does patientprovider race/ethnicity and language concordance matter? *Journal of General Internal Medicine, 25*, 1172–1177.
Venkataraman, R., Nanda, N., Baweja, G., Parikh, N., & Bhatia, V. (2004). Prevalence of diabetes mellitus and related conditions in Asian Indians living in the United States. *The American Journal of Cardiology, 94*(7), 977–980.
Vlaar, E., Admiraal, W., Busschers, W., Holleman, F., Nierkens, V., et al. (2013). Screening South Asians for type 2 diabestes and prediabetes: (1) comparing oral glucose tolerance and haemoglobing A1c test results and (2) comparing the two sets of metabolic profiles of individuals diagnosed with these two tests. *BMC Endocrinology Disorder, 13*, 8.
Wang, E. T., de Koning, L., & Kanaya, A. M. (2010). Higher protein intake is associated with diabetes risk in South Asian Indians: The metabolic syndrome and atherosclerosis in South Asians living in America (MASALA) study. *Journal of the American College of Nutrition, 29*(2), 130–135.

Wang, E., Wong, E., Dixit, A., Fortmann, S., Linde, R., et al. (2011). Type 2 diabetes: Identifying high risk Asian American subgroups in a clinical population. *Diabetes Research and Clinical Practice, 93*(2), 248–254.

Westphal, S. A. (2008). Obesity, abdominal obesity, and insulin resistance. *Clinical Cornerstone, 9*(1), 23–29 discussion 30–31.

Wilkinson, P., Sayer, J., Laji, K., Grundy, C., Marchant, B., Kopelman, P., & Timmis, A. D. (1996). Comparison of case fatality in South Asian and white patients after acute myocardial infarction: Observational study. *BMJ, 312*(7042), 1330–1333. https://doi.org/10.1136/bmj.312.7042.1330.

Wolstein, J., Babey, S. H., & Diamant, A. L. (2015). *Obesity in California*. UCLA Center for Health Policy Research.

World Bank. (2015). *South Asia* [Online]. Retrieved from http://data.worldbank.org/region/sas.

World Health Organization. (2011). *Use of Glycated Haemoglobin (HbA1c) in the diagnosis of diabetes mellitus screening for type 2 diabetes*. World Health Organization. Retrieved from http://www.who.int/diabetes/publications/report-hba1c_2011.pdf

Xavier, D., Pais, P., Devereaux, P., Xie, C., Prabhakaran, D., et al. (2008). Treatment and outcomes of acute coronary syndromes in India (CREATE): A prospective analysis of registry data. *Lancet, 371*(9622), 1435–1442.

Yang, W., Dall, T. M., Halder, P., Gallo, P., Kowal, S. L., et al. (2013a). Economic costs of diabetes in the US in 2012. *Diabetes Care, 36*, 1–14.

Yang, W., Dall, T. M., Halder, P., Gallo, P., Kowal, S. L., et al. (2013b). Economic costs of diabetes in the US in 2012. Supplemental data. *Diabetes Care, 36*, 1–10.

Ye, J., Rust, G., Baltrus, P., & Daniels, E. (2009). Cardiovascular risk factors among Asian Americans: Results from a National Health Survey. *Annals of Epidemiology, 19*(10), 718–723.

Yuen, L., & Wong, V. W. (2015). Gestational diabetes mellitus: Challenges for different ethnic groups. *World Journal of Diabetes, 6*(8), 1024–1032.

Yusuf, S., Hawken, S., Ounpuu, S., Dans, T., Avezum, A., Lanas, F., et al. (2004). Effect of potentially modifiable risk factors associated with myocardial infarction in 52 countries (the INTERHEART study): Case-control study. *Lancet, 364*(9438), 937–952. https://doi.org/10.1016/S0140-6736(04)17018-9.

Yusuf, S., Hawken, S., Ounpuu, S., Bautista, L., Franzosi, M. G., et al. (2005). Obesity and the risk of myocardial infarction in 27,000 participants from 52 countries: A case-control study. *Lancet, 366*(9497), 1640–1649.

Chapter 8
Cancer Risk, Risk Reduction, and Screening and Treatment Access among U.S. South Asians

Francesca Gany, Anuradha Hashemi, and Jennifer Leng

This chapter explores cancer risk, risk reduction, and screening and treatment access among South Asian Americans and describes several biological and lifestyle factors that affect South Asians' cancer risk. This chapter includes the following sections: 1. Epidemiology of Cancer among South Asians in the United States; 2. Genetic Factors and Risk; 3. Infections and Cancer Risk: Human Papilloma Virus (HPV), Hepatitis B (HBV), and Hepatitis C (HCV); 4. Human Microbiome; 5. Water Supply and Arsenic Poisoning in Bangladesh and West Bengal; 6. Air Pollution and Exposure to Particulate Matter; 7. Health Behaviors: Use of Alternative Tobacco Products (ATPs), Diet, Physical Activity, Sleep and Stress; and Health Care Access and Utilization: Pap Testing, Breast, Colorectal, and Oral Cancer Screening, Use of Complementary Medicine, Palliative Care, and Linguistically Responsive Care.

8.1 Epidemiology of Cancer among South Asians in the U.S

There is a lack of nationally representative and disaggregated data on South Asian populations in the U.S. This limits our understanding of cancer risk in South Asian communities in the U.S. However, some data do exist. Data from the National Cancer Institute's Surveillance, Epidemiology, and End Results (SEER) program and from the Centers for Disease Control and Prevention's National Program for Cancer Registries (NPCR) from 2006 to 2010 reported a lower overall cancer incidence rate of 216.8/100,000 in male (compared to 554.1 in non-Hispanic whites)

F. Gany (✉) · A. Hashemi · J. Leng
Memorial Sloan Kettering Cancer Center, Immigrant Health and Cancer, Disparities Center, New York, USA
e-mail: ganyf@mskcc.org; hashemia@mskcc.org; lengj@mskcc.org

M. J. Perera, E. C. Chang (eds.), *Biopsychosocial Approaches to Understanding Health in South Asian Americans*, Cross-Cultural Research in Health, Illness and Well-Being, https://doi.org/10.1007/978-3-319-91120-5_8

and 212.0/100,000 in female (compared to 444.6 in non-Hispanic whites) Asian Indians/Pakistanis compared to the rate of non-Hispanic Whites (Torre et al. 2016). In South Asian immigrant populations, cancer incidence profiles change post-immigration to more closely reflect incidence rates of the general American population (Hossain et al. 2008). Among Indian and Pakistani immigrants in the U.S., prostate and breast cancers are the most common (Hossain et al. 2008).

Existing data also suggests that, although screening rates for breast cancer vary between studies, South Asian women tend to be diagnosed with late stage breast cancer, which can reduce survival. A 2011 analysis of SEER data found that Asian Indian and Pakistani women were 50% more likely to be diagnosed with Stage IV breast cancer than non-Latino White women (Ooi et al. 2011). Asian Indian/ Pakistani women in the U.S. have also been found to be more likely to be diagnosed with breast cancer before age 40 than non-Hispanic White women (16.2% vs 6.2%) (Kakarala et al. 2010). Taken together, despite lower overall incidence in South Asians in the U.S., these findings suggest higher risk of poor cancer-related outcomes among South Asians in the U.S. and a concomitant need for more rigorous screening in this population.

Oral cancer is a major concern among South Asian populations. This is largely due to the prevalent use of smokeless tobacco products, with additional risk conferred by human papilloma virus (HPV) infection. In India and Pakistan, the most common cancer in men is oral cancer and in women is cervical cancer (Hossain et al. 2008). Oral cancer accounts for over 30% of all cancers in India, and India has the highest incidence of oral cavity and pharynx cancers among women (Coelho 2012). This oral cancer risk migrates with diasporic populations and will be discussed further in the sections on HPV infection and alternative tobacco products.

In addition to oral cancer, rates of colon and lung cancer are increasing in the U.S. (Hossain et al. 2008). Among immigrants, this epidemiologic shift is thought to be due to the adoption of new lifestyle practices that can occur after migration, such as decreased physical activity, decreasing childbirth rates, and dietary changes (Hossain et al. 2008). Other countries with large populations of South Asians, including the United Kingdom, have experienced similar cancer incidence trends. This pattern has been noted for breast cancer incidence, which is the leading cancer of all Indian women outside of India, and has been attributed to increased obesity among Asian Indians in the U.K. (Maringe et al. 2013).

8.2 Genetic Factors and Risk

In 2003, the Indian Genome Variation Database (IGVdb) was the first large-scale comprehensive study that was built to catalog and map genetic variation among Indian subpopulations. Single nucleotide polymorphisms (SNPs) were used to identify combinations of genotypes that are associated with cancer risk (Bag et al. 2012). One 2008 case control study with 375 participants found a much greater risk for head and neck cancers (Odds Ratio [OR]: 4.47; 95% Confidence Interval [CI]:

1.62–12.31) for patients that carried a combination of GSTM1 null, GSTT1 null and GSTP1 variations than those that carried the individual variations (Singh et al. 2008). A 2008 international collaborative study between American and Indian investigators found that three sequence variations on 8q24 independently increased prostate cancer risk among North Indians, with OR values equivalent to 1.60, 1.77, and 1.85 for each respective sequence studied (Tan et al. 2008). A recent study emerging from India was the first to find that a mitochondrial D310 instability in breast cancer patients may be indicative of early progression of breast cancer to metastasis (Alhomidi et al. 2013).

The IGVdb was also used to understand interactions between genes and environments, as it relates to cancer risk. A 2005 study among North Indians observed a significant gene-environment interaction that the GSTP1 gene polymorphism combined with tobacco use tremendously increased risk for bladder cancer (OR: 24.06) (Mittal et al. 2005). Genotype combinations were found to be associated with risk of upper digestive tract cancers in another study that assessed patients with a history of smoking, tobacco chewing, and alcohol abuse (Soya et al. 2007). The gene-environment findings to date indicate that engagement in health behaviors that involve tobacco and alcohol use possibly interacts with certain gene expressions to increase cancer risk among South Asian populations. There is a greater need for research on alcohol-related cancers and their genetic contributions, including head and neck and liver cancers. Many reviewed studies have had small sample sizes, which may have generated false-positive associations, and more research is needed in several areas of cancer genetics in South Asian populations.

8.3 Infections and Cancer Risk

In addition to genetic factors, infection and chronic inflammation can increase cancer risk. This section discusses the prevalence of Human Papilloma Virus, Hepatitis B Virus and Hepatitis C Virus among South Asians, and the associated cancer vulnerability. More research is needed to better understand the epidemiology of HPV, Hepatitis B, and Hepatitis C in South Asians in the U.S., and to implement surveillance, outreach, screening, and treatment interventions accordingly. Treatment outcomes among South Asian Americans also need to be further studied.

8.3.1 Human Papilloma Virus (HPV)

The precise epidemiology of HPV-related infections and cancers, including cancer of the cervix and of the head and neck, among South Asian men and women in the U.S. is unknown. HPV, the major cause of cervical cancer, is a significant health concern in South Asia itself, and therefore among South Asian immigrant communities. South Asian countries have a high proportion (26%) of HPV type 18, one of the strains that is most closely associated with cervical cancer (Munoz et al. 2004). In 2012, an estimated 122,844 new cervical cancer cases were diagnosed in India and there were 67,477 cervical cancer deaths, constituting one fourth of the global burden of cervical cancer (Arbyn et al. 2011). Bangladesh, Nepal, and India rank among the countries with the highest cervical cancer mortality rates and incidence rates in Asia (Arbyn et al. 2011). The 9 HPV types implicated in invasive cervical cancer comprise 92.2% (CI: 87.9–95.3) of the HPV infections in India (Arbyn et al. 2011; Kumar et al. 2015). In 2014, a nonavalent HPV vaccine was approved for use in the U.S. that covers HPV types 6, 11, 16, 18, 31, 33, 45, 52, and 58 (Kumar et al. 2015). Widespread vaccine uptake could significantly impact cervical cancer prevention and should be a focus of public health and primary care activities in South Asian immigrant communities. HPV has also been connected to 19 out of 50 cancers of the oropharyngeal tract, including cancers of the tonsil and pharynx and penile and anal cancers (Kumar et al. 2015). The potential link between HPV and such cancers should be further elucidated, particularly the link between oropharyngeal cancers among South Asians in the U.S. in the context of tobacco use.

Although understudied in the U.S., studies from other South Asian diasporic countries, such as the U.K., reveal cultural barriers to HPV infection prevention that may also be relevant among South Asians in the U.S. One major barrier is the link of HPV infection with sexual activity, and the cultural norms against acknowledging such a link. A study of White British, Pakistani, African Caribbean, and Indian women in the U.K. found an overall lack of education around HPV transmission and testing (McCaffery et al. 2003), emphasizing the role of education as a major barrier to prevention. Another study of London-based Muslim women's attitudes towards self-sampling for HPV in the context of cervical cancer screening found that participants were generally positive about cervical cancer screening but acknowledged that some women in their community were reluctant to be screened because of embarrassment, language difficulties, fear, or because they were unmarried and did not want to communicate implicit messages about being sexually active (Szarewski et al. 2009). Women were also concerned about not doing the test correctly, but thought that self-testing might overcome barriers to screening for some women. HPV testing itself and the possibility of testing positive for HPV were also thought to raise potentially difficult issues relating to trust, blame, and fidelity within marriages (Szarewski et al. 2009). The effectiveness of existing HPV vaccination programs for South Asians should be evaluated. Educational outreach specifically to girls and women, in addition to boys and men, about HPV transmission and cervical cancer testing should be considered as an intervention to increase HPV vaccination and HPV-related cancer screening. This topic is described in more detail in the section below on Healthcare Access.

8.3.2 *Hepatitis B Virus (HBV)*

HBV is endemic in South Asian countries, with high rates of current or past infection. A retrospective study in England reported that HBV infection prevalence was 3.1 times higher among South Asians than among non-South Asians (Hahne et al. 2003). The estimated lifetime risk of infection was 1.4% in South Asians and 0.4% in non-South Asians, and the estimated risk of chronic infection was 0.8% in South Asians and 0.02% in non-South Asians (Hahne et al. 2003). South Asian blood donors have been found to have a high frequency of new HBV infections, at a rate 4.3 times higher than that among non-South Asians (Hahne et al. 2003). Further, the incidence of acute HBV infection can be up to 10 times higher in South Asian children than in non-South Asian children (Hahne et al. 2003). Hepatitis B virus (HBV) infection can lead to serious liver damage. Without treatment, about 15–25% of people with HBV die prematurely from cirrhosis, liver failure, or liver cancer (Cohen et al. 2013), indicating a need for awareness of HBV in this group.

In the U.S., it is likely that Hepatitis B infection remains a significant health concern for South Asians, especially for those who have recently emigrated from their countries of origin. Among those of Indian descent, rates have been found to be 1.4–3% in India and 1–6% in the U.S. (Tong et al. 2011), indicating a need to understand changes that occur upon migration to the U.S. that may increase risk. U.S. providers need to be aware of the risk of Hepatitis B infection, and to incorporate screening, and treatment if indicated, into the care of their South Asian patients.

8.3.3 *Hepatitis C Virus (HCV)*

Similar to Hepatitis B, Hepatitis C may increase risk of liver failure, cirrhosis, and cancer. Studies have shown a rate of infection in South Asia of <2% in India and 5% in Pakistan, compared with 1.3% among the overall U.S. population (Nguyen and Nguyen 2013). In a community-based testing program at five sites in England, the overall prevalence of anti-hepatitis C virus (HCV) in people of South Asian origin was 1.6% but varied by country of birth and recent immigrants were at an increased risk of infection (Uddin et al. 2010).

8.4 Human Microbiome

Babies are born with a sterile gastrointestinal (GI) tract but bacteria begin to colonize immediately after birth. The human microbiota consists of more than 10,000 bacterial species that aid humans in normal physiological activities. The microbiota help to create an optimal internal environment via processes including the extraction of energy from food, the release of accessory growth factors, and the stimulation of both innate and adaptive immune systems. Each individual houses a specific set of microorganisms in the gut. Throughout life, bacterial populations can change due to external factors such as geography, socioeconomic status, lifestyle, diet, hygiene, and the use of antibiotics (Sommer and Backhed 2013).

The microbiota has been implicated in both cancer development and cancer prevention (Graham et al. 2009; Zhu et al. 2013). The potential role of microbiota in cancer, whether protective or adverse, is of growing interest and warrants further investigation among South Asians in the U.S., especially considering the change that the microbiota undergo upon migration, with changes in diet and in other environmental factors.

8.5 Water Supply and Arsenic Poisoning in Bangladesh & West Bengal

Arsenic-contaminated water first started appearing in Bangladesh in the 1940s as a result of a global initiative to provide clean water to the country's rural communities by installing tube-wells. These wells were usually placed at a depth of 200 meters to eliminate contamination with illness-causing microorganisms. Evidence of arsenic contamination began surfacing in the early 1990s. Arsenic concentration in tube-well drinking water was >50 ug/L in many regions of Bangladesh (safe arsenic concentration is <10 ug/L, per World Health Organization [WHO] guidelines) (Smith et al. 2000). It has since been estimated that arsenic contamination affects as many as 77 million people in South Asia.

Although contaminated drinking water is the most common cause of arsenic exposure, eating crops irrigated with contaminated groundwater also produces arsenic exposure. Rice cultivated in South Asia, particularly in the West Bengal area, has high levels of arsenic contamination (Halder et al. 2012). Given that rice is a staple of many South Asian diets, South Asians in the U.S. may face an increased risk of arsenic ingestion through consumption of rice and rice products both grown in the U.S. and imported from South Asia.

Chronic arsenic exposure is associated with higher rates of skin, bladder and lung cancer (Ruiz de Luzuriaga et al. 2011). Studies in Bangladesh and West Bengal have investigated arsenic-associated skin cancer, which is common and can be detected early from the distinctive skin lesions. There is a greater risk of arsenic-associated skin cancer for those who smoke, lack proper nutrition, and have greater exposure to sunlight (Ruiz de Luzuriaga et al. 2011). The combined lung, liver and bladder cancer mortality rates of Bangladeshis chronically exposed to arsenic is over two times greater (229.6 per 100,000) than those for the overall Bangladeshi population (103.5 per 100,000) (Ooi et al. 2011). There are not yet data on Bangladeshis living in the U.S. There is a need to study the long-term health effects of prior low to moderate levels of arsenic exposure among Bangladeshi immigrants, who hail from one of the most arsenic-contaminated regions in the world. The detrimental effects of arsenic exposure in their homeland may carry over to Bangladeshi and other South Asian communities in the U.S.

8.6 Air Pollution and Exposure to Particulate Matter

Particulate matter (PM), one of the six most common air pollutants, is a widespread threat to health. PM includes coarse particles, such as sand and large dust particles (referred to as PM10), and fine particles that stem from gases emitted from power plants, industries, and automobiles found in smoke and haze (referred to as PM2.5). These particles can pass through the throat and nose and enter the lungs and can cause serious health effects, including cancer. The association between all-cause, cardiopulmonary, and lung cancer mortality with PM2.5, sulfate particles, and sulfur dioxide has been illustrated (Pope 3rd et al. 2002; Pope et al. 1995).

Air pollution has become a major concern in India in recent years, with majority of the Indian urban population exposed to some of the highest pollutant levels in the world. This is exacerbated by the use of open biomass stoves, which can generate large amounts of PM and of carbon monoxide, hydrocarbons, oxygenated organics, free radicals and chlorinated organics, which have been linked to a host of health problems including lung cancer (Brown et al. 2000; Owens and Randhawa 2004). Air pollution is also a concern for certain South Asians in the U.S. as there is elevated PM exposure among occupations with disproportionate South Asian representation, such as taxi drivers. Professional taxicab driving is a common occupation among South Asians, with over 40% of drivers in New York City, and approximately 20% in Chicago, San Francisco, and Washington DC, originating from South Asia (India, Pakistan, Bangladesh, and Nepal) (Tan et al. 2008). Taxi drivers work long hours (Schaller Consulting 2004) (10–12 hours/day shifts ~6 days/week), most often in heavy traffic. Thus, a large part of their day is spent inside a vehicle cabin where they are potentially exposed to high levels of traffic-related PM. Taxi drivers are already at increased risk for cancer due to a number of other factors, including poor diet and a sedentary lifestyle; exposure to PM exacerbates that risk. Many studies (although none conducted specifically among South Asians in the U.S.) have demonstrated a high prevalence of lung cancer among taxi drivers (Chen et al. 2015).

More research is needed on the health effects of air pollution, specifically PM exposure, among at-risk South Asian occupational groups, including taxi drivers, gas station attendants, and restaurant workers in the U.S. More research is also needed on those exposed to PM though cooking stoves and their occupations in their countries of origin, to determine effective ways to mitigate the impact of the exposure.

8.7 Health Behaviors

8.7.1 Use of Alternative Tobacco Products (ATPs)

The use of alternative tobacco products (ATPs) is prevalent among South Asians. These varied products have names, ingredients, and utilization patterns that differ by South Asian region. Among the most commonly used smokeless South Asian ATPs are paan, gutka, supari, mainpuri, mawa, zarda, khaini, mishri, and gul. Many of these are areca nut-based, contain ground/powdered tobacco and a variety of flavorings, and are consumed orally. Paan, or betel quid, generally refers to areca nut wrapped in a betel leaf, and includes slaked lime, spices, and sometimes tobacco. Gutka, a packaged product, contains powdered/granulated tobacco, areca nut, slaked lime, catechu, and spices, packed in tins or sachets. Dozens of carcinogens are found in smokeless ATPs, including nitrosamines, nitrosamino acids, polycyclic aromatic hydrocarbons, aldehydes, and metals (World Health Organization International Agency for Research on Cancer 2004). Nicotine is the principal addictive agent, and nicotine absorption is linked to an increased risk of oral soft tissue lesions, oral cancer, esophageal cancer, and pancreatic cancer. In 2004, the International Agency for Research on Cancer reported that betel-quid and areca nut are also carcinogens, independent of tobacco, and can cause oral cancer, cancer of the pharynx, and cancer of the esophagus (World Health Organization International Agency for Research on Cancer 2004). In addition to associations with oral, pancreatic, and liver cancers, the use of ATPs imparts increased risk of premature death (Willis et al. 2012).

The high rates of smokeless ATP use in South Asia have been well-documented, and there is strong evidence that ATP use and documented rates of oral cancers is high among diasporic South Asian communities in the U.K., Canada, Malaysia, and South Africa that are outside of South Asia (Auluck et al. 2009; Ramanathan 1979; van Wyk et al. 1993). Yet, there are limited data in the U.S. on this topic, although existing studies suggest that rates of use among South Asians in the U.S. may be similar to rates in South Asia. The 2004 California Asian Indian Tobacco Survey is the only published population-based survey on prevalence of South Asian ATP use, and reported that oral mucosal lesions are present in approximately 60% of current ATP users in the U.S. and that ATP use is the strongest risk factor for the development of oral lesions and leukoplakia (Shulman et al. 1939).

Knowledge and personal views of ATPs among South Asians vary. Use of ATPs is highly culturally and socially linked. ATP use is a popular component of cultural and religious holidays for Hindu and Muslim Asian Indian communities. Studies examining traditional practices and acculturation of South Asians in different communities across California and Chicago have found that ATP use continued to play a traditional role in families' customs and traditions well after migration to the U.S. (Mukherjea et al. 2012). Reasons cited for ATP use among South Asian men and women include social acceptability of ATP use in Pakistani and Bangladeshi communities, a possible low level of awareness of health risks associated with use of

ATPs, and insufficient professional advice and cessation aids (White et al. 2006). Mukherjea et al. (2012) found that use of culturally-linked alternative tobacco products was a symbolic behavior to maintain culture and was an expression of South Asian ethnic identity in a new dominant culture, such as the U.S. (Mukherjea et al. 2012).

Studies on South Asian ATP availability in Western countries found that ATP products were often readily available and loosely regulated, rarely containing warning labels (Longman et al. 2010). Other Western countries with large South Asian immigrant populations have increased surveillance of the popular use of culturally specific tobacco products; however, this has not historically been the case in the U.S. although regulation of ATPs has emerged at state and city levels in recent years. In 2003, New York banned the sale of gutka to minors and legislation on bidis exists in several cities, including New York, Fremont, and Chicago. New York and Fremont ban the sale of bidis to all individuals under the age of 18, while Chicago has totally banned their sale. In addition, lack of merchant awareness of federal and local tobacco regulations can have significant implications for the sale and availability of alternative tobacco products (ATPs). While it is known that the application of warning labels on conventional tobacco packaging and signs in merchant shops increases consumers' awareness of the health risks associated with cigarette use, there is limited comparable literature on merchants' awareness of ATP regulations or the effect of these regulations on consumer's knowledge of health risks.

In the U.S., cessation programs targeting ATP use among South Asians are very limited. Tobacco quit lines, a conventional tobacco product cessation model popular in the U.S., have limited culturally responsive intervention strategies for South Asians because they offer services for conventional smokeless tobacco users (Mukherjea and Modayil 2013). Language and cultural barriers may also prevent South Asians from using these services, and it is unknown if these services would have a similar impact on South Asian populations, even if linguistically and culturally responsive. In a literature review of effective intervention strategies, Mukherjea et al. (2013) suggest that ATP use cessation interventions that are inclusive of cultural and religious leaders are more likely to be effective (Mukherjea and Modayil 2013). Direct messages from community and religious leaders along with educational materials are potentially effective intervention techniques due to the importance and influence of these roles in the community. Mass media campaigns and workplace interventions are strategies that have been used in the U.K. and in India, indicating potential for successful implementation in the U.S. (Mishra et al. 2009; Murukutla et al. 2012). Another U.K.-based program using a community health worker model in ATP cessation programs for South Asians is also a promising intervention method for South Asians in the U.S. (Croucher et al. 2003).

8.7.2 Diet

The relationship between diet and cancer risk is complicated and findings on the association between diet and different types of cancers have not always been consistent. However, it is thought that obesity, concentrated sugars and refined flour products, low fiber intake, consumption of red meat, and imbalance of omega-3 and omega-6 fats may contribute to excess cancer risk, with more compelling evidence for some foods than for others. Changes in dietary patterns have been thought to play a major role in the growing incidence of colon, prostate, and breast cancers among South Asians in the U.S., as well as in the U.K. Researchers in both countries have emphasized that a dietary intake higher in fat, alcohol, and meat than is typical of South Asian diets has been associated with increased cancer risk (Hossain et al. 2008; Maringe et al. 2013).

Vegetarianism is common in South Asia; however, it is unclear if the South Asian vegetarian diet, which varies in components depending on South Asian region, leads to better cardiometabolic health. In some studies, vegetarianism has been linked to reduced risk of breast cancer among South Asians (Dos santos silva et al. 2002; Gathani et al. 2017). However, other studies have found other diet-related variables to be better predictors of breast cancer risk, including macronutrient intake and fruit, vegetable, and legume consumption (Borugian et al. 2004; Farvid et al. 2016). Nutrient consumption and diet can vary by South Asian country and area of the country, indicating a need to disaggregate associations with cancer by South Asian background group.

Dietary interventions must consider the cultural value of food to be effective. In a study of Asian Indians in California, researchers found that Asian Indian patients perceived their doctor's dietary advice as "irrelevant" or "missing the mark" because the advice did not take into account the social and cultural relevance of food (Koenig et al. 2012). Diet was not viewed simply as a behavior, but rather, food was seen as an important means through which Indians maintained a sense of continuity of their cultural identity (National Cancer Institute 2009). In addition, identifying potential dietary risk factors among U.S. South Asians will require a more thorough understanding of diets across the diaspora and immigrant generations.

Developing healthful, culturally tailored dietary guides for the multiplicity of South Asian subpopulations would be salutary if the recommendations were acceptable and implemented. Encouraging substitution of common South Asian diet staples (white rice and white flour) with healthier and relatively culturally acceptable items (barley, brown rice, millet, and couscous) is a potentially significant intervention strategy. Partnering with South Asian restaurants to modify menus to include more nutritious foods would potentially be impactful for South Asian Americans.

8.7.3 Physical Activity

Physical activity may reduce the risk for several types of cancer, including endometrial, breast, and colon cancer. More than 50 studies have found that adults who increase the frequency, duration, or intensity of physical activity can reduce their risk of developing colon cancer by 30 to 40 percent relative to those who are sedentary (Kandula and Lauderdale 2005).

Kandula and Lauderdale analyzed data from the 2001 California Health Interview Survey and found that foreign-born Asians were least likely to participate in leisure-time physical activity and have high levels of physical inactivity compared to US-born individuals (Dave et al. 2015). In South Asian communities, cultural beliefs and practices can discourage physical activity. Physical activity levels are lower among women, older people and people of lower socioeconomic status. Individual participation in regular physical activity can be seen as a violation of the South Asian cultural norm of putting family before self. Pressure on South Asian adults to fulfill social and financial obligations to kin (e.g. long work hours) may place particular demands and constraints on time, leading to a lack of opportunity to participate in physical activity. Limited time and resources can be particularly challenging for lower socioeconomic groups. For young people, lack of encouragement, support from family members, and a cultural emphasis on school and working over exercise, are barriers to participation in recreational sports and physical activity. Traditional gender roles in South Asian communities can also influence physical activity. Religious norms around modesty, avoidance of mixed-sex activity, and fear of going out alone could limit South Asian women's participation in recreational physical activity. Family and community expectations of women to fulfill domestic responsibilities and disapproval of women's activity outside their homes can also be discouraging. In a study in Chicago, physical activity decreased after marriage and having children, and chronic diseases constrained older women from more vigorous activity (Chida et al. 2008).

Among South Asian immigrants, as cancer profiles change to more closely reflect those of their adopted countries, further research is needed on the evolution of health behaviors post immigration and their impact on cancer risk (Hossain et al. 2008). Future interventional research should focus on increasing physical activity levels, including exercise interventions that respond to cultural norms.

8.7.4 Sleep

Sleep deprivation contributes to repeated circadian disruption, and impairment of the immune system, and is potentially linked to cancer-promoting biological mechanisms. The effect of sleep deprivation on cancer risk is especially relevant among night shift workers. The relationship of sleep as it relates to cancer risk in South

Asians in the U.S. has not been specifically studied. Sleep hygiene should be discussed with all patients and community members with impaired sleep behaviors.

8.7.5 Stress

Psychosocial stressors have been linked to an increase in cancer risk. A review in 2008 found 165 studies that found an association between stress and higher cancer incidence, 330 studies found poorer survival in patients with diagnosed cancer, and 53 found higher cancer mortality among those with high stress levels compared to those with lower stress levels (Bhattacharya and Schoppelrey 2004).

Like many immigrant groups, South Asians are susceptible to psychological distress due to migration, subsequent pressures to acculturate, and other social determinants that have a significant impact on functioning and quality of life. Acculturative stress is one such source of psychological distress that can include intergenerational conflict, discrimination, and depression. Qualitative interviews with recent South Asian migrant families in New York City revealed that acculturative stress can impact multiple generational groups, including foreign-born parents and their children (Kaduvettoor-Davidson and Inman 2013). Among South Asian youth in the U.K. and U.S., lower levels of acculturation and discrimination, coupled with high parental expectations and pressure, can lead to increased stress. Kaduvettoor-Davidson and Inman found that, among national samples of first and second generation South Asians in the U.S. ranging from 18 to 83 years old, perceived discrimination was positively and significantly associated with perceived stress (Inman et al. 1999). With respect to gender, culture conflict has been identified as a major source of stress for South Asian women (Brown et al. 2000). Already existing stress can be further exacerbated by a cancer diagnosis.

8.7.6 Health Care Access and Utilization

Many South Asians have poor access to, and utilization of, crucial allopathic healthcare. Lack of insurance coverage, language barriers, perceived discrimination, and cultural and religious/spiritual determinants of healthcare utilization all contribute to this lack of uptake. A higher proportion of South Asians lack health insurance compared with non-Latino Whites, (21% of South Asians v. 14% of non-Latino Whites), a primary determinant of access to healthcare (Owens and Randhawa 2004). Poor utilization of healthcare services by South Asians also reflects linguistic barriers, including limited English proficiency, and lack of adequate interpreter services; cultural discordance with the healthcare system, including religious beliefs and preferences for homeopathy or reliance on home remedies; transportation; prioritization of time and resources to provide for family needs over individual health needs (e.g. by working long hours or supporting/taking care of other family members); and/or reluctance to approach health facilities because of a perception that health services are inappropriate or unsupportive towards immigrants' health concerns.

Cultural and religious values and beliefs can have a significant impact on an individual's decision to seek out healthcare, especially for sensitive or complex issues, including certain types of cancer screening. Among patients who do access healthcare services, unaddressed language and cultural differences may create barriers to regular and periodic utilization of healthcare services, as well as potentially complicate the effective delivery of health promotion and other health messages.

In situations where providers have an inadequate understanding of South Asian patients' needs, an environment of mistrust and lack of respect may be created, which can further hinder the relationship between the patient and provider. Mistrust is often linked to providers' lack of knowledge of South Asian culturally-linked health beliefs. For example, certain South Asians may withhold intimate problems from medical professionals to protect family "izzat," or honor. Cultural responsiveness education of healthcare providers has the potential to address these types of issues and improve the quality of patient-provider interactions (Gomez et al. 2007).

8.7.7 *Pap Testing, Breast, Colorectal, and Oral Cancer Screening*

Cervical cancer screening rates among South Asian women in the U.S. have been found to be significantly lower than among the general U.S. population. 55–65% of South Asians report timely receipt of mammography (i.e. within the past two years) (Islam et al. 2006; Promotion, n.d.), which is significantly below the Healthy People 2020 objectives of 81.1% (Gupta et al. 2002a). In a community sample of South Asian women in Canada, results showed low rates and knowledge of pap smears, which were significantly associated with low levels of formal education and with low acculturation (Boxwala et al. 2010). South Asian women have been found to be more likely to receive mammograms if they perceived breast cancer screening to be useful, and if it was recommended by a primary care provider, indicating the importance of regular access to primary care (Qiu and Ni 2003). For South Asian women who do not adhere to breast and cervical cancer screening guidelines, reasons generally include lack of knowledge of the purpose of screenings, financial and language barriers, and cultural modesty. Culturally appropriate breast cancer education has been shown to improve mammogram rates.

Despite the increased risk of oral cancer faced by South Asians, accessing oral health services remains a low priority in the community. An analysis of the National Health Interview Survey (NHIS) showed that Asian Indians are less likely than other Asians and non-Hispanic whites to have seen a dentist in the prior year (55.6%) (Menon et al. n.d.). The study also found that approximately 60% were unaware of the increased oral cancer risk among South Asians. This limited utilization of oral health services not only impacts the early detection of oral cancer but also the maintenance of oral health.

In a subsample aged 50 years or older from the South Asian Health Descriptor Study in Chicago, 2.2% of participants believed that they were at risk for colorectal cancer; 8% reported a past stool blood test (SBT); and 13.6% had had a sigmoidoscopy or colonoscopy (Gupta et al. 2002b). Language acculturation and medical mistrust were significantly related to SBT completion. Language acculturation, income, living in the United States for more than 5 years, perception of colorectal cancer risk, and past SBT were significantly related to endoscopic cancer screening (Gupta et al. 2002b).

8.7.8 *Use of Complementary Medicine*

According to the WHO, traditional medicine, a term often used interchangeably with complementary and alternative medicine (CAM), is a set of knowledge and practices that are based on beliefs and experience and used to prevent, diagnose, and treat both physiological and psychological illnesses. Immigrants often continue to follow traditional healing practices after migration; their health seeking behavior therefore frequently combines alternative treatment methods with Western medicine. Use of CAM is widespread among South Asians, and encompasses several modalities, including Ayurveda and herbal remedies.

In a study of patterns and perceptions of CAM use among leukemia patients visiting a hematology clinic in north India, 56% of the participants mentioned alternative methods for diagnosis and treatment and only about 4% of the patients informed their medical doctors about this practice (Worth et al. 2009). Potential complications of adverse reactions to CAM and Ayurvedic medicine were not tracked in these studies and the topic has been largely unstudied.

Some South Asian immigrants use imported herbal medicines that are known to be contaminated with harmful substances, including arsenic, which has been linked to several forms of cancer. The New York City Department of Health and Mental Hygiene surveys imported herbal remedies and maintains a comprehensive list of contaminated products that providers may be aware of when working with this population.

8.7.9 *Palliative Care*

The provision of palliative care requires particular sensitivity to language and to patient and family values and caregiving patterns. There is need for palliative care services in South Asian languages, and in a manner which accounts for South Asian cultural values and sense of family duty. A study by Worth et al. (Worth et al. 2009) examined palliative care services through the lenses of both the patient and the health provider (Worth et al. 2009). The study found that services were often inflexible and unable to respond effectively when faced with needs such as culturally appropriate food or gender-specific staff to provide personal care (Worth et al. 2009). The study also revealed that while professionals had the motivation and desire to provide appropriate care, their understanding was often lacking or culturally insufficient (Worth et al. 2009). Yet, the study was not conducted in the U.S., indicating a need for this research.

8.7.10 Linguistically Responsive Care

Several federal and state policies aimed at addressing linguistic and cultural barriers to patient care in recent decades may benefit South Asians. Title VI of the Civil Rights Act of 1964 prohibited discrimination on the basis of national origin, which can extend to language preference, and required healthcare providers and benefit agencies to take "reasonable steps" to ensure that patients have "meaningful access" to their healthcare. An executive order mandated by President Clinton in 2000 specified the legal requirement for service agencies that receive federal funding, including those related to healthcare, to develop a system for persons with limited English proficiency (LEP) to access their services. Although adherence to these policies and the quality of language services varies widely across the U.S., the laws in New York State offer more detailed provisions for ensuring that limited English proficient patients can access interpretation services. The New York State Patients' Bill of Rights requires interpreters and translations of important forms or instructions to be made regularly available for language groups that comprise more than one percent of a hospital's service area population, as determined by the U.S. Census. Lack of adequate medical interpretation services for South Asian communities remains a major barrier to healthcare access and utilization. Miscommunication due to linguistic differences and subsequent perceived ineffectiveness of medical consultations, frequently due to inappropriate use of family members as interpreters, creates barriers to accurate understanding of medical instructions and health messages. Education on the rights of patients to access care in their preferred language, and on how to work effectively with qualified medical interpreters, is needed for medical providers, the broader healthcare community, and for community members themselves. Furthermore, providers should work to build trust with South Asian patients by providing patient-centered care that enables patients to feel culturally and personally respected.

Unfortunately, given the wide diversity of languages spoken across South Asian subgroups, and the variable adherence to these policy protections, much vigilance will be needed to assure adequate language access services.

8.8 Conclusion

There is a tremendous need to disaggregate health care access and health outcomes data by characteristics such as South Asian country of origin, length of stay in the U.S., language proficiency, SES status, and occupational risk among others. Each of the lifestyle behaviors explored in this chapter require further integrated research that affect policy and community alike. Community-engaged research methods, which bring together researchers, stakeholders, patients, and community members, can be used to develop and then test intervention models aimed at initiating and maintaining healthful behaviors among South Asian populations. Potential agents include coaches, community health workers, peers, and families; potential settings include religious centers, health care systems, community-based organizations, restaurants, and workplaces; and potential audiences could vary across genders, generations, languages, faiths, and socio-economic status. Once successful interventions are identified, South Asian community leaders and institutions should use their position as culturally and linguistically competent influencers to implement them. South Asian community members should be educated about health insurance access, primary care, and medical homes. Primary care providers need to be trained in patient centered care, eliciting a patient's Health Belief Model to elicit beliefs about health that may impact cancer risk and outcomes, and how to work with interpreters in the presence of language discordance. Health services research needs to be conducted to examine health systems barriers to and facilitators of care, and to ensure that protections already in place for linguistic minorities are enforced, especially in light of the tremendous linguistic diversity of the South Asian community.

References

Alhomidi, M. A., Vedicherla, B., Movva, S., Rao, P. K., Ahuja, Y. R., & Hasan, Q. (2013). Mitochondrial D310 instability in Asian Indian breast cancer patients. *Tumour Biology, 34*(4), 2427–2432.

Arbyn, M., Castellsague, X., de Sanjose, S., Bruni, L., Saraiya, M., Bray, F., Ferlay, J. (2011). Worldwide burden of cervical cancer in 2008. *Annals of oncology : official journal of the European Society for Medical Oncology*, *22*(12), 2675–2686. Epub 2011/04/08. doi: https://doi.org/10.1093/annonc/mdr015. PubMed PMID: 21471563.

Auluck, A., Hislop, G., Poh, C., Zhang, L., Rosin, M. P. (2009). Areca nut and betel quid chewing among south Asian immigrants to western countries and its implications for oral cancer screening. *Rural and Remote Health,9*(2), 1118. Epub 2009/05/19. PubMed PMID: 19445556; PubMed Central PMCID: PMCPmc2726113.

Bag, A., Jyala, N. S., Bag, N. (2012). Indian studies on genetic polymorphisms and cancer risk. *Indian Journal of Cancer*, *49*(1), 144–162. Epub 2012/07/31. doi: https://doi.org/10.4103/0019-509x.98941. PubMed PMID: 22842182.

Bhattacharya, G., Schoppelrey, S. L. (2004). Preimmigration beliefs of life success, postimmigration experiences, and acculturative stress: South Asian immigrants in the United States. *Journal of Immigrant Health*, *6*(2), 83–92. Epub 2004/03/12. doi: https://doi.org/10.1023/b:joih.0000019168.75062.36. PubMed PMID: 15014225.

Borugian, M. J., Sheps, S. B., Kim-sing, C., et al. (2004). Insulin, macronutrient intake, and physical activity: Are potential indicators of insulin resistance associated with mortality from breast cancer? *Cancer Epidemiol Biomarkers Prevention, 13*(7), 1163–1172.

Boxwala, F. I., Bridgemohan, A., Griffith, D. M., Soliman, A. S. (2010). Factors associated with breast cancer screening in Asian Indian women in metro-Detroit. *Journal of immigrant and minority health, 12*(4), 534–543. Epub 2009/07/25. doi: https://doi.org/10.1007/s10903-009-9277-0. PubMed PMID: 19629691; PubMed Central PMCID: PMCPmc4276127.

Brown, E. R., Ojeda, V. D., Wyn, R., & Levan, R. (2000). Racial and ethnic disparities in access to health insurance and health care. *UCLA Center for Health Policy Research.*

Chen, G., Wan, X., Yang, G., & Zou, X. (2015). Traffic-related air pollution and lung cancer: A meta-analysis. *Thorac Cancer, 6*(3), 307–318.

Chida, Y., Hamer, M., Wardle, J., Steptoe, A. (2008). Do stress-related psychosocial factors contribute to cancer incidence and survival? *Nature clinical practice Oncology, 5*(8), 466–475. Epub 2008/05/22. doi: https://doi.org/10.1038/ncponc1134. PubMed PMID: 18493231.

Coelho, K. R. (2012). Challenges of the oral cancer burden in India. *Journal of cancer epidemiology, 2012*, 701932. Epub 2012/10/25. doi: https://doi.org/10.1155/2012/701932. PubMed PMID: 23093961; PubMed Central PMCID: PMCPmc3471448.

Cohen, C., Caballero, J., Martin, M., Weerasinghe, I., Ninde, M., Block, J.. (2013).Eradication of hepatitis B: A nationwide community coalition approach to improving vaccination, screening, and linkage to care. *Journal of community health, 38*(5),799–804. Epub 2013/05/30. doi: https://doi.org/10.1007/s10900-013-9699-4. PubMed PMID: 23715963.

Croucher, R., Islam, S., Jarvis, M. J., Garrett, M., Rahman, R., Shajahan, S., Howells, G. (2003). Oral tobacco cessation with UK resident Bangladeshi women: A community pilot investigation. *Health Education Research, 18*(2),216–223. Epub 2003/05/06. PubMed PMID: 12729180.

Dave, S. S., Craft, L. L., Mehta, P., Naval, S., Kumar, S., Kandula, N. R. (2015). Life stage influences on U.S. south Asian women's physical activity. *American journal of health promotion : AJHP, 29*(3),e100–e108. Epub 2014/04/11. doi: https://doi.org/10.4278/ajhp.130415-QUAL-175. PubMed PMID: 24717067.

Dos santos silva, I., Mangtani, P., Mccormack, V., Bhakta, D., Sevak, L., & Mcmichael, A. J. (2002). Lifelong vegetarianism and risk of breast cancer: A population-based case-control study among south Asian migrant women living in England. *International Journal of Cancer., 99*(2), 238–244.

Farvid, M. S., Chen, W. Y., Michels, K. B., Cho, E., Willett, W. C., & Eliassen, A. H. (2016). Fruit and vegetable consumption in adolescence and early adulthood and risk of breast cancer: Population based cohort study. *BMJ, 353*(i2343).

Gathani, T., Barnes, I., Ali, R., et al. (2017). Lifelong vegetarianism and breast cancer risk: A large multicentre case control study in India. *BMC Women's Health, 17*(1), 6.

Gomez, S. L., Tan, S., Keegan, T. H., Clarke, C. A. (2007). Disparities in mammographic screening for Asian women in California: A cross-sectional analysis to identify meaningful groups for targeted intervention. *BMC Cancer, 7*(201). Epub 2007/10/27. doi: https://doi.org/10.1186/1471-2407-7-201. PubMed PMID: 17961259; PubMed Central PMCID: PMCPmc2198916.

Graham, D. Y., Lu, H., Yamaoka, Y. (2009). African, Asian or Indian enigma, the east Asian helicobacter pylori: Facts or medical myths. *Journal of digestive diseases, 10*(2), 77–84. Epub 2009/05/12. doi: https://doi.org/10.1111/j.1751-2980.2009.00368.x. PubMed PMID: 19426388; PubMed Central PMCID: PMCPmc2846403.

Gupta, A., Kumar, A., Stewart, D. E. (2002a). Cervical cancer screening among south Asian women in Canada: The role of education and acculturation. *Health Care for Women International, 23*(2), 123–134. Epub 2002/03/01. doi: https://doi.org/10.1080/073993302753429004. PubMed PMID: 11868960.

Gupta, M., Shafiq, N., Kumari, S., Pandhi, P. (2002b). Patterns and perceptions of complementary and alternative medicine (CAM) among leukaemia patients visiting haematology clinic of a north Indian tertiary care hospital. *Pharmacoepidemiology and drug safety, 11*(8), 671–676. Epub 2003/01/07. doi: https://doi.org/10.1002/pds.782. PubMed PMID: 12512243.

Hahne, S., Ramsay, M., Soldan, K., Balogun, K., Mortimer, P. (2003). Hepatitis B incidence among south Asian children in England and Wales: Implications for immunisation policy. *Archives of disease in childhood, 88*(12), 1082–1083. Epub 2003/12/13. PubMed PMID: 14670774; PubMed Central PMCID: PMCPmc1719373.

Halder, D., Bhowmick, S., Biswas, A., Mandal, U., Nriagu, J., Mazumdar, D. N., Chatterjee, D., Bhattacharya, P. (2012). Consumption of brown rice: A potential pathway for arsenic exposure in rural Bengal. *Environmental science & technology, 46*(7), 4142–4148. Epub 2012/02/23. doi: https://doi.org/10.1021/es204298a. PubMed PMID: 22352724.

Hossain, A., Sehbai, A., Abraham, R., & Abraham, J. (2008). Cancer health disparities among Indian and Pakistani immigrants in the United States: A surveillance, epidemiology, and end results-based study from 1988 to 2003. *Cancer, 113*(6), 1423–1430. Epub 2008/08/13. https://doi.org/10.1002/cncr.23686.

Inman, A. G., Constantine, M. G., & Ladany, N. (1999). *Cultural value conflict: An examination of Asian Indian women's bicultural experience. Asian and Pacific islander Americans: Issues and concerns for counseling and psychotherapy* (pp. 31–41).

Islam, N., Kwon, S. C., Senie, R., Kathuria, N. (2006). Breast and cervical cancer screening among south Asian women in new York City. *Journal of immigrant and minority health, 8*(3), 211–221. Epub 2006/06/23. doi: https://doi.org/10.1007/s10903-006-9325-y. PubMed PMID: 16791531.

Kaduvettoor-Davidson, A., & Inman, A. G. (2013). South Asian Americans: Perceived discrimination, stress, and Well-being. *Asian American Journal of Psychology., 4*(3), 155.

Kakarala, M., Rozek, L., Cote, M., Liyanage, S., Brenner, D. E. (2010). Breast cancer histology and receptor status characterization in Asian Indian and Pakistani women in the U.S.–a SEER analysis. *BMC Cancer, 10*, 191. Epub 2010/05/13. doi: https://doi.org/10.1186/1471-2407-10-191. PubMed PMID: 20459777; PubMed Central PMCID: PMCPmc2873947.

Kandula, N. R., Lauderdale, D. S. (2005). Leisure time, non-leisure time, and occupational physical activity in Asian Americans. *Annals of epidemiology, 15*(4), 257–265. Epub 2005/03/23. doi: https://doi.org/10.1016/j.annepidem.2004.06.006. PubMed PMID: 15780772.

Koenig, C. J., Dutta, M. J., Kandula, N., Palaniappan, L. (2012). All of those things we don't eat: A culture-centered approach to dietary health meanings for Asian Indians living in the United States. *Health Communication, 27*(8), 818–828. Epub 2012/03/01. doi: https://doi.org/10.1080/10410236.2011.651708. PubMed PMID: 22364189; PubMed Central PMCID: PMCPmc4324757.

Kumar, S., Biswas, M., Jose, T. (2015). HPV vaccine: Current status and future directions. *Medical journal, Armed Forces India, 71*(2), 171–177. Epub 2015/04/11. doi: https://doi.org/10.1016/j.mjafi.2015.02.006.; PubMed PMID: 25859081 PubMed Central PMCID: PMCPmc4388981.

Longman, J. M., Pritchard, C., Mcneill, A., Csikar, J., & Croucher, R. E. (2010). Accessibility of chewing tobacco products in England. *Journal of Public Health (Oxf), 32*(3), 372–378.

Maringe, C., Mangtani, P., Rachet, B., Leon, D. A., Coleman, M. P. (2013). dos Santos Silva I. Cancer incidence in south Asian migrants to England, 1986–2004: Unraveling ethnic from socioeconomic differentials. *International journal of cancer, 132*(8), 1886–1894. Epub 2012/09/11. doi: https://doi.org/10.1002/ijc.27826. PubMed PMID: 22961386.

McCaffery, K., Forrest, S., Waller, J., Desai, M., Szarewski, A., Wardle, J. (2003). Attitudes towards HPV testing: A qualitative study of beliefs among Indian, Pakistani, African-Caribbean and white British women in the UK. *British journal of cancer, 88*(1), 42–46. Epub 2003/01/31. doi: https://doi.org/10.1038/sj.bjc.6600686. PubMed PMID: 12556957; PubMed Central PMCID: PMCPmc2376794.

Menon, U., Szalacha, L., Prabhughate, A., Kue, J. (2014). Correlates of colorectal cancer screening among south Asian immigrants in the United States. *Cancer Nursing, 37*(1), E19–E27. Epub 2013/05/02. doi: https://doi.org/10.1097/NCC.0b013e31828db95e. PubMed PMID: 23632468.

Mishra, G. A., Shastri, S. S., Uplap, P. A., Majmudar, P. V., Rane, P. S., Gupta, S. D.(2009). Establishing a model workplace tobacco cessation program in India. Indian journal of occupational and environmental medicine,*13*(2), 97–103. Epub 2010/04/14. doi: https://

doi.org/10.4103/0019-5278.55129. PubMed PMID: 20386628; PubMed Central PMCID: PMCPmc2847335.

Mittal, R. D., Srivastava, D. S., A, M., B. M. (2005). Genetic polymorphism of drug metabolizing enzymes (CYP2E1, GSTP1) and susceptibility to bladder cancer in North India. *Asian Pacific journal of cancer prevention : APJCP 6*(1), 6–9. Epub 2005/03/23. PubMed PMID: 15780023.

Mukherjea, A., Modayil, M. V. (2013). Culturally specific tobacco use and south Asians in the United States: A review of the literature and promising strategies for intervention. *Health promotion practice, 14*(5 Suppl), 48s–60s. Epub 2013/05/22. doi: https://doi.org/10.1177/1524839913485585. PubMed PMID: 23690257.

Mukherjea, A., Morgan, P. A., Snowden, L. R., Ling, P. M., Ivey, S. L. (2012). Social and cultural influences on tobacco-related health disparities among south Asians in the USA. *Tobacco control, 21*(4), 422–428. Epub 2011/06/29. doi: https://doi.org/10.1136/tc.2010.042309. PubMed PMID: 21708814; PubMed Central PMCID: PMCPmc3292671.

Munoz, N., Bosch, F. X., Castellsague, X., Diaz, M., de Sanjose, S., Hammouda, D., Shah, K. V., Meijer, C. J. (2004). Against which human papillomavirus types shall we vaccinate and screen? The international perspective. *International journal of cancer, 111*(2), 278–285. Epub 2004/06/16. doi: https://doi.org/10.1002/ijc.20244. PubMed PMID: 15197783.

Murukutla, N., Turk, T., Prasad, C. V., Saradhi, R., Kaur, J., Gupta, S., Mullin, S., Ram, F., Gupta, P. C., Wakefield, M. (2012). Results of a national mass media campaign in India to warn against the dangers of smokeless tobacco consumption. *Tobacco control 21*(1), 12–17. Epub 2011/04/22. doi: https://doi.org/10.1136/tc.2010.039438. PubMed PMID: 21508418.

National Cancer Institute. (2009). *Physical activity and cancer* Available from: https://www.cancer.gov/about-cancer/causes-prevention/risk/obesity/physical-activity-fact-sheet

Nguyen, L. H., Nguyen, M. H. (2013). Systematic review: Asian patients with chronic hepatitis C infection. *Alimentary Pharmacology & Therapeutics,37*(10), 921–936. Epub 2013/04/06. doi: https://doi.org/10.1111/apt.12300. PubMed PMID: 23557103.

Ooi, S. L., Martinez, M. E., Li, C. I. (2011). Disparities in breast cancer characteristics and outcomes by race/ethnicity. Breast cancer research and treatment, *127*(3), 729–738. Epub 2010/11/16. doi: https://doi.org/10.1007/s10549-010-1191-6. PubMed PMID: 21076864; PubMed Central PMCID:PMCPmc3081535.

Owens, A., Randhawa, G. (2004). It's different from my culture; they're very different': Providing community-based, 'culturally competent' palliative care for south Asian people in the UK. *Health & Social Care in the Community*, *12*(5), 414–421. Epub 2004/09/18. doi: https://doi.org/10.7748/cnp2004.04.3.3.8.c113. PubMed PMID: 15373820.

Pope, C. A., 3rd, Thun, M. J., Namboodiri, M. M., Dockery, D. W., Evans, J. S., Speizer, F. E., Heath, C. W., Jr. (1995). Particulate air pollution as a predictor of mortality in a prospective study of U.S. adults. American journal of respiratory and critical care medicine, *151*(3 Pt 1), 669–674. Epub 1995/03/01. doi: https://doi.org/10.1164/ajrccm/151.3_Pt_1.669. PubMed PMID: 7881654.

Pope, C. A., 3rd, Burnett, R. T., Thun, M. J., Calle, E. E., Krewski, D., Ito, K., Thurston, G. D. (2002). Lung cancer, cardiopulmonary mortality, and long-term exposure to fine particulate air pollution. *JAMA*, *287*(9), 1132–1141. Epub 2002/03/07. PubMed PMID: 11879110; PubMed Central PMCID: PMCPmc4037163.

Promotion. (n.d.). *OoDPaH. Healthy People 2020 [cited 2016 December 9].* Available from: https://www.healthypeople.gov/.

Qiu, Y., Ni, H. (2003). Utilization of dental care services by Asians and native Hawaiian or other Pacific islanders: United States, 1997–2000. *Advance Data*, *2003*(336), 1–11. Epub 2003/06/21. PubMed PMID: 12815937.

Ramanathan, K. (1979). Oral precancerous conditions in peninsular Malaysia. *The Medical journal of Malaysia*, *33*(3), 216–221. Epub 1979/03/01. PubMed PMID: 522725.

Ruiz de Luzuriaga, A. M., Ahsan, H., Shea, C. R. (2011). Arsenical keratoses in Bangladesh--update and prevention strategies. *Dermatologic Clinics,29*(1), 45–51. Epub 2010/11/26. doi: https://doi.org/10.1016/j.det.2010.09.003. PubMed PMID: 21095527.

Schaller Consulting. (2004). *The changing face of taxi and limousine drivers: U.S., large states and metro areas and new York City*. Brooklyn, NY.

Shulman, J. D., Beach, M. M., Rivera-Hidalgo, F. (2004). The prevalence of oral mucosal lesions in U.S. adults: Data from the third National Health and nutrition examination survey, 1988-1994. *Journal of the American Dental Association(1939),135*(9), 1279–1286. Epub 2004/10/21. PubMed PMID: 15493392.

Singh, M., Shah, P. P., Singh, A. P., Ruwali, M., Mathur, N., Pant, M. C., Parmar, D. (2008). Association of genetic polymorphisms in glutathione S-transferases and susceptibility to head and neck cancer. *Mutation research, 638*(1–2), 184–194. Epub 2007/11/24. doi: https://doi.org/10.1016/j.mrfmmm.2007.10.003. PubMed PMID: 18035380.

Smith, A. H., Lingas, E. O., Rahman, M. (2000). Contamination of drinking-water by arsenic in Bangladesh: A public health emergency. *Bulletin of the World Health Organization 78*(9), 1093–1103. Epub 2000/10/06. PubMed PMID: 11019458; PubMed Central PMCID: PMCPmc2560840.

Sommer, F., Backhed, F. (2013). The gut microbiota–masters of host development and physiology. *Nature reviews Microbiology,11*(4),227–238. Epub 2013/02/26. doi: https://doi.org/10.1038/nrmicro2974. PubMed PMID: 23435359.

Soya, S. S., Vinod, T., Reddy, K. S., Gopalakrishnan, S., Adithan, C. (2007). Genetic polymorphisms of glutathione-S-transferase genes (GSTM1, GSTT1 and GSTP1) and upper aerodigestive tract cancer risk among smokers, tobacco chewers and alcoholics in an Indian population. *European journal of cancer (Oxford, England : 1990),43*(18), 2698–2706. Epub 2007/08/21. doi: https://doi.org/10.1016/j.ejca.2007.07.006. PubMed PMID: 17707637.

Szarewski, A., Cadman, L., Ashdown-Barr, L., Waller, J. (2009). Exploring the acceptability of two self-sampling devices for human papillomavirus testing in the cervical screening context: A qualitative study of Muslim women in London. *Journal of medical screening, 16*(4), 193–198. Epub 2010/01/08. doi: https://doi.org/10.1258/jms.2009.009069. PubMed PMID: 20054094.

Tan, Y. C., Zeigler-Johnson, C., Mittal, R. D., Mandhani, A., Mital, B., Rebbeck, T. R., Rennert, H. (2008). Common 8q24 sequence variations are associated with Asian Indian advanced prostate cancer risk. *Cancer epidemiology, biomarkers & prevention : a publication of the American Association for cancer research, cosponsored by the American society of preventive oncology. 17*(9), 2431–2435. Epub 2008/09/05. doi: https://doi.org/10.1158/1055-9965.epi-07-2823. PubMed PMID: 18768513; PubMed Central PMCID: PMCPmc3074274.

Tong, M. J., Pan, C. Q., Hann, H. W., Kowdley, K. V., Han, S. H., Min, A. D., Leduc, T. S. (2011). The management of chronic hepatitis B in Asian Americans. *Digestive diseases and sciences, 56*(11), 3143–3162. Epub 2011/09/22. doi: https://doi.org/10.1007/s10620-011-1841-5. PubMed PMID: 21935699.

Torre, L. A., Sauer, A. M., Chen, M. S., Kagawa-singer, M., Jemal, A., & Siegel, R. L. (2016). Cancer statistics for Asian Americans, native Hawaiians, and Pacific islanders, 2016: Converging incidence in males and females. *CA: A Cancer Journal for Clinicians, 66*(3), 182–202.

Uddin, G., Shoeb, D., Solaiman, S., Marley, R., Gore, C., Ramsay, M., Harris, R., Ushiro-Lumb, I., Moreea, S., Alam, S., Thomas, H. C., Khan, S., Watt, B., Pugh, R. N., Ramaiah, S., Jervis, R., Hughes, A., Singhal, S., Cameron, S., Carman, W. F., Foster, G. R. (2010). Prevalence of chronic viral hepatitis in people of south Asian ethnicity living in England: The prevalence cannot necessarily be predicted from the prevalence in the country of origin. *Journal of viral hepatitis, 17*(5), 327–335. Epub 2009/12/17. doi: https://doi.org/10.1111/j.1365-2893.2009.01240.x. PubMed PMID: 20002307.

van Wyk, C. W., Stander, I., Padayachee, A., Grobler-Rabie, A. F. (1993). The areca nut chewing habit and oral squamous cell carcinoma in south African Indians. A retrospective study. *South African medical journal = Suid-Afrikaanse tydskrif vir geneeskunde, 83*(6), 425–429. Epub 1993/06/01. PubMed PMID: 8211462.

White, M., Bush, J., Kai, J., Bhopal, R., & Rankin, J. (2006). Quitting smoking and experience of smoking cessation interventions among UK Bangladeshi and Pakistani adults: The views of community members and health professionals. *Journal of epidemiology and community health., 60*(5), 405–411 Epub 2006/04/15.

Willis, D., Popovech, M., Gany, F., Zelikoff, J. (2012). Toxicology of smokeless tobacco: Implications for immune, reproductive, and cardiovascular systems. *Journal of toxicology and environmental health Part B, Critical reviews, 15*(5), 317–331. Epub 2012/08/03. doi: https://doi.org/10.1080/10937404.2012.689553. PubMed PMID: 22852812.

World Health Organization International Agency for Research on Cancer. (2004). *Betel-quid and Areca-nut chewing and some Areca-nut-derived nitrosamines*. Lyon.

Worth, A., Irshad, T., Bhopal, R., Brown, D., Lawton, J., Grant, E., Murray, S., Kendall, M., Adam, J., Gardee, R., Sheikh, A. (2009). Vulnerability and access to care for south Asian Sikh and Muslim patients with life limiting illness in Scotland: Prospective longitudinal qualitative study. *BMJ(Clinical research ed), 338*, b183. Epub 2009/02/05. doi: https://doi.org/10.1136/bmj.b183. PubMed PMID: 19190015 PubMed Central PMCID: PMCPmc2636416.

Zhu, Q., Gao, R., Wu, W., Qin, H. (2013). The role of gut microbiota in the pathogenesis of colorectal cancer. *Tumour Biology : The journal of the International Society for Oncodevelopmental Biology and Medicine, 34*(3), 1285–1300. Epub 2013/02/12. doi: https://doi.org/10.1007/s13277-013-0684-4. PubMed PMID: 23397545.

Chapter 9
Mental Health Conditions among South Asians in the United States

Pratyusha Tummala-Narra and Anita Deshpande

South Asian immigrants and their children face acculturative stress, and specifically numerous challenges in the U.S., such as loss, separation, alienation, and anxiety about the new cultural environment, challenges with English language communication, immigration status, financial limitations, family and intergenerational stress, and discrimination. Stress related to acculturation, trauma, and discrimination has been linked with negative mental health outcomes, including depression, anxiety, and substance abuse, among South Asians in the U.S. This chapter delineates the impact of immigration, acculturation, and trauma on mental health conditions among first and second generation South Asians in the U.S. Additionally, we address barriers to the identification of mental health problems, issues of access to adequate care, and provide recommendations for culturally informed mental health interventions.

9.1 South Asians in the United States

As of 2010, South Asian individuals represent approximately 20% of the overall Asian American population in the United States (Inman et al. 2014; U.S. Census Bureau 2010). According to the 2010 U.S. Census, the Asian Indian population has increased by approximately 62% since 2000, and is currently the second largest Asian group in the U.S., with approximately 3.18 million people (Chandras et al. 2013; U.S. Bureau of Census 2010). There is notable diversity with regard to cultural, religious, and linguistic backgrounds among South Asians due to differences

P. Tummala-Narra (✉) · A. Deshpande
Counseling, Developmental & Educational Psychology, Boston College, Chestnut Hill, MA, USA
e-mail: tummalan@bc.edu

M. J. Perera, E. C. Chang (eds.), *Biopsychosocial Approaches to Understanding Health in South Asian Americans*, Cross-Cultural Research in Health, Illness and Well-Being, https://doi.org/10.1007/978-3-319-91120-5_9

across national origin and region. Additionally, there are significant variations in immigration status (e.g., temporary visa, refugee, asylum seeker, undocumented, dependent, permanent resident, U.S. citizen) among South Asians in the U.S. that are often related to reasons for migration (e.g., seeking employment or education, joining family members, escaping political and religious persecution or natural disaster) (Inman and Tummala-Narra 2014).

Immigration from South Asian countries to the United States should be understood as occurring across multiple waves over time, with the sociopolitical climates of both the United States and individuals' countries of origin playing a significant role in shaping their reasons for migration (Inman et al. 2015). The first notable wave of South Asians who immigrated to the U.S. (1899–1917) consisted mostly of Sikh men from the British Indian province of Punjab who sought out work within the railroad, lumber and agriculture industries (Bhatia 2007; Leonard 1997). The second major influx of South Asians did not occur until the U.S. government implemented the Immigration and Naturalization Act in 1965, almost 50 years after the passage of the Chinese Exclusion Act (Inman and Tummala-Narra 2010). In contrast to the Punjabi immigrants of the nineteenth and early twentieth centuries, South Asian immigrants who arrived to the U.S. in the 1960s and 70s had origins in various parts of India, Pakistan, Bangladesh, Sri Lanka, Afghanistan and Nepal (Leonard 1997). Majority of these South Asians were English proficient, highly skilled professionals seeking to expand their professional expertise and opportunities within the areas of medicine, engineering, science and academia (Bhatia 2007; Leonard 1997). By the mid-1980s, the primary reason for immigration shifted towards family reunification in addition to seeking vocational opportunities (e.g., small businesses). Another shift in the South Asian immigration to the U.S. occurred during the 1990s and 2000s when opportunities within the emerging software industry opened to this community (Sharma and Tummala-Narra 2014).

Over the past two decades, increasing numbers of South Asian immigrants in the U.S. have fled political, religious, and caste-based conflicts within their countries of origin. Further, recent South Asian immigration reflects an increasing number of older adults who live with their children and grandchildren who have settled in the U.S, and international students in U.S. colleges and universities (Institute of International Education 2011; Tummala-Narra et al. 2012). These different waves of immigration have contributed to considerable diversity among South Asian communities in the U.S., with implications for education, social class, and cultural, religious, and generational perspectives.

9.2 Acculturation

The term *acculturation* refers to "the extent to which individuals have maintained their culture of origin or adapted to the larger society" (Phinney 1996, p. 921). Research indicates that while South Asians typically immigrate to the U.S. in pursuit of the "American Dream" (Bhattacharya and Schoppelrey 2004), they often encounter unexpected post-migration changes in gender roles and family structure and dynamics, and spiritual practices, all of which can both buffer against or contribute to psychological distress.

9.2.1 Gender Roles and Family Structure

Traditional relational dynamics among many South Asian families are shaped within a patriarchal context, where gender roles are delineated by specific expectations of men and women (Inman and Tewari 2003; Kallivayalil 2010). Men are typically seen as the heads of their households, and therefore, expected to prioritize their education and career so that they may adequately provide economically for and make decisions on behalf of their families (Inman and Tewari 2003). In some families, education and career are seen as secondary goals for South Asian women as their responsibilities as caregivers within the home are expected to come first (Dasgupta 1998; Inman and Tewari 2003; Kallivayalil 2010). Women may experience pressure to ensure children's cultural and religious socialization in the context of immigration, even as parents and extended family in the country of origin are no longer readily accessible to support child rearing (Tummala-Narra 2013). Further, financial strain and the desire to secure greater economic security contribute to changes in the work lives of men and women. Although men are increasingly involved in their children's lives, many women are employed and often expected to be primary caretakers for the children. Many women grapple with multiple demands both within and outside of their homes.

In addition to negotiating gender roles, South Asian immigrants can encounter shifts in family dynamics due to the differences in acculturation across different generations (Khanna et al. 2009; Tummala-Narra 2013). It has been noted that first generation South Asians (born and raised outside of the U.S. and migrated to U.S. as adults) experience themselves as "allocentric," reflecting an emphasis on the family unit as an integral part of conceptions of the self (Farver et al. 2002, p. 340). Traditional South Asian family dynamics operate within a collectivistic framework, where family needs are prioritized over individual needs. Commitment to meeting family needs is maintained by a hierarchical system of organized family roles based upon age, birth order, and gender (Das and Kemp 1997; Inman and Tewari 2003; Roland 1996). This emphasis on collectivism manifests in family interactions, including a sense of reciprocal caregiving between parents and children, where parents tend to care for their children well into adulthood and children attend to their parents' needs in older adulthood (Inman and Tewari 2003). From a worldview that emphasizes an individualistic orientation, the closeness among traditional South Asian family members can be misperceived as evidence of enmeshment where older adolescent and adult children are seen as having a diminished sense of agency (Inman and Tewari 2003). South Asian immigrants and their children often struggle with navigating across divergent cultural contexts that approach family relationships in unique ways, which can contribute to anxiety concerning separation and the potential of losing a sense of family connection and unity.

9.2.2 Religious and Spiritual Practices

Acculturation further involves religious and spiritual practices. South Asians are affiliated with diverse religious philosophies including Hinduism, Islam, Christianity, Sikhism, Buddhism, Jainism, Zoroastrianism, and Judaism (Leonard 1997). The ways in which South Asian immigrants engage in religious and spiritual practices have evolved over time as the growth of South Asian communities resulted in established places of worship and spiritual centers. Prior to 1965, South Asian immigrants had little to no access to community gatherings and worship, and as such, most individuals practiced their religion within their homes and some individuals disconnected from their religious affiliations (Leonard 1997; Sharma and Tummala-Narra 2014). By the 1970s, the second major wave of South Asian immigrants created opportunities for public religious gatherings for people who shared religion and national origin. This was evident in the establishment of Hindu temples, Islamic mosques, Sikh gurdwaras, and Buddhist viharas. Over the next several decades, these religious institutions opened their doors to individuals from various countries of origin who shared the same religious beliefs (Leonard 1997).

Religious institutions often serve as “the means to create community and to transmit homeland culture and values to children and thus are critical sites shaping the identity construction processes of immigrants and their descendants” (Kurien, p. 438, 2005). Engaging in religious and spiritual practices offers many South Asians a positive sense of connection with communities reminiscent of their countries of origin, and serves as a buffer against stress associated with acculturation, such as racism-related stress. South Asian immigrants may also turn to their beliefs in fate or a higher power when attempting to make meaning of life events and transitions. For example, when South Asian immigrants experience disappointment concerning pre-migration hopes and post-migration experiences, engaging in religious and spiritual practices offers a way to bear emotional stress accompanying these experiences (Sharma et al. 2015; Tummala-Narra et al. 2013).

9.3 Acculturative Stress

The immigrant experience has been conceptualized as one that involves mourning for the loss and separation from loved ones and for a familiar cultural context (Ainslie 2011; Akhtar 2011). The process of acculturation can be particularly stressful for racial and ethnic groups who experience starker contrasts between culture of origin and new cultural context (Kanukollu and Mahalingam 2011). *Acculturative stress* refers to the psychological burden resulting from *adapting* to a new culture

(Berry 2003; Roysircar and Maestas 2002; Tummala-Narra et al. 2012). Acculturative stress among South Asians in the U.S. has been linked to mental health problems, such as depression (Masood et al. 2009; Tummala-Narra et al. 2012). Acculturative stress for South Asians, similar to many other immigrant groups in the U.S., can be produced through a number of factors, such as language and communication barriers, family and intergenerational stress, and discrimination (Inman and Tewari 2003; Tummala-Narra 2013).

9.3.1 Language and Communication Barriers

Many first-generation South Asians face challenges with English proficiency and fluency, and communication. South Asian immigrants have typically been raised in countries where they have exposure to English. However, it is important to keep in mind that there is considerable variation with regard to English exposure across regions (e.g., rural vs. urban), education, and socioeconomic status. In fact, in contrast with the model minority stereotype (Petersen 1966; Kanukollu and Mahalingam 2011), significant numbers of South Asian immigrants have little access to English-based education in their countries of origin, and face economic struggles pre- and post-migration. More than half of immigrants from Bangladesh in Southern California, for example, live below 200% of the poverty line, and problems with English proficiency contribute to reduced access to healthcare and social and legal services (Asian Pacific American Legal Center of Southern California 2005; Choudhury et al. 2009). Language barriers are also evident among many older adults who migrate to the U.S. later in life. Many older adults experience a sense of "role loss" (Becker et al. 2003, p. S151; Blair 2012), as they experience shifts in power, respect, and authority within their families post-migration. Among these subgroups of South Asians, language and communication barriers contribute to social isolation and psychological distress (Blair 2012; Tummala-Narra et al. 2013).

South Asian immigrants who arrive as children or adolescents to the U.S. often struggle with social and academic issues at school, and have little access to translators or bilingual education in schools. Additionally, there is considerable variation in how well South Asian students acquire academic English skills, and in accessing adequate educational supports in their transition to U.S. schools (American Psychological Association 2012). Some South Asian children and adolescents linguistically and culturally translate for their parents and/or extended family (e.g., aunts, uncles, grandparents), and often play a key role in family members' access to health care. Studies indicate that while carrying the role of translating is experienced as stressful, adolescents recognize the significance of supporting family members, and develop a sense of self-efficacy as a function of providing such support (American Psychological Association 2012; Lueck and Wilson 2010; Tummala-Narra 2016).

9.3.2 Family and Intergenerational Stress

Family and marital conflict, along with the loss of extended family support, have been found to be associated with physical and mental health problems (e.g., depressive symptomology) among South Asian families (Leung et al. 2011; Masood et al. 2009). For some families, economic stress and unemployment further contribute to conflict and psychological distress (Leung et al. 2011). The family context has been noted to be a contributor to both resilience and stress among South Asian families (Masood et al. 2009). On one hand, family support is often critical to individuals' identification of and coping with mental health problems. On the other hand, mental health problems may reflect dysfunctional and/or conflictual family dynamics (Almeida 2005).

Intergenerational conflicts in South Asian families are often rooted in an array of stressors outside of the home, such as those related to language, lack of social support, financial struggles, and discrimination. Different members of the family experience acculturation in unique ways, contributing to distinct worldviews and challenges in communication and understanding across generations (Akhtar 2011; Tummala-Narra 2016). For first- and second-generation South Asians (born and raised in the U.S.) who have, at least in part, internalized Euro-American cultural values, familial disagreement and conflict can emerge over a number of life decisions concerning romantic partnerships (e.g. dating, marriage), academic achievement, and career choice (Khanna et al. 2009). For second-generation children and adolescents, negotiating different cultural contexts can be challenging as their efforts to engage with and develop a bicultural identity may be perceived by their parents and other family members as "too Americanized." As a way to cope with this conflict, children and adolescents may develop a dual sense of self, where they adapt to home, school, and neighborhood environments by modifying their behaviors in each context in order to maintain a sense of belonging and minimize conflict with loved ones (Tummala-Narra et al. 2016). It is important to note that a sense of acceptance within the host culture has been found to be associated with lower acculturative stress (Inman et al. 2014).

Research indicates that families in which parents tend to be separated from mainstream U.S. context experience more conflict between parents and adolescents. In fact, large gaps in acculturative styles (e.g., *acculturation gaps)* between those of parents and adolescents have been related to lower self-esteem and greater anxiety among adolescents (Farver et al. 2002). Additionally, some studies indicate that Asian Indian women with less supportive family environments experience more internal conflict related to sex roles, and the negotiation of diverging demands within and outside of one's home contributes to *cultural values conflict*, or negative emotional experience produced in efforts to manage conflictual expectations and values (Inman 2006; Kaduvettoor-Davidson and Inman 2012).

Acculturation gaps (Prathikanti 1997) are thought to shape individuals' interpersonal relationships, both within and outside of the family. For example, second-generation adolescents and young adults often experience their worlds within and outside of their homes as alienated from each other, and therefore can face challenges in developing an integrated sense of self. Further, in the face of acculturation gaps, first-generation parents may also experience more psychological distance from their children, or deepen their sense of connection with their cultural heritage in the hope of bridging a loss of continuity for themselves and their children. It has also been noted that many South Asian parents overemphasize academic achievement, sometimes placing excessive pressure on their children to excel in schools and in the workplace (Roysircar et al. 2010). At the same time, both first- and second-generation parents emphasize education and connection to one's ethnic and/or religious community as a way of coping with competition and discrimination in mainstream U.S. context (Inman et al. 2014).

9.3.3 Discrimination

Throughout the history of South Asian immigration to the U.S., racial, ethnic, and religious discrimination has been a part of South Asians' experiences (Das and Kemp 1997). Over the past decade, there has been growing awareness of the negative impact of racism and discrimination directed against South Asians in the U.S. With the rise of anti-immigrant sentiment related to the terrorist attacks of 9/11 and ongoing threats to national security, many South Asians, particularly Muslims and those perceived to be Muslim, have been targets of murder, physical violence, verbal harassment, and other forms of discrimination (e.g., deportation, profiling, vandalism of places of worship) (Ahluwalia and Pellettiere 2010; Inman et al. 2014). Stereotypes of South Asians span a broad range, including conceptions of South Asians as terrorists with radical ideology, as exotic, as submissive, and as model minorities who are academically and professionally successful with minimal experiences of social and psychological stress, (Patel 2007). These stereotypes have important implications for individuals' sense of identity, self-esteem, and belonging in mainstream U.S. context. In fact, although developing a strong sense of ethnic identity (i.e. connection with one's ethnic heritage and community) may protect one from various types of acculturative stress, studies indicate that a stronger ethnic identity may not be sufficient to protect against racism-related stress (Inman et al. 2014; Smith and Silva 2011; Sodowsky et al. 1995; Tummala-Narra et al. 2011).

Some research has also indicated that first- and second-generation South Asians may experience race and racism in unique ways (Inman et al. 2014; Inman et al. 2015). Nevertheless, racism-related stress among both first- and second-generation South Asians has been associated with negative effects on self-esteem and on mental health, such as depression, anxiety, and suicidal ideation, among South Asians in the U.S. (Kaduvettoor-Davidson and Inman 2013; Miller et al. 2011; Rahman and Rollock 2004; Tummala-Narra et al. 2012). Additionally, greater internalization of not only negative stereotypes but also "positive" stereotypes (e.g., model minority) has been associated with higher levels of psychological distress and negative attitudes concerning help-seeking (Gupta et al. 2011). The internalization of the model minority stereotype is also thought to interfere with positive ethnic identity development, as individuals face overwhelming pressure to meet high educational and professional goals, often at the cost of psychological well-being (Gupta et al. 2011).

Many South Asians in the U.S. experience multiple forms of discrimination and marginalization. Specifically, individuals who suffer various types of minority stress such as racism, sexism, heterosexism, homophobia, ableism, and classism are among the most vulnerable to psychological distress (Sandil et al. 2015). When South Asian women and men experience marginalization within and outside of their ethnic and religious communities, they may cope with their feelings of isolation and alienation by hiding aspects of their identities in different contexts. For example, the opportunity to openly discuss sexual identity is typically unavailable in many South Asian communities in which lesbian, gay, bisexual, transgender, or queer (LGBTQ) identities are either dismissed or pathologized. It has also been noted that identifying with these identifies is viewed by many South Asians as a "Western disease" (Choudhury et al. 2009, p. 250). These perceptions contribute to an impossible bind when negotiating sexual, ethnic, and religious identities. Additionally, internalized homophobia has implications for sexual behavior. One such example is evident in the lives of some South Asians who have same-sex relationships while being married to an opposite-sex spouse in order to manage family and community responsibilities (Choudhury et al. 2009). At the same time, LGBTQ South Asians struggle with racism within mainstream LGBTQ communities (Sandil et al. 2015). Multiple marginalization can result in under-reporting of emotional stress and mental health problems and service utilization (Choudhury et al. 2009).

9.4 Mental Health Issues

The various types of acculturative stress implicated in the process of immigration are important to consider when approaching mental health issues among South Asians in the U.S. Each of these stressors discussed thus far, along with pre-migration and post-migration cultural beliefs and explanations concerning mental health, affects individuals', families', and communities' conceptualizations of mental health and mental health treatment and recovery processes. In the following sections, we discuss the prevalence of mental health problems and traumatic stress, culturally-based explanations of illness and healing, and underutilization of services and barriers to mental health care.

9.4.1 *Prevalence of Mental Health Problems and Traumatic Stress*

Depictions of South Asians as a successful minority group in the U.S. have masked mental health problems such as depression and suicidality, and psychosocial concerns such as domestic and sexual violence and AIDS among South Asians (Masood et al. 2009). In fact, there is a paucity of epidemiological studies that have examined the prevalence of mental health problems, such as depression, anxiety, bipolar disorder, post-traumatic stress disorder, eating disorders, substance abuse, psychotic disorders, and suicide within South Asian communities in the U.S. There is also minimal data on the prevalence of dementia and related disorders among South Asians, and most assessment measures for dementia that exist for Asian Americans have been validated with East Asian Americans (Fujii 2011; Sayegh et al. 2013). Prevalence of mental health problems and developmental disabilities across gender and age groups (children, adolescents, emerging adults, adults, older adults) is also virtually absent. A recent content analysis of psychological research with South Asian Americans (Inman et al. 2014) indicated that mental health issues have not received adequate attention by researchers possibly due to mental health stigma and related reluctance to report mental health problems within South Asian communities, and due to the model minority myth and the related perception that mental health issues are less significant.

Epidemiological data concerning the prevalence of mental health problems within South Asian countries is inadequate for a number of reasons (e.g., lack of representation across regions, varying definitions of illness, lack of standardized indicators of illness, incomplete reporting) (Baxter et al. 2013). It is also important to recognize that pre-migration mental health history, including culture specific or culture-bound syndromes, and family history of mental illness can be highly relevant to post-migration psychological health and help-seeking behavior. For example, in India, several culture specific syndromes have been documented, such as *Suudu* which involves painful urination and heat in the pelvic area among men and women, and *Dhat* which involves severe anxiety and somatic symptoms associated with sexual impotence (passing of white discharge or semen in urine) (Chhabra and Bhatia 2008). Clinicians trained in the United States may be unfamiliar with these syndromes and their presentation, and may need to secure adequate consultation to make accurate diagnostic assessments.

Further, it is important to consider potential differences in mental health across immigrant generations. Over the past decade, majority of studies in the U.S. examining differences in prevalence of mental health problems across generation have indicated that first generation (foreign born) immigrants tend to have better mental health outcomes when compared with the second generation (U.S. born) (Alegría et al. 2008; García-Coll and Marks 2012; Abe-Kim et al. 2007). Research concerning this *immigrant paradox* among South Asians is still in its infancy. However, researchers and clinicians should consider that the expression and reporting of psychological distress may at least in part account for differences in prevalence across immigrant generation (American Psychological Association 2012).

Although literature on prevalence rates of mental health problems among South Asians living in the U.S. is limited, researchers from the United Kingdom (U.K.) and Canada have begun to examine the pervasiveness of mental health illness among South Asian populations within their communities. Surveying the research being conducted in these countries may help to provide a better sense of what South Asian Americans are encountering with regards to mental health concerns and inform future empirical investigations seeking to attain these much needed statistics in the U.S.

9.4.2 Depression and Suicidal Ideation and Behavior

Research with South Asians in the U.K. and Canada has largely focused on the prevalence of depression among South Asians, with the findings from these studies being somewhat mixed. In one study conducted in the U.K. (Bhui et al. 2004), researchers examined and compared the prevalence of depressive symptoms between Punjabi and English primary care attendees. This investigation revealed significantly higher rates of depressive symptoms among Punjabi participants when compared to their English counterparts. The findings from this study also revealed that depression rates were particularly high among South Asian women and those diagnosed with a physical disability. More recently, researchers (Williams et al. 2015) sought to compare the prevalence rates of depression between South Asian, White European and Black Caribbean older adults living in the West London area of England. The results from this study were consistent with the previously cited study, revealing significantly higher rates of depression, almost twofold, among first generation South Asian immigrants when compared to their White European counterparts.

In contrast to the above findings, other studies have found relatively lower rates of depressive symptoms within the South Asian community when compared to the broader population (Berthoud and Nazroo 1997; Hussain and Cochrane 2004; Ineichen 2012). In 2014, researchers in Canada (Islam et al. 2014) examined mental health outcomes among South Asian immigrant and South Asian Canadian-born populations. This investigation revealed that prevalence rates for mood disorders such as depression did not seem to vary significantly among these populations, but rather, the researchers found higher prevalence rates of anxiety and psychosocial stress among South Asian immigrants when compared to Canadian-born South Asians. These findings raise a number of factors that potentially account for these discrepancies including underreporting depressive symptoms due to stigma, conceptualizing mental health problems as a physical condition and overlooking within group differences such as variance in generational status, time period of migration, socioeconomic status, and acculturative status (Bhui et al. 2004; Hussain and Cochrane 2004; Rastogi et al. 2014; Williams et al. 2015). Most research concerning mental health with South Asians in the U.S. has focused on Asian Indian populations (Inman et al. 2014; Masood et al. 2009). A few studies have examined the prevalence of depression among Asian Indians, and have found that depression may be more prevalent among Asian Indians when compared with other Asian American groups, and that Asian Indians may be less apt to identify depressive and anxious symptoms and seek help (Conrad and Pacquiao 2005; Leung et al. 2011). Other studies have noted that Asian Indian older adults are vulnerable to depressive symptomology, particularly those with lower English proficiency (Diwan et al. 2004; Sayegh et al. 2013; Tummala-Narra et al. 2013). In the U.S., some studies have noted a growing risk of suicidal ideation and behavior among some Asian American subgroups, but there are few recent studies focused specifically on suicidality among South Asians in the U.S. (Chu et al. 2011). Patel and Gaw (1996), in a review of suicide among immigrants from the Indian subcontinent, noted higher rates of suicide among young South Asian women immigrants when compared with South Asian men immigrants and with young women in mainstream contexts, and disproportionately higher rates of suicide among Hindu immigrants.

9.4.3 Interpersonal Violence

Research with South Asians in the U.S. has also focused on experiences of interpersonal violence. It is worth noting that majority of these studies have focused on domestic violence or intimate partner violence suffered by South Asian women. The prevalence of intimate partner violence among South Asians has been estimated to be greater than that occurring in other cultural groups (Abraham 2000; Inman et al. 2014). In fact, according to a study conducted in the early 2000s (Raj and Silverman 2003), approximately 40% of South Asian women in the greater Boston area reported experiencing physical and/or sexual violence in an intimate partner relationship in which they were involved at the time of the study. Other studies have estimated prevalence rates of 30–50% of intimate partner violence among South Asian women (Fingeld-Connett and Johnson 2013). Intimate partner violence within South Asian families has been thought to be connected to patriarchal norms and acculturative stress (Ahmad et al. 2004; Kallivayalil 2010; Singh 2009). As such, South Asian women have been noted to remain longer with their abusive partners, and tend to have limited access to resources (Fingeld-Connett and Johnson 2013). Some women have difficulty coping with the lack of financial resources, education, and immigration status, placing them in a vulnerable position in relation to their abusive partners. Many women also struggle with a belief that they are responsible for the success of their marriage and for keeping their children together with the father, and for upholding the family's reputation within their ethnic and/or religious communities (Anitha 2011; Kallivayalil 2010). The possibility of rejection by their families and communities, forced separation from children, and deportation, may all be realistic consequences of speaking out about abusive behavior (Fingeld-Connett and Johnson 2013). These realities are sometimes overlooked by mental health professionals who may emphasize the importance of agency and self-reliance for survivors without a consideration for cultural, social, and economic factors (Yoshihama et al. 2012).

More recently, scholars have called attention to the problem of sexual violence (occurring outside of intimate partner relationships) within South Asian communities. While the prevalence of child sexual abuse among South Asians in the U.S. is unknown, practitioners are aware of their female and male South Asian clients' experiences with childhood sexual abuse. The topic of sexual abuse is highly stigmatized in most communities, as the purity and honor of girls and women is held to be tantamount to the family's standing within the broader community. Kanukollu and Mahalingam (2011) have eloquently described the ways in which silence concerning sexual abuse within families and communities can serve to protect the idealized identities (e.g., model minority identity) of South Asian communities. At the same time, such idealization comes at a psychosocial cost to female and male survivors of sexual abuse, many of whom remain silent about their traumatic experiences and never receive support.

The effects of interpersonal violence, such as intimate partner violence and sexual violence, are profound, spanning a broad range of problems including poor physical health, depression, post-traumatic stress, anxiety, eating disorders, substance abuse, and suicidal ideation (Inman et al. 2014). The silence around interpersonal violence within South Asian communities, and the stress associated with migration can increase survivors' vulnerability to mental health problems. Further, culturally-embedded conceptualizations of violence and abuse, approaches to coping with violence, and access to culturally informed services influence survivors' disclosure of the abuse and help seeking (Ahmad et al. 2004; Anitha 2011). It is also important to consider that interpersonal violence among South Asians sometimes occurs in the context of family dislocation due to political and religious violence and persecution, war, trafficking, and natural disasters. There is a scarcity of information regarding the additive effects of community and political trauma and interpersonal violence among South Asians in the U.S. However, many South Asian survivors of trauma contend with multiple types of traumatic events, some of which may be experienced as more acceptable to disclose to others within and outside of their communities.

9.4.4 Culturally-Based Explanations of Illness and Healing

The expression of psychological distress can vary considerably across cultural contexts. The terms used to describe distress may not be commensurate with Western, Euro-American labels of distress (e.g., sad, depressed). For example, the National Asian Women's Health Organization (National Asian Women's Health Organization 1996) presented data from interviews with South Asian women in California who described their mental health concerns by using terms such as guilt, pressure, isolation, and stress (Leung et al. 2011). Additionally, South Asian immigrants may find it challenging to translate painful emotional experiences from their heritage language to English, and may find that some terms are untranslatable across languages (Akhtar 2011; Tummala-Narra 2016). According to some research, individuals from non-Western and non-White backgrounds experiencing depression report somatic problems more often than individuals from Western and/or White backgrounds (Karasz et al. 2007). Expressions of psychological distress are often situated within culturally-embedded explanations of mental illness, and this is evident in culture-bound or culture-specific syndromes that are characterized by somatic and psychological symptoms (DSM-V, American Psychiatric Association 2013). Kleinman (1986) contrasted somatization as an expression of distress from "psychologization." The latter is thought to be congruent with Western, Euro-American middle class conceptualizations. It has been suggested that people in several Asian countries tend to emphasize somatic suffering over emotional suffering, and as such, believe that they could be helped through medical treatment (Karasz et al. 2007). The lack of overt attention to emotional suffering (e.g., depression) by individuals then can certainly influence not only help-seeking behavior, but also providers' ability to identify mental health problems (Kirmayer et al. 1993).

In South Asian contexts, it is often the case that somatic symptoms, rather than verbal expressions of psychological stress, are identified as acceptable forms of expressing distress, particularly for women. In fact, some research indicates that South Asian women tend to report higher somatic symptomology when compared with men and with White, Euro-American women (Karasz et al. 2007). Among both South Asian women and men, religious and spiritual beliefs (e.g., possession by evil spirits, destiny or fate, karma resulting from past lives) or the belief in the family or individual being cursed guide understandings of psychotic disorders (Kumar and Nevid 2010; Leung et al. 2011). Mental illness carries a stigma for many South Asians. Consequently, it is often the case that both awareness of and treatment of mental illness is kept private within families in an effort to maintain family reputation and honor, and connection with ethnic and religious communities (Leung et al. 2011).

South Asian immigrants may be more likely to conceptualize severe mental health symptoms as a disease with biological origins that requires professional intervention (Karasz 2005; Kumar and Nevid 2010). Although mild to moderate depressive and anxious symptoms may not be perceived as mental health problems in South Asian cultural contexts, more severe mental health problems such as bipolar disorder and psychotic disorders are often recognized as mental disorders that should be addressed through professional treatment and/or religious practices (Thara et al. 2004). In a study of perceptions of major depression and schizophrenia with Asian Indians in the U.S., Kumar and Nevid (2010) found that a case vignette of schizophrenia presented to participants elicited stronger endorsement of biological explanations when compared with a case vignette of major depression. Scholars have also noted that many South Asians regard certain conditions such as cognitive decline in older adults as normative (Sayegh et al. 2013). These findings call attention to the potential influence of causal explanations of mental health problems on stigma and attitudes toward help-seeking (Kumar and Nevid 2010).

Many South Asians in the U.S. tend to approach healing from psychological distress by turning to spiritual and religious leaders in their communities, engaging in spiritual practices (e.g., prayer) and traditional health practices. For example, some Asian Indian immigrants and their children practice yoga, meditation, Reiki, and use homeopathy and Ayurvedic medicine as a way of coping with stress related to physical and mental health problems (Ahmad et al. 2004; Tewary 2005). Such healing practices reflect a cultural emphasis on the interrelationship between the mind and the body, and on achieving a sense of balance that is thought to promote physical and psychological health. Although access to traditional healing has grown over the past decade, primarily in urban areas of the U.S., South Asians who are able to travel to their countries of origin on a regular basis have increased access to these traditional healing practices as an alternative, or in addition, to Western, Euro-American approaches (e.g., psychotherapy, psychopharmacology). In fact, extended family members in the country of origin sometimes offer assistance in access to traditional healing practices. Although many South Asians are reluctant to burden family members and friends with their mental health issues, family support is an important source of support in healing from mental health concerns. Collectivistic coping strategies, such as sharing emotional struggles related to loss and challenges of acculturation with close family members and friends, have been found to be effective methods of coping with stress among South Asians in the U.S. (Yeh et al. 2006).

9.4.5 Underutilization of Mental Health Services and Barriers to Adequate Care

South Asians in the U.S. underutilize mental health services when compared with the general U.S. population, and when they do seek help from mental health professionals, it is often the case that their concerns have reached greater severity or crisis levels (Loya et al. 2010). Many individuals underestimate the need for help, and prefer confiding in people outside of formal systems of care (Chu et al. 2011). Additionally, South Asians tend to prefer consulting with general physicians about psychological issues rather than mental health professionals (Leung et al. 2011). A common course of entry into mental health services is through referral by primary care physicians to psychiatrists, psychologists, social workers, and other mental health professionals. Studies have indicated that service use may vary across immigrant generation, with U.S. born Asian Americans using mental health services more than foreign born Asians and Asian Americans (Abe-Kim et al. 2007). Although scholars (Frey and Roysircar 2006) have noted that acculturation may be associated with greater utilization of resources among South Asians in the U.S., data regarding service utilization across the first and second generation more specifically remains inconclusive.

South Asians in the U.S. face multiple barriers in securing adequate mental health care. For both the first and second generation, the problems of stigma and silence surrounding issues of mental health and illness and interpersonal violence prohibit many individuals and families from seeking help (Loya et al. 2010). The problem of stigma is compounded by the model minority notion which contributes to the perception that one should not require professional help for psychological issues (Gupta et al. 2011; Kanukollu and Mahalingam 2011). It is important to consider that many South Asians are unaware of mental health services that may be available to them, or how these services may be helpful to them. Psychiatric and psychological treatments offered in mental health service systems in the U.S. are unfamiliar to many South Asian immigrants. There are also concerns about whether a Western-trained, non-South Asian mental health professional would be able to understand one's cultural background, values, and perspectives. For example, a South Asian immigrant who is experiencing marital conflict may be concerned about a practitioner's ability to recognize both his/her personal needs and family obligations and responsibilities. In a different case, a second-generation South Asian American may be concerned about a practitioner pathologizing his/her emotional closeness and sense of interdependence with his/her family members. It is important to note, however, that some South Asians prefer to work with non-South Asian mental health professionals, due to concerns about privacy and disclosure of issues considered taboo (e.g., sex, sexuality, violence) within their families and communities. Individuals who have experienced discrimination and/or marginalization within their ethnic and/or religious communities may also be more likely to seek help from non-South Asian practitioners.

Language barriers further impede help-seeking among South Asians. Most mental health settings do not have access to bilingual practitioners or to interpreters for South Asian languages. Additionally, even when a patient is proficient or fluent in English, he/she may prefer to communicate at least periodically with the practitioner in his/her heritage language. Bilingual and multilingual individuals experience memory, emotion, and identity uniquely in different languages, and therefore, may find it important to move back and forth between languages with practitioners (Akhtar 2011). In the case of interpersonal violence and other forms of trauma, processing traumatic material in the heritage language and in English can be critical to the recovery process (Tummala-Narra 2016).

Economic challenges and social inequality challenge some South Asians' abilities to access adequate care (Tewary 2005). For example, individuals may not have access to transportation to services, or they may not have access to childcare or to time away from their jobs to keep appointments with mental health professionals. Additionally, many South Asian immigrants in the U.S. provide financial support to families in their countries of origin and, as such, prioritize family economic and educational needs over their personal mental health needs. Societal perceptions of South Asians as a privileged, non-marginalized minority in the U.S. can contribute to systemic neglect of mental health needs within these communities, including a lack of funding for culturally informed interventions. Mental health professionals should be aware that experiences of discrimination based on race, ethnicity, gender, language, religion, social class, sexual orientation and identity, and dis/ability is a significant barrier to seeking help. Further, for most undocumented South Asians, the threat of deportation becomes a prohibitive factor in service utilization (American Psychological Association 2012).

9.5 Recommendations for Culturally Informed Interventions

Culturally informed interventions that are multifaceted (e.g., clinical, community) are essential for addressing the mental health needs of South Asian individuals, families and communities in the U.S. Although over the past two decades, culturally informed services aimed to provide support to Asian Americans have been developing in a few urban areas in the U.S., most mental health services have yet to prioritize and implement culturally informed care to South Asians. Ongoing training and consultation is required for practitioners, researchers, and educators to address bias, communication problems, and misdiagnosis. There should be more attention directed toward developing appropriate assessment measures used in evaluating psychopathology and resilience (American Psychological Association 2012). It is also important that practitioners recognize the diversity within South Asian communities with regard to language, culture, religion, geographic origin, circumstances of immigration, acculturation, social class, sexual orientation, dis/ability, immigration (documentation) status, and immigrant generation (first, second, third) when conducting assessment, formulating diagnosis and treatment plan, and in implementing an intervention. South Asians also experience intersections of various aspects of identities (e.g., gender, religion, race, sexual orientation, dis/ability) in a multitude of ways, often involving internal and interpersonal conflict. Practitioners can help South Asian patients to address the ways in which they may feel conflicted about their loyalties to different communities with which they identify, and the psychological stress experienced in the face of potential loss, separation, or rejection by one or more of these communities (Tummala-Narra 2014).

Clinical interventions typically involve psychological testing, psychotherapy, crisis counseling, and psychopharmacology. Culturally informed psychotherapeutic interventions with South Asians are guided by various theoretical approaches (e.g., cognitive-behavioral, family systems, humanistic, psychodynamic). Each of these approaches, while distinct in its conceptualization of psychological issues and therapeutic techniques, shares an emphasis on the influence of sociocultural context on individual and family life. Each approach also attends to the impact of sociopolitical context (e.g., immigration policy, war, terrorism) and systemic injustice (e.g., sexism, racism, homophobia, classism, ableism) on mental health problems.

We recommend that culturally based expressions of distress and explanations of mental health problems, ways of coping with stress, and the use of indigenous healing practices be explored by the practitioner. Culturally informed practice further examines the role of stigma on an individual's experiences of mental health problems and relationships with family and friends. Interventions that include family members, friends, and spiritual mentors or leaders, when appropriate, are often helpful in reducing stigma and misunderstandings concerning mental health care (Leung et al. 2011). Practitioners should attend to the daily challenges of navigating multiple cultural and linguistic contexts, economic stress, experiences of discrimination, and isolation within and outside of one's ethnic and/or religious communities. Culturally informed care should also attend to pre- and post-migration traumatic stress, marital and family conflict, and intergenerational conflict. We underscore the importance of practitioners to engage in their own self-examination with regard to their conscious and unconscious biases and assumptions concerning South Asians in the U.S. (Tummala-Narra 2016). It is important to recognize that stereotypes about cultural groups typically operate on an unconscious level (Dovidio 2009), and are sometimes enacted in the relationship between a therapist and a patient. Therefore, practitioners should engage in open and active learning concerning the experiences of different cultural groups within and outside of their work environments, such that they will be able to develop accurate conceptualizations of their patients' lives.

In addition to clinical interventions, culturally informed community-based and outreach interventions are critical for addressing the mental health needs of South Asians in the U.S. (Chu et al. 2011). As most South Asians have a preference for seeking help from informal sources of support (e.g., family, friends), interventions that create dialogue among peers and across generational lines is especially important in building awareness about factors that contribute to psychological distress (e.g., acculturative stress, discrimination, trauma, separation from loved ones, family conflicts, identity conflicts), dispelling myths about mental illness and suicide, reducing stigma, identifying mental health problems, and accessing appropriate mental health care. As many South Asians seek the help of physicians when coping with physical and psychological stress, developing awareness of mental health issues among primary care physicians through education and outreach activities would also facilitate the identification of mental health problems. Increasingly, South Asian community-based interventions, such as domestic violence shelters, legal advocacy services, programs for older adults, women's discussion groups, youth groups, and political advocacy groups, have been emerging and becoming more visible within South Asian communities in the U.S., with promising outcomes for mental health (Blair 2012; Tummala-Narra et al. 2013). However, outreach, education, and open dialogue within and across South Asian communities remains underdeveloped and understudied in the mental health professions. In the future, more in-depth efforts within the mental health professions must be taken in order to address mental health problems among South Asians in the U.S., including further research, training, and education and more sophisticated and nuanced conceptualizations of South Asians' social and psychological experiences, with attention to both psychopathology and resilience. Further, resources should be directed toward further education, dialogue, de-stigmatization, and community-based advocacy for mental health concerns within South Asian communities.

References

Abe-Kim, J., Takeuchi, D. T., Hong, S., Zane, N., Sue, S., Spencer, M. S., Appel, H., Nicadao, E., & Algería, M. (2007). Use of mental health-related services among immigrant and US-born Asian Americans: Results from the national Latino and Asian American study. *American Journal of Public Health, 97*(1), 91–98. https://doi.org/10.2105/AJPH.2006.098541.

Abraham, M. (2000). Isolation as a form of marital violence: The South Asian immigrant experience. *Journal of Social Distress & the Homeless, 9*, 221–236. https://doi.org/10.1023/A:1009460002177.

Ahluwalia, M. K., & Pellettiere, L. (2010). Sikh men post-9/11: Misidentification, discrimination, and coping. *Asian American Journal of Psychology, 1*(4), 303–314. https://doi.org/10.1037/a0022156.

Ahmad, F., Riaz, S., Barata, P., & Stewart, D. E. (2004). Patriarchal beliefs and perceptions of abuse among South Asian immigrant women. *Violence Against Women, 10*(3), 262–282.

Ainslie, R. (2011). Immigration and the psychodynamics of class. *Psychoanalytic Psychology, 28*(4), 560–568. https://doi.org/10.1037/a0025262.

Akhtar, S. (2011). *Immigration and acculturation: Mourning, adaptation, and the next generation*. Lanham: Jason Aronson.

Alegria, M., Chatterji, P., Wells, K., Cao, Z., Chen, C., Takeuchi, D., et al. (2008). Disparity in depression treatment among racial and ethnic minority populations in the United States. *Psychiatric Services, 59*(11), 1264–1272. https://doi.org/10.1176/appi.ps.59.11.1264.

Almeida, R. (2005). Asian Indian families: An overview. In M. McGoldrick, J. Giordano, & N. Garcia-Preto (Eds.), *Ethnicity & family therapy* (pp. 377–393). New York: Guilford.

American Psychological Association. (2012). *Crossroads: The psychology of immigration in the new century, report of the APA presidential task force on immigration*. Washington, DC: Author.

American Psychiatric Association. (2013). *Diagnostic and statistical manual of mental disorders* (5th ed.). Washington, DC: Author.

Anitha, S. (2011). Legislating gender inequalities: The nature and patterns of domestic violence experienced by South Asian women with insecure immigration status in the United Kingdom. *Violence Against Women, 17*, 1260–1285.

Asian Pacific American Legal Center of Southern California. (2005). *The diverse face of Asians and Pacific Islanders in California*. Los Angeles: APALC.

Baxter, A. J., Patton, G., Scott, K. M., Degenhardt, L., & Whiteford, H. A. (2013). *Global epidemiology of mental disorders: What are we missing?* https://doi.org/10.1371/journal.pone.0065514.

Becker, G., Beyene, Y., Newsom, E., & Mayen, N. (2003). Creating continuity through mutual assistance: Intergenerational reciprocity in four ethnic groups. *The Journals of Gerontology, Series B: Psychological Sciences & Social Sciences, 58*(3), S151–S159.

Berry, J. W. (2003). Conceptual approaches to acculturation. In *Acculturation: Advances in theory, measurement, and applied research* (pp. 17–37). https://doi.org/10.1037/10472-004.

Berthoud, R., & Nazroo, J. (1997). The mental health of ethnic minorities. *New Community, 23*, 309–324.

Bhatia, S. (2007). *American karma: Race, culture, and identity in the Indian diaspora*. New York: New York University Press.

Bhattacharya, G., & Schoppelrey, S. L. (2004). Preimmigration beliefs of life success, Postimmigration experiences, and acculturative stress: South Asian immigrants in the United States. *Journal of Immigrant Health, 6*(2), 83–92. https://doi.org/10.1023/b:joih.0000019168.75062.36.

Bhui, K., Bhugra, D., Goldberg, D., Sauer, J., & Tylee, A. (2004). Assessing the prevalence of depression in punjabi and english primary care attenders: The role of culture, physical illness and somatic symptoms. *Transcultural Psychiatry, 41*(3), 307–322. https://doi.org/10.1177/1363461504045642.

Blair, T. R. (2012). "Community ambassadors" for South Asian elder immigrants: Late-life acculturation and the roles of community health workers. *Social Science & Medicine, 75*(10), 1769–1777. https://doi.org/10.1016/j.socscimed.2012.07.018.

Chandras, K. V., Chandras, S. V., & DeLambo, D. A. (2013). Counseling Asian-American Indians from India: Implications for training multicultural counselors. Resource document. American counseling Association's VISTAS 2013 quarterly electronic monograph. http://www.counseling.org/docs/vistas/counseling-asian-americanindians-from-india–implications-for-training-multicultural-counselors.pdf. Accessed 1 December 2015.

Chhabra, V., & Bhatia, R. G. (2008). Cultural bound syndromes in India. *Delhi Psychiatry Journal, 11*(1), 15–18.

Choudhury, P. P., Badhan, N. S., Chand, J., Chhugani, S., Choksey, R., Husainy, S., Lui, C., & Wat, E. C. (2009). Community alienation and its impact on help-seeking behavior among LGBTIQ South Asians in Southern California. *Journal of Gay & Lesbian Social Services, 21*(2–3), 247–266. https://doi.org/10.1080/10538720902772196.

Chu, J. P., Hsieh, K., & Tokars, D. A. (2011). Help-seeking tendencies in Asian American with suicidal ideation and attempts. *Asian American Journal of Psychology., 2*(1), 25–38. https://doi.org/10.1037/a0023326.

Conrad, M. M., & Pacquiao, D. E. (2005). Manifestation, attribution, and coping with depression among Asian Indians from the perspectives of health care practitioners. *Journal of Transcultural Nursing, 16*(1), 32–40. https://doi.org/10.1177/1043659604271239.

Das, A. K., & Kemp, S. F. (1997). Between two worlds: Counseling south Asian Americans. *Journal of Multicultural Counseling and Development, 25*(1), 23–33. https://doi.org/10.1002/j.2161-1912.1997.tb00313.x.

Dasgupta, S. D. (1998). Gender roles and cultural continuity in the Asian Indian immigrant community in the U.S. *Sex Roles, 38*(11–12), 953–974. https://doi.org/10.1023/A:1018822525427.

Diwan, S., Jonnalagadda, S. S., & Gupta, R. (2004). Differences in the structure of depression among older Asian Indian immigrants in the United States. *Journal of Applied Gerontology, 23*(4), 370–384. https://doi.org/10.1177/0733464804270584.

Dovidio, J. F. (2009). Racial bias, unspoken but heard. *Science, 326*(5960), 1641–1642. https://doi.org/10.1126/science.1184231.

Farver, J. A. M., Narang, S. K., & Bhadha, B. R. (2002). East meets west: Ethnic identity, acculturation, and conflict in Asian Indian families. *Journal of Family Psychology, 16*(3), 338–350. https://doi.org/10.1037/0893-3200.16.3.338.

Fingeld-Connett, D., & Johnson, E. D. (2013). Abused South Asian women in westernized countries and their experiences seeking help. *Issues in Mental Health Nursing, 34*, 863–873.

Frey, L. L., & Roysircar, G. (2006). South Asian and East Asian international students' perceived prejudice, acculturation, and frequency of help resource utilization. *Journal of Multicultural Counseling and Development, 34*, 208–222.

Fujii, D. (2011). *The neuropsychology of Asian-Americans*. New York: Taylor & Francis.

García-Coll, C., & Marks, A. (Eds.). (2012). *The immigrant paradox in children and adolescents: Is becoming American a developmental risk?* Washington, DC: American Psychological Association Press.

Gupta, A., Szymanski, D. M., & Leong, F. T. (2011). The "model minority myth": Internalized racialism of positive stereotypes as correlates of psychological distress, and attitudes toward help-seeking. *Asian American Journal of Psychology, 2*(2), 101–114. https://doi.org/10.1037/a0024183.

Hussain, F., & Cochrane, R. (2004). Depression in South Asian women living in the UK: A review of the literature with implications for service provision. *Transcultural Psychiatry, 41*(2), 253–270. https://doi.org/10.1177/1363461504043567.

Ineichen, B. (2012). Mental illness and suicide in British South Asian adults. *Mental Health, Religion & Culture, 15*(3), 235–250. https://doi.org/10.1080/13674676.2011.643861.

Inman, A. G. (2006). South Asian women: Identities and conflicts. *Cultural Diversity & Ethnic Minority Psychology, 12*(2), 306–319. https://doi.org/10.1037/1099-9809.12.2.306.

Inman, A., & Tewari, N. (2003). The power of context: Counseling South Asians within a family context. In G. Roysircar, D. Sandhu & V. Bibbins (Eds.), *Multicultural competencies: A guidebook of practices* (pp. 97–107). Alexandria: AMCD.
Inman, A. G., & Tummala-Narra, P. (2010). Clinical competencies in working with immigrant communities. In J. Cornish, L. Nadkarni, E. Rodolfa, & B. Schreier (Eds.), *Handbook of Multicultural Counseling Competencies* (pp. 117–152). New York: Wiley.
Inman, A. G., & Tummala-Narra, P. (2014). Immigration and human rights. In M. Miville & A. Ferguson (Eds.), *The Handbook of race-ethnicity and gender in psychology* (pp. 87–109). New York: Springer.
Inman, A. G., Devdas, L., Spektor, V., & Pendse, A. (2014). Psychological research on south Asian Americans: A three-decade content analysis. *Asian American Journal of Psychology, 5*(4), 364–372 (2006). https://doi.org/10.1037/a0035633.
Inman, A. G., Tummala-Narra, P., Kaduvettoor-Davidson, A., Alvarez, A. N., & Yeh, C. J. (2015). A qualitative exploration of the role of race and racism for first generation Asian Indians. *The Counseling Psychologist, 43*(2), 217–247.
Institute of International Education (2011). *Institute of International Education: Opening minds to the world (Annual Report).* http://www.iie.org/Who-WeAre/AnnualReport/~/media/Files/Corporate/AR/2010-IIE-Annual-Report.ashx. Accessed 1 December 2015.
Islam, F., Khanlou, N., & Tamim, H. (2014). South Asian populations in Canada: Migration and mental health. *BMC Psychiatry, 14*, 154.
Kaduvettoor-Davidson, A., & Inman, A. G. (2012). Predictors of cultural values conflict for Asian Indian women. *Journal of Multicultural Counseling and Development, 40*, 2–10.
Kaduvettoor-Davidson, A., & Inman, A. G. (2013). South Asian Americans: Perceived discrimination, stress, and well-being. *Asian American Journal of Psychology, 4*(3), 155–165.
Kallivayalil, D. (2010). Narratives of suffering of South Asian immigrant survivors of domestic violence. *Violence Against Women, 16*(7), 789–811.
Kanukollu, S. N., & Mahalingam, R. (2011). The idealized cultural identities model on help-seeking and child sexual abuse: A conceptual model for contextualizing perceptions and experiences of south Asian Americans. *Journal of Child Sexual Abuse, 20*(2), 218–243. https://doi.org/10.1080/10538712.2011.556571.
Karasz, A., Dempsey, K., & Fallek, R. (2007). Cultural differences in the experience of everyday symptoms: A comparative study of South Asian and European American women. *Culture, Medicine, & Psychiatry, 31*, 473–497.
Khanna, A., McDowell, T., Perumbilly, S., & Titus, G. (2009). Working with Asian Indian American families: A Delphi study. *Journal of Systemic Therapies, 28*(1), 52–71. https://doi.org/10.1521/jsyt.2009.28.1.52.
Kirmayer, L. J., Robbins, J. M., Dworkind, M., & Yaffe, M. J. (1993). Somatization and the recognition of depression and anxiety in primary care. *American Journal of Psychiatry, 150*(5), 734–741. https://doi.org/10.1176/ajp.150.5.734.
Kleinman, A. (1986). *Social origins of distress and disease: Depression, neurasthenia, and pain in modern China.* New Haven: Yale University Press.
Kumar, A., & Nevid, J. S. (2010). Acculturation, enculturation, and perceptions of mental disorders in Asian Indian immigrants. *Cultural Diversity and Ethnic Minority Psychology, 16*(2), 274–283. https://doi.org/10.1037/a0017563.
Kurien, P. (2005). Being young, brown and Hindu. *Journal of Contemporary Ethnography, 34*(4), 434–469.
Leonard, K. I. (1997). *The south Asian Americans.* Westport: Greenwood Press.
Leung, P., Cheung, M., & Tsui, V. (2011). Asian Indians and depressive symptoms: Reframing mental health help-seeking behavior. *International Social Work, 55*(1), 53–70. https://doi.org/10.1177/0020872811407940.
Loya, F., Reddy, R., & Hinshaw, S. P. (2010). Mental illness stigma as a mediator of differences in Caucasian and South Asian college students' attitudes toward psychological counseling. *Journal of Counseling Psychology, 57*(4), 484–490. https://doi.org/10.1037/a0021113.

Lueck, K., & Wilson, M. (2010). Acculturative stress in Asian immigrants: The impact of social and linguistic factors. *International Journal of Intercultural Relations, 34*, 47–57. https://doi.org/10.1016/j.ijintrel.2009.10.004.

Masood, N., Okazaki, S., & Takeuchi, D. T. (2009). Gender, family, and community correlates of mental health in South Asian Americans. *Cultural Diversity and Ethnic Minority Psychology, 15*(3), 265–274. https://doi.org/10.1037/a0014301.

Miller, M. J., Yang, M., Farrell, J. A., & Lin, L. (2011). Racial and cultural factors affecting the mental health of Asian Americans. *American Journal of Orthopsychiatry, 81*(4), 489–497. https://doi.org/10.1111/j.1939-0025.2011.01118.x.

National Asian Women's Health Organization. (1996). Emerging communities: *A health needs assessment of South Asian women in 3 California counties*. http://www.nawho.org/atf/cf/BC9650E6-A7EB-483F-A210-CC3E0D7445A6NAWHOEmerg.pdf. Accessed 1 December 2015.

Patel, N. (2007). The construction of south-Asian-American womanhood. *Women & Therapy, 30*(3/4), 51–61. https://doi.org/10.1300/j015v30n04_05.

Patel, S. P., & Gaw, A. C. (1996). Suicide among immigrants from the Indian subcontinent: A review. *Psychiatric Services, 47*(5), 517–521.

Petersen, W. (1966, December 26). Success story of one minority group in the U.S. U.S. News and World Report, pp 73–78.

Phinney, J. S. (1996). When we talk about American ethnic groups, what do we mean? *American Psychologist, 51*(9), 918–927. https://doi.org/10.1037//0003-066x.51.9.918.

Prathikanti, S. (1997). East Indian American families. In E. Lee (Ed.), *Working with Asian Americans: A guide for clinicians* (pp. 79–100). New York: Guilford Press.

Rahman, O., & Rollock, D. (2004). Acculturation, competence, and mental health among south Asian students in the United States. *Journal of Multicultural Counseling and Development, 32*, 130–142.

Raj, A., & Silverman, J. G. (2003). Immigrant South Asian women at greater risk for injury from intimate partner violence. *American Journal of Public Health, 93*(3), 435–437. https://doi.org/10.2105/ajph.93.3.435.

Rastogi, P., Khushalani, S., Dhawan, S., Goga, J., Hemanth, N., Kosi, R., Sharma, R. K., Black, B. S., Jayaram, G., & Rao, V. (2014). Understanding clinician perception of common presentations in South Asians seeking mental health treatment and determining barriers and facilitators to treatment. *Asian Journal of Psychiatry, 7*, 15–21. https://doi.org/10.1016/j.ajp.2013.09.005.

Roland, A. (1996). *Cultural pluralism and psychoanalysis: The Asian and North American experience*. New York: Routledge.

Roysircar, G., & Maestas, M. L. (2002). Assessing acculturation and cultural variables. In *Asian American Mental Health* (pp. 77–94). https://doi.org/10.1007/978-1-4615-0735-2_6.

Roysircar, G., Carey, J. C., & Koroma, S. (2010). Asian Indian college students' science and math preferences: Influences of cultural contexts. *Journal of Career Development, 36*(4), 324–347.

Sandil, R., Robinson, M., Brewster, M. E., Wong, S., & Geiger, E. (2015). Negotiating multiple marginalizations: Experiences of South Asian LGBQ individuals. *Cultural Diversity and Ethnic Minority Psychology, 21*(1), 76–88. https://doi.org/10.1037/a0037070.

Sayegh, P., Kellough, J., Otilingam, P. G., & Poon, C. Y. (2013). South Asian and middle Eastern American older adults: Dementia, mood disorders, and anxiety disorders. *Clinical Gerontologist, 36*(3), 216–240. https://doi.org/10.1080/07317115.2013.767873.

Sharma, A., & Tummala-Narra, P. (2014). Psychotherapy with Hindus. In P. S. Richards & A. E. Bergin (Eds.), *Handbook of Psychotherapy and Religious Diversity* (2nd ed., pp. 321–345). Washington, D.C.: American Psychological Association Press.

Singh, A. A. (2009). Helping south Asian immigrant women use resilience strategies in healing from sexual abuse: A call for a culturally relevant model. *Women and Therapy, 32*(4), 361–376.

Smith, T. B., & Silva, L. (2011). Ethnic identity and personal Well-being of people of color: A meta-analysis. *Journal of Counseling Psychology, 58*(1), 42–60. https://doi.org/10.1037/a0021528.

Sodowsky, G. R., Kwan, K. L., & Pannu, R. (1995). Ethnic identity of Asians in the United States. In J. G. Ponterotto, J. M. Cases, L. A. Suzuki, & C. M. Alexander (Eds.), *Handbook of multicultural counseling* (pp. 123–154). Thousand Oaks: Sage.

Tewary, S. (2005). Asian Indian immigrant women: A theoretical perspective on mental health. *Journal of Human Behavior in the Social Environment, 11*(1), 1–22. https://doi.org/10.1300/J137v11n01_01.

Thara, R., Padmavati, R., & Srinivasan, T. (2004). Focus on psychiatry in India. *British Journal of Psychiatry, 184*, 366–373.

Tummala-Narra, P. (2013). Psychotherapy with south Asian women: Dilemmas of the immigrant and first generations. *Women & Therapy, 36*(3–4), 176–197. https://doi.org/10.1080/02703149.2013.797853.

Tummala-Narra, P. (2016). *Psychoanalytic theory and cultural competence in psychotherapy*. Washington, DC: American Psychological Association.

Tummala-Narra, P., Inman, A. G., & Ettigi, S. (2011). Asian Indians' responses to discrimination: A mixed-method examination of identity, coping, and self-esteem. *Asian American Journal of Psychology, 2*(3), 205–218.

Tummala-Narra, P., Alegria, M., & Chen, C. (2012). Perceived discrimination, acculturative stress, and depression among South Asians: Mixed findings. *Asian American Journal of Psychology., Special Issue: Secondary analysis of the National Latino and Asian American Study (NLAAS) Dataset-Part I, 3*(1), 3–16.

Tummala-Narra, P., Sathasivam-Rueckert, N., & Sundaram, S. (2013). Voices of older Asian Indian immigrants: Mental health implications. *Professional Psychology: Research and Practice, 44*(1), 1–10. https://doi.org/10.1037/a0027809.

Tummala-Narra, P., Deshpande, A., & Kaur, J. (2016). South Asian adolescents' experiences of acculturative stress and coping. *American Journal of Orthopsychiatry, 86*(2), 194–211 https://doi.org/10.1037/ort0000147.

U.S. Bureau of Census. (2010). *Population projections of the United States by age, sex, race and Hispanic origin: 1992 to 2050*. Washington, DC: Government Printing Office.

Williams, E. D., Tillin, T., Richards, M., Tuson, C., Chaturvedi, N., Hughes, A. D., & Stewart, R. (2015). Depressive symptoms are doubled in older British South Asian and black Caribbean people compared with Europeans: Associations with excess co-morbidity and socioeconomic disadvantage. *Psychological Medicine, 45*(9), 1861–1871. doi:https://doi.org/10.1017/S0033291714002967.

Yeh, C. J., Inman, A., Kim, A. B., & Okubo, Y. (2006). Asian American families' collectivistic coping strategies in response to 9/11. *Cultural Diversity and Ethnic Minority Psychology, 12*, 134–148.

Yoshihama, M., Ramakrishnan, A., Hammock, A. C., & Khaliq, M. (2012). Intimate partner violence prevention program in an Asian immigrant community:Integrating theories, data, and community. *Violence Against Women, 18*(7), 763–783. https://doi.org/10.1177/1077801212455163.

Part IV
Barriers to Promoting Health in South Asian Americans

Chapter 10
Issues in Counseling South Asian Americans

Farah A. Ibrahim and Jianna R. Heuer

The present chapter considers variables that may enhance counseling Sou h Asian Americans (SAAs) on health-related issues. The primary concerns in heal -related counseling are prevention of chronic diseases, psychoeducation, and a erence to management schedules for chronic diseases. Cultural factors, and gene tional status appear to be important in designing and conducting interventions fo both health promotion and chronic disease management.

The chapter begins with a brief summary of chronic diseases th SAAs appear to be susceptible to, and the rationale for this susceptibility as ident ed in the literature; these include Coronary Heart Disease (CAD), Type II iabetes Mellitus (T2DM), Oral and Breast cancers, and comorbid psychological orders. This will be followed by cultural factors that may influence health behav and adherence to disease management requirements.The last segment of the apter will address issues that may increase compliance with health promotio d disease management information.

F. A. Ibrahim (✉)
University of Colorado-Denver, Denver, Colorado, U
e-mail: Farah.Ibrahim@ucdenver.edu

J. R. Heuer
Private Practice, New York City, NY, USA

M. J. Perera, E. C. Chang (eds.), *Biopsychos pproaches to Understanding Health in South Asian Americans*, Cross-C esearch in Health, Illness and Well-Being, https://doi.org/10.1007/97 9-91120-5_10

10.1 Chronic Health Conditions among SAAs

10.1.1 Organic Medical Conditions

Previous chapters have addressed South Asian Americans' vulnerability to chronic diseases and weight gain. Common chronic health conditions faced by South Asians in the United States and in their countries of origin are chronic degenerative diseases such as CAD, specifically atherosclerosis and T2DM (Palaniappan et al. 2010; Raj 2011). Risk factors for CAD among South Asians include: cigarette smoking, diabetes mellitus, hypertension, high LDL cholesterol and low HDL cholesterol levels, obesity (BMI greater than 25), lack of physical activity, family history of premature heart disease, and age. Among men and women, the susceptibility is higher in men older than 45 years of age, and in women older than 55 years of age (Sikand 2011). Risk factors for T2DM among South Asians include: older age, obesity, family history, physical inactivity, and dietary habits, which includes a high percentage of saturated fat, and low consumption of fruits and vegetables. Both in culture o origin and among immigrants, South Asian populations have higher incidence an prevalence of these two diseases than white populations (Abate and Chandalia)01; Gujral et al. 2013; Misra 2011; Simmons et al. 1989). Higher rates of these tw iseases are evident in immigrant South Asian populations in Australia, Europe, Nor America, and in Asian countries.

Interesting the risk factors that are common for white populations are not always similar nong South Asian populations. For both T2DM and cardiovascular disease, risk fa rs include: Metabolic syndrome (Metabolic syndrome is characterized by a clus of cardiovascular disease (CVD) risk factors, including abdominal obesity, eleva blood glucose, dyslipidemia, and high blood pressure [Ford 2005; Garber 200 hypertension, and obesity (Lovegrove 2007; McKeigue et al. 1992; Tan et al. 2). Higher concentrations of plasma triglycerides and lower concentrations of l density lipoprotein cholesterol than whites have been reported in over 50% South Asians in the US and UK (Gupta et al. 2004; Laws et al. 1994; Tziomalo al. 2008). The single most important component of metabolic syndrome among uth Asians is insulin resistance. Insulin resistance is a condition in which the produces insulin but does not use it effectively. When people have insulin resi ce, glucose builds up in the blood instead of being absorbed by the cells, lea to type 2 diabetes or pre-diabetes (National Institute of Diabetes and Digestive Kidney Diseases (NIDDK) 2014). Metabolic syndrome is evident in South ns at a much younger age, compared with white Europeans, and SAAs typica velop the disease 5–10 years earlier and at a lower BMI (Misra 2011; Misra and m 2007; Sattar and Gill 2015). Other risk factors for South Asians include: ex ody fat, abdominal obesity, high waist-to-hip ratio, normal waist circumferen gher intra-abdominal fat, and high truncal subcutaneous fat (Misra and Vikran 7).

Recent research has highligh e increase in fast food intake among third ion South Asian American h is a risk factor for cardiovascular disease

(Becerra et al. 2014). In general, economic, social, and lifestyle conditions are considered to be risk factors for chronic diseases, however in the case of South Asians it appears that both genetic and environmental factors are involved (Barnett et al. 2006). Lifestyle changes due to urban living, technological changes, and affluence have resulted in greater susceptibility to these disorders (Bharmal 2012; Lesser et al. 2014). Lifestyle changes and disease management are critical factors in promoting health among SAA.

10.1.2 Comorbid Psychological Disorders

Mental health issues related to living with chronic diseases are quite common. The literature identifies depression, anxiety, and nonspecific psychological disorders specifically related to T2DM (Gonzalez et al. 2011; Kessler et al. 2001; Li et al. 2009; Mezuk et al. 2008). Information about comorbid disorders with chronic diseases among ethnic non-dominant populations, and specifically among SAA is not readily available.

Depression is fairly common among South Asians in their cultures of origin (Ali 2014; Lin et al. 1985). Nazroo (2001) found that in UK the symptoms of depression were high among SAA immigrants compared to the nonimmigrant population, and depression was higher among immigrant SAA women compared to immigrant SAA men. However, in comparing South Asians to White Americans, depression rates appear much lower (Ahmed and Bhugra 2007; Jackson-Triche et al. 2000). Ahmed and Bhugra (2007) note that a common problem for ethnic minorities is the under diagnosis of depression in the Western world (Ballenger et al. 2001; Lecrubier 2001; Sartorius et al. 1996). A primary reason is that Western explanatory models of depression differ from other cultures, and how they may define depression, or what depression means, and how it is expressed in non-Western cultures. Wheeler and Izzard (1997) identified the difference between individualism and collectivism, and how socialization in these contexts influences behavior in addressing personal problems: In Western societies the goal is to instigate change in the individual's situation and, in Eastern societies, it is important to maintain personal-familial-social equilibrium by learning to adjust, or accepting fate.

Somatic symptom disorders also appear to be common among Asian populations in general, and South Asians in particular (Ali 2014; Hsu 1999; Kirmayer and Young 1998). South Asian Americans tend to express psychological distress with somatic symptoms, potentially related to tacit cultural prohibitions against verbalizing psychological distress (Ali 2014). Research has also identified somatic symptoms common among immigrants making geographic transitions (Lin et al. 1985). Ali (2014) notes that since most medical personnel ignore somatic symptoms when they cannot find any physical cause, clients frequently turn to religious leaders, family, or traditional healers. Additionally, the anxiety and depression that accompanies chronic disorders could also be the cause for nonspecific somatic symptoms (DiMatteo et al. 2000; Katon et al. 1984; Kessler et al. 1985; Kessler et al. 2001).

Katon et al. (1984) identified depression as a result of dealing with chronic illness. Njobvu et al. (1999) note that stress from work, life, language issues, could be associated with somatic symptoms.

There are several reasons for depression and somatic symptoms among immigrant populations; primary is the issue of culture loss and bereavement (loss of family and friends, familiar environment, etc.,) upon moving to a country that is far away from one's home country (Bhugra 2004; Bhugra and Becker 2005; Henry et al. 2005). Additionally, rules of conduct and expectations of behavior shift as one moves from collectivism to a culture that emphasizes individualism (Rogers-Sirin et al. 2014). Adjustment to all these changes and cultural losses can be challenging. Coupled with the cultural norm in South Asia to deal with adversity with stoicism, the adjustment process can lead to internalizing psychological pain, resulting in depression and somatic symptoms. These cultural and social challenges, along with the losses associated with of migration lead to acculturative stress (Rogers-Sirin et al. 2014). Managing acculturative stress is critical for South Asian immigrants, especially given that they are at high-risk for certain chronic disorders that are exacerbated by stress, as well as poor diet, racism and exclusion, and other social and environmental conditions that worsen physical health (Fenton and Sadiq-Sangster 1996; Lesser et al. 2014).

10.2 Factors to Consider in Treating SAAs

10.2.1 Client/Patient Factors

Bhugra and Mastrogianni (2004) identify culture as the learned, shared beliefs, values, attitudes and behaviors characteristic of a society or population. Ibrahim and Heuer (2016) note that culture is learned through the socialization process, and that it influences individual values, beliefs and assumptions, worldview, and modes of problem-solving and decision-making. Cultural psychiatry specifies that culture influences the sources, symptoms and the idioms of distress; including explanatory models, coping mechanisms, and help-seeking behavior, as well as the social response to distress, and to disability (Hussain and Cochrane 2002; Kirmayer 2001).

There are several pitfalls in working with cultural differences within the health domain, and these include: An assumption of shared definitions and meaning of illness constructs across languages, which can marginalize the impact of cultural and religious beliefs of the patient or client (Kleinman 1987). Kirmayer (2001) notes that in cultures where conflict, stress, anxiety, or depression are not publicly discussed, people tend to somaticize; whereas in cultures where these issues are openly addressed, there is a tendency to "psychologize" (p. 23). For example, there is considerable diversity among South Asian subgroups in their culture and religion, which influences their idioms of illness and health. Individuals in South Asia who were exposed to Western culture during the colonization of the subcontinent by the

British, may tend to psychologize their issues, whereas people in remote areas, such as the The Havik Brahmins, tend to use somatization (Nichter 1981). Fenton and Sadiq-Sangster (1996) state that very few studies with culturally different populations have focused on their perspective on mental illness. For example, South Asian Pathan women saw physical and mental illness on a continuum and always considered physical reasons for psychological issues, and also considered it fate, therefore nothing could be done about psychological pain (Currer 1986). Generic cultural information about South Asians may not apply to an individual, and it may be necessary to focus on the client's explanation and probe for understanding of what the health issue is, how it is understood and defined, and what would help (Ali 2014; American Psychiatric Association 2013b). Using an instrument such as the Cultural Identity Check List (Ibrahim 2008), cultural identity can be analyzed by exploring ethnicity, gender identification, sexual orientation, disability status, religion/spirituality, along with educational level of client and immediate family members, ability, social class, region the person grew up in, and were s/he lives now.

10.2.2 Acculturation Status

Health professionals must also understand acculturation status of patients as this is a complex process, given the generational differences among the SAA populations. Pumariega et al. (2005) note "increasingly, the process of cultural transition is being recognized as much as a psychological process as a sociological one, with significant implications for the mental health of immigrants" (p. 584). Along with the stress of acculturation and adaptation to a foreign culture, immigrants of color are subjected to exclusion, emotional and psychological abuse of racism, and rejection (Pascoe and Richman 2009). Perceived discrimination is linked to greater obesity, hypertension, greater likelihood of breast cancer, substance abuse, depression, anxiety and self-reported health problems (Ibrahim and Ohnishi 2001; Paradies 2006; Williams and Mohammad 2009; Williams et al. 2003). Since 2001, due to the terrorist attack on the US, South Asians have been subjected to increased instances of racism, exclusion, and discrimination, increasing their stress, due to prejudice (Ibrahim and Dykeman 2011; Tummala-Narra et al. 2011). Williams and Mohammad (2009) note that in general stressful experiences do not increase vulnerability to mental and physical illness, however, when stressors are unpredictable and uncontrollable, they are especially harmful to health.

Pascoe and Richman (2009) state that stress created by prejudice, exclusion, and discrimination may leave individuals with less energy or resources for making healthy behavior choices. Research supports this contention that perceived discrimination is related to health behaviors that have clear links to disease outcomes, e.g., smoking (Landrine and Klonoff 1996), alcohol and substance abuse (Bennett et al. 2005; Martin et al. 2003; Yen et al. 1999), as well as nonparticipation in behaviors that promote good health, such as cancer screening, diabetes management, and condom use (McSwan 2000; Ryan et al. 2008; Yoshikawa et al. 2004).

Frequently, the immigrant generation retains its primary culture to a large extent, especially if interaction is limited with the larger cultural system, such as for older adults who came to the U.S. with their adult children. Phinney and Ong (2007) postulated that immigrant ethnic identity development may involve two parallel dimensions: ethnic identity i.e., maintenance of cultural heritage, values, and practices; and a national identity, adoption of mainstream cultural assumptions, and ways of being. The relationship between the two dimensions varies, requiring professionals to understand the role of ethnic and national identities in an individual. A strong ethnic identity is associated with positive mental health (Phinney and Ong 2007; Smith and Silva 2011). Most US-educated South Asians tend to develop a bicultural identity and are able to negotiate mainstream culture effectively, in work and social settings. However, when they return home their identity often shifts back to culture of origin. This shift has elements of border-crossing phenomenon, and can create stress and discomfort (Marsico and Varzi 2016; Simão 2012). First and second generation immigrants are bicultural because of their immigrant parent's influence, and tend to value cultural assumptions of mainstream society over South Asian culture in social and work environments, they have not had as extensive an exposure to the cultural assumptions of their parents, except for secondhand information, and have been exposed to US culture from birth through school, peers, community, media, etc.; this factor is also considered a reason for chronic illnesses due to a preference for Western diet high in carbohydrates, red meat, and junk food (Patel 2012; Thakore-Dunlap and Van Velsor 2014). Given the variations in acculturation level, it is imperative that a health professional is able to assess, and understand the cultural identity and acculturation status of SAA clients. Research shows that migration is also a key determinant of increased risk of chronic diseases for South Asians, especially since migration has not led to increased risk of chronic disease among other ethnic groups, such as the Afro-Caribbean people (Pascoe and Richman 2009). Although, the reasons are not clear, since more research is needed, it is obvious that the stress of migration, along with the propensity for T2DM and other chronic diseases, the South Asian diet preference, may be important to be highly aggressive in implementing meaningful interventions to support health and reduction of stress among South Asians (Lakhanpaul et al. 2014; Lesser et al. 2014).

10.2.3 Health Care Provider Factors

Another barrier may be an overemphasis on the socially constructed meaning of ethnicity and race among health professionals without a full understanding of what an overarching ethnic term, such as South Asian, means to a South Asian client/patient (Bhopal et al. 1997: Parkes et al. 1997). Several researchers have identified that the terms South Asian, or Asian may not be what individuals from South Asia personally identify with, since differences in South Asia are defined regionally, e.g. Punjabi, Marathi, Bengali, etc. In addition, there are several different languages in

South Asia; there are approximately 300 languages and/or dialects in the Indian subcontinent (Mosely and Asher 1994).

Another possible limitation for Western-educated health professionals is the lack of understanding about the differences between Western and Eastern conception of mind and body as separate or holistic, which influences verbal expression of symptoms, the meaning of health and ill-health, and the ability of the health professional to understand what is communicated (Hussain and Cochrane 2002; Wilson and Maccarthy 1994). Speaking from a holistic perspective, the South Asian client/patient may explain their symptoms in a manner that addresses both mind and body and use local idioms of distress. For example, he/she may point to the chest, (i.e., the core area where emotional pain is experienced and expressed) and state that is where the pain is located. Yet, this does not necessarily mean it is a heart condition, as psychological pain of grief and loss is believed to be experienced in the area around the heart among South Asians (Currer 1986; Fenton and Sadiq-Sangster 1996; Ibrahim et al. 1997; Krause 1989).

Wheeler and Izzard (1997) focusing on the individual-community interaction of Western and Eastern cultures note that health professionals in the West understand their role to bring about change in an individual's situation, meanwhile in the East the role of the healer is to align the individual with collective values, the goal is to help the client to adjust to a situation. This factor influences whether the illness is ignored or treated. Collectivism, family duty, and role of an individual all influence how the client/patient will respond to health concerns. Providing for the family may be more important than taking the time to exercise and manage a diet regimen to combat impending or ongoing cardiovascular disease (Wheeler and Izzard 1997).

To promote good health and management of chronic health conditions it is important to understand the cultural beliefs and acculturation status of the individual, and how health or disease management is perceived. It is critical that cultural beliefs are understood within the context of acculturation status. Health providers must be cautious in assuming that simply knowing about culture of origin of a cultural group that they are knowledgeable about a specific client's cultural values and beliefs in promoting health and disease management. The psychological literature presents a general perspective on cultural assumptions of South Asian Americans, however these may not be sensitive to individual and regional cultural variations and the application of general information to a specific client may result in cultural oppression and malpractice (Dana 1998).

It is helpful in working with South Asian clients is to understand the client's acculturation level, i.e., Assimilation, Integration, Separation, and Marginalization are four acculturation strategies proposed by Berry (1997). Acculturation is perceived as having a positive or a negative effect on health (Njobvu et al. 1999). Similarity to host culture facilitates adaptation and results in Integration, in this strategy, an individual maintains pride in his/her/zir cultural identity, and functions effectively in host culture, as an accepted immigrant. Cultural and racial differences can result in rejection and exclusion in host culture (Pascoe and Richman 2009). This can lead to three other acculturation strategies, i.e., Assimilation, shedding culture of origin, without learning the new culture, or Separation, where the hold on culture of origin is maintained along with avoiding interaction with host culture; the third outcome is Marginalization. This occurs when cultural issues have not been resolved, and there is little interest in connecting with host culture due to exclusion or discrimination, along with disaffection with culture of origin (Berry 1997).

10.2.4 Common Cultural Assumptions

South Asians similar to other Asian cultures are highly collectivistic and influenced by Confucian principles of ordered positions of family members, with filial piety (Ibrahim and Ingram 2007; Ibrahim et al. 1997). Religion and spirituality play a significant role in the lives of South Asians, and religious beliefs tend to be stronger among immigrants than in successive generations (Haeri 1997; Ibrahim et al. 1997; Wilson and Maccarthy 1994). Although the core beliefs that are transmitted intergenerationally may not be evident to later generations, they are often maintained without conscious recognition (Ibrahim 2015; Ibrahim and Heuer 2016; Ibrahim et al. 1997; Walsh and McGoldrick 2004). Religious leaders may be sought for medical and psychological problems, and using prayer and religious verses cited by a religious leader can be seen as helpful and is a common practice in South Asia, and among recent immigrants (Ibrahim 2014). Somatization among South Asians may be attributed to spiritual beliefs, such as possession by a bad spirit, which would require a spiritual intervention instead of intervention by a Western-educated health professional (Cochrane and Sasidharan 1996); Hussain and Cochrane 2002; Ibrahim and Dykeman 2011).

Both religious and spiritual leaders may be employed in conjunction with Western medicine approaches (Hussain and Cochrane 2002). Another variable to consider when working with South Asians is to understand their indigenous healing system which include: Ayurvedic medicine, meditation, and yoga (Ali 2014). On the Indian subcontinent the first intervention is usually with Ayurvedic medicine. It is considered less intrusive and does not have the side effects of allopathic medicine (Patel et al. 2015). Ali (2014) notes that primary care medical professionals must discuss traditional (cultural) treatments and whether a patient is already being treated using Ayurvedic medicine, which includes natural ingredients but can interact with allopathic medicines.

Ali (2014) considers somatization also may occur due to cultural prohibitions against speaking about emotional distress, or discomfort, etc., due to the value of stoicism, and fear of stigmatization. The majority of South Asians visit a primary care physician for somatic problems (Atri et al. 1996; Balarajan et al. 1989). More acculturated individuals are likely to report more physical symptoms for psychological problems than less acculturated individuals, these findings are based on adjusted scores for psychological distress, medical conditions, and disability (Alegria et al. 2004). It also reflects acculturation and lack of recognition of culturally acquired behavior among highly acculturated individuals. Although the stereotype of somatization exists for South Asians, it is important to conduct a full medical evaluation before referring them for mental health services. For instance, the anxiety underlying somatic problems can be related to symptoms of emerging physical disorders (Ali 2014).

Another cultural value among South Asians is modesty. For example, as a result of modesty, women may not feel comfortable exercising in public facilities, possibly leading to lack of exercise (Ali 2014). Lack of exercise results in obesity and functions as a predisposition for cardiovascular disease and T2DM (Qiu et al. 2012). Other factors related to lack of physical exercise noted by patients is lack of time, collective orientation (taking care of others is more important than taking care of oneself), pain, tiredness, and depressive symptoms (Palaniappan et al. 2010; Qiu et al. 2012).

10.3 Making Interventions/Treatment with SAAs Culturally Sensitive

10.3.1 Making Medical Interventions Culture-Specific

To move beyond the impasse in reaching across cultural boundaries to convey the gravity of the situation of chronic diseases, it is important to use a communication model that is responsive to the cultural identity and context of the client (Betsch et al. in press; Ibrahim and Heuer 2016). Betsch et al., introduced the concept of culture-sensitive health communication, and define it as "the deliberate and evidence-informed adaptation of health communication to the recipient's cultural background in order to increase knowledge, to improve preparation for medical decision making, and to enhance the persuasiveness of messages in health promotion" (p. 3). Alden et al. (2014) assert that there is a gap in medical decision-making that is specific to differences in culture and the effect of cultural differences on the efficacy of health promotion programs. Alden et al. (2014) recommend that the process of communicating health promotion information should take into account the cultural identity and cultural context of an individual to enhance the effectiveness of medical interventions, e, g., incorporating a South Asian Punjabi patient's cultural beliefs, assumptions, and dietary preferences when making specific recommendations for medication and dietary restrictions (Misra 2011). Recent research indicates that the supportive sociocultural context, i.e., support from family and the community was very influential in adherence to medical recommendations for South Asian immigrants in Britain. Social support needs to be considered a critical variable in adherence to medication and health management (Patel et al. 2015). Similar recommendations, to have supportive networks, including familial and community are seen as a strength for psychological interventions (Ibrahim and Arredondo 1986; Ivey et al. 2008).

10.3.2 Culturally Responsive Communication

To facilitate cross-cultural communication, the recommended process in counseling and psychotherapy involves educating mental health professionals to first understand one's own cultural identity, worldview (values, beliefs, and assumptions), the context in which one was socialized, one's acculturation level to mainstream U.S. culture, and one's privilege and oppression (Ibrahim and Heuer 2016). In addition, it is recommended that professionals take the Implicit Attitude Test ([IAT], 2011; https://implicit.harvard.edu/implicit/) to recognize implicit biases that health professionals may hold, as a result of growing up in a hierarchical society (Ibrahim and Heuer 2016).

The next step involves learning to conduct the cultural assessments (cultural identity evaluation, worldview, acculturation status, privilege and oppression) to prepare to work in a diverse society. The final step is to learn about all the cultures (dominant and non-dominant) within this society, and to specifically focus on the hierarchies in the social system, access to opportunities, and challenges that people face due to their position in the system. Further, there is an emphasis on learning a communication strategy that is flexible and reflects the mode of communication used by the client (Ibrahim 2010; Ibrahim and Heuer 2016; Ivey et al. 2018). This requires a systematic training process that facilitates a health professionals' ability to understand the contexts clients' live in, to understand and accept their way of life, and to communicate this understanding effectively and with sensitivity. The central element of this process is to recognize, understand, and acknowledge their own way of being, cultural assumptions, biases and stereotypes, and to recognize their ability to understand the "other." Formal cultural assessments can be useful in recognizing cultural differences, and reduces the chance of making assumptions about clients' cultural identity, worldview, acculturation status, privilege and oppression. As professionals we assume that we have a sense of a client's culture, beliefs, and context, however, what we actually have is a generic understanding about a culture, and we do not understand the variations within a culture. Given the diversity among South Asian Americans (generational and developmental), it is imperative that health promotion professionals undergo intensive training and education that focuses on enhancing sensitivity, increasing knowledge, and skills to work with a culturally diverse clientele (Ibrahim 2010; Ibrahim and Heuer 2016).

10.3.3 Enhancing Sensitivity to Cultural Differences

To enhance cultural sensitivity professionals must undergo training and education, which includes experiential training. (Ibrahim and Heuer 2016; Pedersen and Ivey 2003; Ratts et al. 2015). To begin with, if professionals took the IAT they could learn about their implicit attitudes. In general, when we work in health-related professions, we assume that we care about people and therefore we are doing good work. The IAT generally creates dissonance between what we believe about ourselves when we are confronted with the results and they show us that growing up in a hierarchical society, we unconsciously hold biased assumptions about people, especially about vulnerable populations based on gender, sexual orientation, disability, religion, veteran and migration status (Banaji and Greenwald 1995; Banaji and Hardin 1996).

The experiential component helps individuals understand unconscious bias, and explore feelings. Further, it provides the opportunity to explore this with a group of peers. This exploration eventually includes experiential training with an emphasis on management of biases, especially when working with vulnerable populations (Pedersen and Ivey 2003). Additionally, experiential exercises are incorporated to understand how privilege and oppression functions in hierarchical social systems (Ibrahim 2010; Ibrahim and Heuer 2016). We tend to have a blind spot on these issues and there is an assumption that people are not taking care of themselves because they are choosing not to, or resistant. It is our responsibility to understand the contextual barriers that our clients and patients face, instead of assuming it is resistance (Ibrahim and Heuer 2016; Ivey et al. 2008). We should work toward helping them with options, referrals to appropriate agencies and sources that can help in overcoming environmental and societal barriers (ACA Advocacy Competencies 2003). It is critical for health professionals to be committed to social justice, given the oppression that cultural and non-dominant groups, including; women, LGBT, people with disabilities, immigrant, alternate religious communities face. The level playing field hypothesis is passé because we have increased our awareness about the challenges that people face in hierarchical social systems (ACA Advocacy Competencies 2003). These concerns have also been incorporated in the ethical principles of major mental health professional association, e.g. The American Counseling Association (2014), the American Psychological Association (2010), American Association of Marriage and Family Therapy (2015), American Psychiatric Association (2013a), National Association of Social Workers (2008). Incorporating cultural and social justice concerns in ethical codes and competency statements is not enough, professional associations and accrediting bodies or health-related fields need to develop and mandate training protocols to enhance sensitivity and competence in working with a diverse clientele (Ratts et al. 2015).

10.3.4 Specific Recommendations for South Asians: Chronic Disease Management

The psychological literature does not provide specific guidelines for chronic disease management for South Asians. Brown et al. (2002) conducted research with family physicians who work with patients with T2DM in UK. Brown et al. (2002) identified distinct facilitators and barriers to managing T2DM in three domains: patient, physician, and systemic factors. The three factors were related, however, education about the disease was important for all three domains. Brown et al. (2002) note that although this study focused on T2DM, the results are relevant for management of all chronic diseases. Education about appropriate dietary practices in order to lower the risk of chronic disease among South Asian immigrants is also emphasized by Jonnalagadda and Diwan (2002). They note that there is a need for in-depth examination of dietary and nutrient intake of this population to better understand the impact of their diet habits and practices on chronic disease risk, to allow health care providers to better meet the health care needs of this community.

Considering patient factors, the World Health Organization (WHO 2003) identified five interrelated factors that affect adherence to treatment regimen for chronic diseases. The WHO report notes that assuming that the patient is the only one who has responsibility for adhering to the treatment regimen is a misunderstanding. They recommend a multidisciplinary coordinated approach to helping people with chronic diseases. This includes: (a) socioeconomic factors (poverty, illiteracy, unemployment, unstable living conditions, lack of support systems, etc.); (b) patient-related factors (ability of patients to follow the prescribed regimen); (c) treatment-related factors (complexity of the medical regimen, duration of treatment, previous treatment failures, frequent changes in treatment, the immediacy of beneficial effects, side-effects, and the availability of medical support to deal with the side effects); (d) condition related factors (illness-related demands faced by the patient); and (e) health-system related factors (effect of health care team and system-related factors on adherence).

Although, general information for enhancing cross-cultural interventions exists, there is limited information about facilitating adherence to chronic disease treatment for South Asian immigrants. Our goal in this section is to formulate some meaningful guidelines to assist South Asian American clients from a cultural perspective to enhance adherence to a medical regimen for chronic disorders. However, it is important to note that generic recommendations do not apply to specific individuals from a cultural group; therefore, care is needed when considering cultural issues specific to a cultural subgroup (Groce 1992; Groce and Zola 1993). Exploring cultural assumptions instead of assuming that a specific South Asian patient would be identical to any description of South Asians found in the literature is very important. Considering all available resources, we propose the following recommendations for a culturally-informed understanding of the South Asian client/patient profile:

1. An important consideration when working with South Asians is the sociocultural context (primary family, extended family, and community of expatriate South Asians (Patel et al. 2015). This environment can be both a facilitator and a challenge in adherence to chronic disease. Sociocultural environment can facilitate recovery by supporting the person in maintaining proper diet and exercise. Collectivism, and duty to be a good family member or kin, can lead to denying personal self-management needs in order to take care of others as providers, and care-takers, etc., (Betsch et al. in press; Wheeler and Izzard 1997).

2. Incorporate indigenous, religious, cultural and social justice considerations about medicine and healing in the therapeutic process (Anderson et al. 2010; Kessler et al. 2013). Considering the benefits of yoga and meditation, and the fact that it is culturally meaningful, incorporate them in the ongoing disease management protocol (Ali 2014; Davidson et al. 2003). Betsch et al., note that to provide effective health communication empirical and theoretical understanding of culture is indispensable. One cultural belief that can be a challenge is fatalism (Ali 2014).
3. Understand the role of stigma and its influence on adherence to the treatment regimen (Ali 2014; Weiss and Ramakrishna 2006; WHO 2003). Illness-related stigma is a critical cultural barrier for South Asians. It is considered the biggest threat to the next generation and their matrimonial prospects. Before considering marriage, South Asians investigate mental and physical disorders in a family for several generations before proposing marriage, to allay fears that the disorders may be transmitted to later generations (Weiss and Ramakrishna 2006).
4. Focus on listening to the client's explanation of the symptoms, and what would help (Castillo 1997; Kleinman 1987). Self-reflection for the health professional on personal beliefs, life experiences, and explanatory models is critical, along with looking at potentially biased attitudes. Confronting and the ability to recognize our personal beliefs and remaining open to the beliefs, life experiences and explanatory models of others, and reflecting on one's own reactions to people and their settings is imperative (Anderson et al. 2010).
5. Recognize the psychological implications of chronic disease (Gonzalez et al. 2011). Specifically, depression and anxiety are common comorbid disorders with chronic diseases. Specifically, with South Asians somatic symptoms are an indication of psychological distress, and possibly of emerging chronic disease (Ali 2014; Fenton and Sadiq-Sangster 1996).
6. Approach clients with sensitivity and care and understand their strengths and challenges (Ivey et al. 2009). To build trust, which is essential for medical interventions, it is necessary to be sincere and respectful toward patients. If there are cultural language barriers, arrangements should be made prior to the first encounter for a medical translator to lay the foundation for a trusting relationship (Anderson et al. 2010).
7. Understand the interacting factors that influence adherence to chronic disease maintenance (WHO 2003), these include: Socioeconomic issues, health care team and system-related factors, condition-related factors, and therapy-related factors (Brown et al. 2002; WHO 2003).
8. Anderson et al. (2010) emphasize recognizing the power differential between the provider and the patient/family, especially with diverse clients, in this case recent immigrants who come from a distinctly different cultural environments to enhance adherence to treatment management.

10.4 Conclusion

This chapter focuses on issues in counseling while working with South Asian immigrants and their progeny in the management of chronic diseases. A brief overview of chronic diseases among South Asian immigrants was presented. Cultural beliefs and assumptions influencing perceptions of illness and cure including spiritual, religious, and Ayurvedic medicine were reviewed; along with the effect of migration and acculturation. Generic South Asian culture was also explored to understand general assumptions of the cultural group. In addition, psychological implications of chronic diseases were also presented. Specific information on enhancing cross-cultural communication between health professionals from a Western individualistic culture and South Asian patients with chronic illness was presented to facilitate adherence to treatment regimen. Finally, the chapter ends with specific guidelines for working with South Asian patients with chronic diseases.

References

Abate, N., & Chandalia, M. (2001). Ethnicity and type 2 diabetes: Focus on Asian Indians. *Journal of Diabetes and its Complications, 15*(6), 320–327.

Ahmed, K., & Bhugra, D. (2007). Depression across ethnic minority cultures: Diagnostic issues. *World Cultural Psychiatry Review*, 47–56 Retrieved from: http://www.wcprr.org.

Alden, D. L., Friend, J., Schapira, M., & Stiggelbout, A. (2014). Cultural targeting and tailoring of shared decision making technology: A theoretical framework for improving the effectiveness of patient decision aids in culturally diverse groups. *Social Science & Medicine, 105*, 1–8.

Alegria, M., Takeuchi, D., Canino, G., Duan, N., Shrout, P., Meng, X. L., et al. (2004). Considering context, place and culture: The national latino and asian american study. *International Journal of Methods in Psychiatric Research, 13*(4), 208–220.

Ali, S. (2014). Identification and approach to treatment of mental health disorders in Asian American populations. In S. Parekh (Ed.), *The Massachusetts General Hospital textbook on diversity and cultural sensitivity in mental health, current clinical psychiatry* (pp. 31–59). New York: Springer Science+Business Media.

American Association of Marriage and Family Therapy. (2015). *Code of ethics*. Alexandria: American Association of Marriage and Family Therapy.

American Counseling Association (ACA). (2003). *Advocacy competencies*. Alexandria: American Counseling Association.

American Counseling Association (ACA). (2014). *Ethical code*. Alexandria: American Counseling Association.

American Psychiatric Association. (2013a). *The principles of medical ethics with annotations especially applicable to psychiatry*. Arlington: American Psychiatric Association www.psychiatry.org. Accessed 24 June 2015.

American Psychiatric Association. (2013b). *The diagnostic and statistical manual of mental disorders (DSM-5*, 5th). Arlington: American Psychiatric Association.

American Psychological Association. (2010). *Ethical principles of psychologists and code of conduct*. Washington, DC: American Psychological Association.

Anderson, N. L. R., Boyle, J. S., Davidhizar, R. E., Giger, J. N., McFarland, M. R., Papadopoulos, T., Purnell, L., Spector, R., Tilki, M., & Wehbe-Alamah, H. (2010). Cultural health assessment. *Journal of Transcultural Nursing, 21*(Supplement I), 3075–3365.

Atri, J., Falshaw, M., Livingstone, A., & Robson, J. (1996). Fair shares in healthcare? Ethnic and socioeconomic influences on recording of preventive care in selected inner London general practices. *British Medical Journal, 312*, 614–617.

Balarajan, R., Yuen, P., & Soni, R. V. (1989). Ethnic differences in general practitioner consultations. *British Medical Journal, 299*, 958–960.

Ballenger, J. C., Davidson, J. R., Lecrubier, Y., Nutt, D. J., Kirmayer, L. J., Lepine, J. P., Lin, K. M., Tajima, O., & Ono, Y. (2001). Consensus statement on transcultural issues in depression and anxiety from the international consensus group on depression and anxiety. *Journal of Clinical Psychiatry, 62*(S13), 47–55.

Banaji, M. R., & Greenwald, A. G. (1995). Implicit gender stereotyping in judgments of fame. *Journal of Personality and Social Psychology, 68*, 181–198.

Banaji, M. R., & Hardin, C. D. (1996). Automatic stereotyping. *Psychological Science, 7*, 136–141.

Barnett, A. H., Dixon, A. N., Bellary, S., Hanif, M. W., O'Hare, J. P., Raymond, N. T., et al. (2006). Type 2 diabetes and cardiovascular risk in the UK South Asian community. *Diabetologia, 49*, 2234–2246.

Becerra, M. B., Herring, P., Marshak, H. H., Banta, J. E. (2014). Generational differences in fast food intake among South-Asian Americans: Results from a population-based survey. *Preventing Chronic Disease, 11*. Retrieved from: https://www.cdc.gov/pcd/issues/2014/14_0351.htm

Bennett, G. G., Wolin, K. Y., Robinson, E. L., Fowler, S., & Edwards, C. L. (2005). Perceived racial/ethnic harassment and tobacco use among African American young adults. *American Journal of Public Health, 95*(2), 238–240. https://doi.org/10.2105/AJPH.2004.037812.

Berry, J. W. (1997). Immigration, acculturation, and adaptation. *Applied Psychology: An International Review, 46*(1), 5–68.

Betsch, C., Bohm, R., Butler, R., Haase, N., Hermann, B., Igarashi, T., et al. (in press). Improving medical decision making and health promotion through culture-sensitive health communication – An agenda for science and practice. *Medical Decision-making* (accepted July 2015).

Bharmal, N. H. (2012). *Acculturation and religiosity as moderators of cardiovascular disease risk among South Asians in the United States*. Doctoral dissertation, UCLA. http://escholarship.org/uc/item/3g07b107. Accessed 15 June 2016.

Bhopal, R. S., Phillimore, P., & Kohli, H. S. (1997). Inappropriate use of the term asian: An obstacle to ethnicity and health research. *Journal of Public Health Medicine, 13*, 244–245.

Bhugra, D. (2004). Migration, distress and cultural identity. *British Medical Bulletin, 69*, 1–13.

Bhugra, D., & Mastrogianni, A. (2004). Globalisation and mental disorders. Overview with relation to depression. *British Journal of Psychiatry, 184*, 10–20.

Bhugra, D., & Becker, M. A. (2005). Migration, cultural bereavement, and cultural identity. *World Psychology, 4*(1), 18–24 http://www.ncbi.nlm.nih.gov/pmc/articles/PMC1414713/pdf/wpa040018.Pdf. Accessed 10 June 2016.

Brown, J. B., Harris, S. B., Webster-Bogaert, S., Wetmore, S., Faulds, C., & Stewart, M. (2002). The role of patient, physician and systemic factors in the management of type 2 diabetes mellitus. *Family Practice, 19*(4), 344–349. https://doi.org/10.1093/fampra/19.4.344.

Castillo, R. J. (1997). *Culture and mental Illness: A client-centered approach*. Pacific Grove, CA: Brooks/Cole.

Cochrane, R., & Sasidharan, S. V. (1996). Mental health and ethnic minorities: A review of the literature and implications for services. In W. Ahmed, T. Sheldon, & O. Stuart (Eds.), *Ethnicity and Health*. New York: NHS Centre for Reviews and Dissemination (Report 5).

Currer, C. (1986). Concepts of mental well- and ill-being: The case of Pathan mothers in Britain. In C. Currer & M. Stacey (Eds.), *Concepts of health, illness and disease: A comparative perspective* (pp. 236–251). Leamington Spa: Berg.

Dana, R. J. (1998). *Understanding cultural identity in intervention and assessment*. Thousand Oaks, CA: Sage.

Davidson, R. J., Kabat-Zinn, J., Schumacher, J., Rosenkranz, M., Muller, D., Santorelli, S. F., Urbanowski, F., Harrington, A., Bonus, K., & Sheridan, J. F. (2003). Alterations in brain and immune function produced by mindfulness meditation. *Psychosomatic Medicine, 65*, 564–570.

DiMatteo, D. R., Lepper, H. S., & Croghan, T. W. (2000). Depression is a risk factor for noncompliance with medical treatment: Meta-analysis of the effects of anxiety and depression on patient adherence. *JAMA Internal Medicine, 160*(14). https://doi.org/10.1001/archinte.160.14.2101.

Fenton, S., & Sadiq-Sangster, A. (1996). Culture, relativism and the expression of mental distress: South Asian women in Britain. *Sociology of Health & Illness, 18*(1), 66–85.

Gonzalez, J. S., Esbitt, S. A., Schneider, H. E., Osborne, P. J., & Kupperman, E. G. (2011). Psychological issues in adults with Type 2 Diabetes. In S. Pagoto (Ed.), *Psychological co-morbidities of physical illness: A behavioral medicine perspective*. New York: Springer Science Business Media. https://doi.org/10.1007/978-1-4419-0029-6_2.

Ford, E. S. (2005). Risks for all-cause mortality, cardiovascular disease, and diabetes associated with the metabolic syndrome: A summary of the evidence. *Diabetes Care, 28*, 1769–1778.

Garber, A. J. (2004). The metabolic syndrome. *Medical Clinics of North America, 88*, 837–846.

Groce, N. (1992). Comparative and cross-cultural issues. *Disability Studies Quarterly, 10*(1), 1–39.

Groce, N., & Zola, I. K. (1993). Multiculturalism, chronic illness, and disability. *Pediatrics, 91*(5), 1048–1055 http://www.ncbi.nlm.nih.gov/pubmed/8479830. Accessed 10 June 2016.

Gujral, U. P., 1 R. Pradeepa, I. R., Weber, M. B., Venkat Narayan, K.M. & Mohan, V. (2013). Type 2 diabetes in south asians: Similarities and differences with white Caucasian and other populations. Annals of the New York Society of Sciences, 1281, 51–63.

Gupta, R., Deedwania, P. C., Gupta, A., Rastogi, S., Panwar, R. B., & Kothari, K. (2004). Prevalence of metabolic syndrome in an Indian urban population. *International Journal of Cardiology, 97*(2), 257–261.

Haeri, N. (1997). *The Sociolinguistic Market of Cairo: Gender, Class and Education*. London and New York: Kegan Paul International.

Henry, H. M., Stiles, W. B., & Biran, M. W. (2005). Loss and mourning in immigration: Using the assimilation model to assess continuing bonds with native culture. *Counselling Psychology Quarterly, 18*(2), 109–119. https://doi.org/10.1080/09515070500136819.

Hsu, S. (1999). Somatisation among asian refugees and immigrants as a culturally-shaped illness behaviour. *Annals of the Academy of Medicine, Singapore, 28*(6), 841–845.

Hussain, F. A., & Cochrane, R. (2002). Depression in South Asian women: Asian women's beliefs on causes and cures. *Mental Health, Religion & Culture, 5*(3), 285–311.

Ibrahim, F. A. (2008). *The cultural identity check list (revised)*. Denver, CO: Copy written document.

Ibrahim, F. A. (2010). Innovative teaching strategies for group work: Addressing cultural responsiveness and social justice. *Journal for Specialists in Group Work, 35*(3), 271–280.

Ibrahim, F. A. (2014, June). *Counseling South Asian Americans and International Students*. Invited two-day training for Texas A&M College Counseling World Conference. College Station, TX.

Ibrahim, F. A. (2015, January). *Counseling South Asian American immigrants. Presentation at the APA National Multicultural Counseling Summit*. GA: Atlanta.

Ibrahim, F. A., & Arredondo, P. M. (1986). Ethical standards for cross-cultural counseling: Counselor preparation, practice, assessment, and research. *Journal of Counseling and Development, 64*, 349–352.

Ibrahim, F. A., & Dykeman, C. (2011). Muslim-Americans: Cultural and spiritual assessment for counseling. *Journal of Counseling and Development, 89*, 387–396.

Ibrahim, F. A., & Heuer, J. R. (2016). *Cultural and social justice counseling: Client specific interventions*. New York: Springer Business+Science Media.

Ibrahim, F. A., & Ingram, M. A. (2007). Counseling South Asian international students. In R. Singaravelu & M. Pope (Eds.), *Counseling international students* (pp. 195–211). Alexandria: ACA Press.

Ibrahim, F. A., & Ohnishi, H. (2001). PTSD and the minority experience. In D. Pope-Davis & H. Coleman (Eds.), *Intersection of race, class, and gender in multicultural counseling* (pp. 89–126). Thousand Oaks: Sage.

Ibrahim, F. A., Ohnishi, H., & Sandhu, D. (1997). Asian-American identity development: South Asian Americans. *Journal of Multicultural Counseling and Development, 25*, 34–50.

Implicit Association Test (IAT). (2011). http://implicit.harvard.edu. Accessed 24 June 2016.
Ivey, A. E., Pedersen, P. B., & Ivey, M. B. (2008). Group Microskills: Culture-centered group process and strategies. Alexandria: American Counseling Association.
Ivey, A. E., Ivey, M. B., & Zalaquett, C. (2018). *Intentional interviewing and counseling: Facilitating client development in a multicultural world.* Boston, MA: Cengage.
Jackson-Triche, M. E., Sullivan, G. J., Wells, K. B., Rogers, W., Camp, P., & Mazel, R. (2000). Depression and health-related quality in ethnic minorities seeking care in general medical settings. *Journal of Affective Disorders, 58*, 89–97.
Jonnalagadda, S. S., & Diwan, S. (2002). *A Brown Paper: The Health of South Asians in the United States*. Retrieved from: http://www.sapha.org/pages.php?id=42
Katon, W., Ries, R. K., & Kleinman, A. (1984). The prevalence of somatization in primary care. *Comprehensive Psychiatry, 25*, 208–215.
Kessler, L. G., Cleary, P. D., & Burke, J. D., Jr. (1985). Psychiatric disorders in primary care: Results of a follow-up study. *Archives of General Psychiatry, 42*, 583–587.
Kessler, R. C., Berglund, P. A., Bruce, M. L., Koch, J. R., Lask, E. M., Leaf, P. J., et al. (2001). The prevalence and correlates of untreated serious mental illness. *Health Services Research, 36*, 987–1007.
Kessler, C., Wischnewsky, M., Michalsen, A., Eisenmann, C., & Melzer, C. (2013). Ayurveda: Between religion, spirituality, and medicine. *Evidence-Based Complementary and Alternative Medicine*. https://doi.org/10.1155/2013/952432.
Kirmayer, L. J. (2001). Cultural variations in the clinical presentation of depression and anxiety: Implications for diagnosis and treatment. *Journal of Clinical Psychiatry, 62*, 22–28.
Kirmayer, L. J., & Young, A. (1998). Culture ad somatization: Clinical epidemiological and ethnographic perspectives. *Psychosomatic Medicine, 60*, 420–430.
Kleinman, A. (1987). Anthropology and psychiatry: The role of culture in cross-cultural research in illness. *British Journal of Psychiatry, 151*, 447–454.
Krause, I. B. (1989). Sinking heart: A Punjabi communication of distress. *Social Science and Medicine, 29*(4), 563–567.
Lakhanpaul, M., Bird, F., Manikam, L., Culley, L., Perkins, G., Hudson, N., Wilson, J., & Hudson, M. (2014). A systematic review of barriers and facilitators to improving asthma management in South Asian children. *Biomedical Central Public Health, 14*, 403 http://www.biomedcentral.com/1471-2458/14/403.
Landrine, H., & Klonoff, E. A. (1996). The schedule of racist events: A measure of racial discrimination and a study of its negative physical and mental health consequences. *Journal of Black Psychology, 22*(2), 144–168.
Laws, A., Jeppesen, J. L., Maheux, P. C., Schaaf, P., Ida Chen, Y. D., & Reaven, G. (1994). Resistance to insulin-stimulated glucose uptake and dyslipidemia in Asian Indians. *Arteriosclerosis and Thrombosis, 14*(6), 917–922.
Lecrubier, Y. (2001). Prescribing patterns for depression and anxiety worldwide. *Journal of Clinical Psychiatry, 62*, 31–36.
Lesser, I. A., Gasevic, D., & Lear, S. A. (2014). The association between acculturation and dietary patterns of south Asian immigrants. *PLoS One, 9*(2), e88495. https://doi.org/10.1371/journal.pone.0088495.
Li, C., Ford, E. S., Zhao, G., Strine, T. W., Dhingra, S., Barker, L., et al. (2009). Association between diagnosed diabetes and serious psychological distress among U.S. adults: The behavioral risk factor surveillance system, 2007. *International Journal of Public Health, 54*, S43–S51.
Lin, H. B., Carter, W. B., & Kleinman, A. M. (1985). An exploration of somatization among Asian refugees and immigrants in primary care. *American Journal of Public Health, 75*(9), 1080–1084.
Lovegrove, J. A. (2007). CVD risk in south Asians: The importance of defining adiposity and influence of dietary polyunsaturated fat. *Proceedings of the Nutrition Society, 66*, 286–298.
Marsico, G., & Varzi, A. (2016). Psychological and social borders: Regulating relationships. In J. Valsiner, G. Marsico, N. Chaudhary, T. Sato, & V. Dazzani (Eds.), *Psychology as a sci-*

ence of human being: The Yokohama Manifesto, Annals of Theoretical Psychology (Vol. 13, pp. 327–335). Geneva: Springer.

Martin, J. K., Tuch, S. A., & Roman, P. M. (2003). Problem drinking patterns among African Americans: The impacts of reports of discrimination, perceptions of prejudice, and "risky" coping strategies. *Journal of Health and Social Behavior, 44*(3), 408–425.

McKeigue, P. M., Pierpoint, T., Ferrie, J. E., & Marmot, M. G. (1992). Relationship of glucose intolerance and hyperinsulinaemia to body fat pattern in south Asians and Europeans. *Diabetologia, 35*, 785–791.

McSwan, K. L. (2000). The impact of sexism on older women's mental and physical health (Doctoral dissertation, Loma Linda University). *Dissertation Abstracts International, 61*(6B), 3323.

Mezuk, B., Eaton, W. W., Albrecht, S., & Golden, S. H. (2008). Depression and type 2 diabetes over the lifespan: A meta-analysis. *Diabetes Care, 31*(12), 383–390.

Misra, R. (2011). Epidemiology, risks, and complications of type 2 diabetes mellitus. In R. Misra (Ed.), *Indian foods: AAPI Guide to nutrition health and diabetes* (2nd ed., pp. 6–10). Chennai: Allied Publishers Private. Ltd.

Misra, A., & Vikram, N. K. (2007). Metabolic syndrome in children and adolescents: Problems in definition, and ethnicity-related determinants. *Diabetes and Metabolic Syndrome: Clinical Research and Reviews, 1*(2), 121–126.

Mosely, C., & Asher, R. E. (1994). *Atlas of the world languages*. London: Routledge.

National Association of Social Workers. (2008). *Code of ethics*. Washington, DC: National Association of Social Workers.

National Institute of Diabetes and Digestive and Kidney Diseases (NIDDK). (2014). *Insulin resistance and prediabetes*. http://www.niddk.nih.gov/health-information/health-topics/Diabetes/insulin-resistance-prediabetes/Pages/index.aspx. Accessed 15 June 2016.

Nazroo, J. Y. (2001). South Asian people and heart disease: an assessment of the importance of socioeconomic position. *Ethnicity & Disease, 11*, 401–411.

Nichter, M. (1981). Idioms of distress: Alternatives in the expression of psychosocial distress: A case study from South Asia. *Culture, Medicine, and Psychiatry, 5*(4), 379–408.

Njobvu, P., Hunt, I., Pope, D., & MacFarlane, G. (1999). Pain amongst ethnic minority groups of South Asian descent in the United Kingdom. *Rheumatology, 38*, 1184–1187.

Palaniappan, L.P., Araneta, M. R. G., Assimes, T. L., Barrett-Connor, E. L., Carnethon, M. R., Criqui, M. H., Fung, G. L., Narayan, K. M. V., Patel, H., Taylor-Piliae, R. E., Wilson, P. W. F., Wong, N. D. (2010). *AHA health advisory. Call to action: Cardiovascular disease in Asian Americans*. http://circ.ahajournals.org/content/122/12/1242.full. Accessed 14 September 2015.

Paradies, Y. (2006). A systematic review of empirical research on self- reported racism and health. *International. Journal of Epidemiology, 35*(4), 888–901.

Parkes, C. M., Laungani, P., & Young, B. (1997). *Death and bereavement across cultures*. London: Routledge.

Pascoe, E. A., & Smart Richman, L. (2009). Perceived discrimination and health: a meta-analytic review. *Psychological Bulletin, 135*(4), 531–554. https://doi.org/10.1037/a0016059.

Patel, J. (2012). To assimilate or to acculturate? *Experience and Other Evidence Essays*. University of Maryland English Department. http://www.english.umd.edu/interpolations/3460. Accessed 8 June 2016.

Patel, N. R., Chew-Graham, C., Bundy, C., Kennedy, A., Blickem, C., & Reeves, D. (2015). Illness beliefs and the sociocultural context of diabetes self-management in British South Asians: A mixed methods study. *BMC Family Practice, 16*, 58–69. https://doi.org/10.1186/s12875-015-0269-y.

Pedersen, P. B., & Ivey, A. E. (2003). Culture-centered exercises to teach basic group skills. *Canadian Journal of Counselling, 37*(3), 197–204.

Phinney, J. S., & Ong, A. D. (2007). Conceptualization and measurement of ethnic identity: Current status and future directions. *Journal of Counseling Psychology, 54*, 271–281.

Pumariega, A. J., Rothe, E., & Pumariega, J. B. (2005). Mental health of immigrants and refugees. *Community Mental Health Journal, 41*(5), 581–597. https://doi.org/10.1007/s10597-005-6363-1.

Qiu, S., Sun, Z., Cai, Z., Liu, L., & Yang, B. (2012). Improving patients' adherence to physical activity in diabetes mellitus: A review. *Diabetes Metabolism Journal, 36*, 1–5. https://doi.org/10.4093/dmj.2012.36.1.1 Accessed 8 October 2015.

Raj, S. (2011). Introduction. In R. Misra (Ed.), *Indian foods: AAPI guide to nutrition health and diabetes* (2nd ed., pp. 1–5). Chennai: Allied Publishers Private. Ltd.

Ratts, M. J., Singh, A. A., Nassar-McMillan, S., Butler, S. K., & McCullough, J. R. (2015). *Multicultural and social justice counseling competencies*. http://www.multiculturalcounseling.org/index.php?option=com_content&view=article&id=205:amcd-endorses-multicultural-and-social-justice-counselingcompetencies&catid=1:latest&Itemid=123. Accessed 24 June 2016.

Rogers-Sirin, L., Ryce, P., & Sirin, S. R. (2014). Acculturation, acculturative stress, and cultural mismatch and their influences on immigrant children and adolescents' well-being. In R. Dimitrova et al. (Eds.), *Global perspectives on well-being in immigrant families* (pp. 11–30). New York: Springer Science+Business Media.

Ryan, A. M., Gee, G. C., & Griffith, D. (2008). The effects of perceived discrimination on diabetes management. *Journal of Health Care for the Poor and Underserved, 19*, 149–163.

Sartorius, N., Üstün, T., Lecrubier, Y., & Wittchen, H. U. (1996). Depression comorbid with anxiety: Results from the WHO study on psychological disorders in primary health care. *British Journal of Psychiatry, 168*(30), 38–43.

Sattar, N., & Gill, J. M. R. (2015). Type 2 diabetes in migrant south Asians: Mechanisms, mitigation, and management. *The Lancet Diabetes and Endocrinology, 3*(12), 1004–1115. https://doi.org/10.1016/S2213-8587(15)00326-5.

Sikand, G. (2011). In R. Misra (Ed.), *Indian foods: AAPI guide to nutrition health and diabetes* (2nd ed., pp. 11–22). Chennai: Allied Publishers Private. Ltd.

Simão, L. M. (2012). The other in the self: A triadic unit. In J. Valsiner (Ed.), *The Oxford handbook of culture and psychology* (pp. 403–420). New York: Oxford University Press.

Simmons, D., Williams, D. R. R., & Powell, M. J. (1989). Prevalence of diabetes in a predominantly Asian community: Preliminary findings of the coventry diabetes study. *British Medical Journal, 298*, 18–21.

Smith, T. B., & Silva, L. (2011). Ethnic identity and personal well-being of people of color. A meta-analysis. *Journal of Counseling Psychology, 58*, 42–60.

Tan, C., Chew, S., & Tai, E. (2004). The metabolic syndrome: An Asian perspective. *International Congress Series, 1262*, 546–549.

Thakore-Dunlap, U., & Van Velsor, P. (2014). Group counseling with South Asian immigrant girls: Reflections and commentary of a group facilitator. *The Professional Counselor, 4*(5), 505–518.

Tummala-Narra, P., Inman, A. G., & Ettigi, S. P. (2011). Asian Indians' responses to discrimination: A mixed-method examination of identity, coping, and self-esteem. *Asian American Journal of Psychology, 2*(3), 205–218.

Tziomalos, K., Weerasinghe, C. N., Mikhailidis, D. P., & Seifalian, A. M. (2008). Vascular risk factors in South Asians. *International Journal of Cardiology, 128*, 5–16.

Walsh, F., & McGoldrick, M. (2004). *Living beyond loss: Death in the family (2nd., Ed.)*. New York: W. W. Norton.

Weiss, M. G., & Ramakrishna, J. (2006). Health-related stigma: Rethinking concepts and interventions. *Psychology Health Medicine, 11*(3), 277–287. https://doi.org/10.1080/13548500600595053.

Wheeler, S., & Izzard, S. (1997). Psychodynamic counsellor training—Integrating differences. *Psychodynamic Counselling, 3*, 401–417.

Williams, D. R., & Mohammed, S. A. (2009). Discrimination and racial disparities in health: Evidence and needed research. *Journal of Behavioral Medicine, 32*, 20–47.

Williams, D. R., Neighbors, H. W., & Jackson, J. S. (2003). Racial/ethnic discrimination and health: Findings from community studies. *American Journal of Public Health, 93*(2), 200–208.
Wilson, M., & Maccarthy, B. (1994). Consultation as a factor in the low rate of mental health service use by Asians. *Journal of Psychological Medicine, 20*, 113–119.
World Health Organization (WHO). (2003). *Adherence to long term therapies: Evidence for action*. Geneva: World Health Organization.
Yen, I. H., Ragland, D. R., Grenier, B. A., & Fisher, J. M. (1999). Workplace discrimination and alcohol consumption: Findings from the San Francisco muni health and safety study. *Ethnicity & Disease, 9*(1), 70–80.
Yoshikawa, H., Wilson, P. D., Chae, D. H., & Cheng, J. (2004). Do family and friendship networks protect against the influence of discrimination on mental health and HIV risk among Asian and Pacific Islander gay men? *AIDS Education and Prevention, 16*(1), 84–100.

Chapter 11
South Asian American Health Research and Policy

Chandak Ghosh

11.1 Introduction

Governmental policies specifically addressing the health needs of South Asian Americans remain non-existent at the federal and state levels. Despite the recent understanding that South Asians Americans are among the fastest growing ethnicities in the United States, movement to understand their health needs through governmental mechanisms has been limited. There are many reasons for this: As governmental policies are created mainly by effective advocacy and because of large population size, South Asian Americans have demonstrated neither in the United States historically. According to the 2010 U.S. Census, more than 3.4 million South Asians live in the U.S., so they account for only 1% of the population. Seventy-to-eighty percent are foreign-born, with nearly 50% remaining non-US citizens, giving less impetus for U.S. legislators to act (South Asian Americans Leading Together – SAALT & Asian American Federation 2012). There are few South Asian Americans in positions of leverage to impact policy changes. South Asian Americans find speaking with one voice to advocate for policies and research problematic. Coming to the United States from different, often rival, countries, cultures, languages, religions, castes, and social classes, they tend not see themselves as part of the same ethnic group. Finally, the stereotype of the South Asian Americans being doctors or computer engineers supports and maintains the "model minority" myth that Asian Americans do not have major health or healthcare access issues because most are educated, wealthy, and well-connected (Lin-Fu 1993). SAALT (2009), however, shows that South Asian Americans are affected by health conditions at rates higher

C. Ghosh (✉)
U.S. Department of Health and Human Services, Human Resources and Services Administration, New York, NY, USA
e-mail: CGhosh@hrsa.gov

M. J. Perera, E. C. Chang (eds.), *Biopsychosocial Approaches to Understanding Health in South Asian Americans*, Cross-Cultural Research in Health, Illness and Well-Being, https://doi.org/10.1007/978-3-319-91120-5_11

than would be expected for the population size. These include heart disease, diabetes, cancer (prostate, colorectal, lung, breast, ovarian, uterine), tuberculosis, HIV/AIDS, mental health (suicide, stigma in seeking professional help, acculturation difficulties). South Asian Americans also face language access barriers when seeing healthcare professionals and encountering public health messages. Nearly all of these health conditions are preventable and medically treatable. Science-driven governmental health policies would be the most effective tools to create uniformity in targeting South Asian Americans with public health campaigns, screening for disease, and developing culturally-appropriate referral mechanisms for treatment.

With the creation of the term "Asian American, Native Hawaiian, and other Pacific Islanders," (AAHNOPI) or its previous iteration "Asian Americans and Pacific Islanders" (AAPI), Americans with Asian heritage joined as a political and social force to establish a solid presence and advocate for health initiatives centered on their needs. Representing more than 50 ethnic groups and speaking more than 100 languages, AANHOPI make up 6 percentage (20.3 million) of the American population (U.S. Census 2016). Their growth rate predicts a doubling to 43 million or 9.3% of the population by 2060 (Colby and Ortman 2014). This leverage has made policymakers take notice. Unfortunately, South Asian Americans feel excluded from the "AANHOPI" term (Bijlani 2005), although, at 3.8 million residents, 18.7% of all Asian Americans, Indians are in the top three most populous Asian American groups (U.S. Census 2016). South Asians and East Asians are historically and culturally distinct (Lam and Palsane 1997). However, as "AANHOPI" is gaining acceptance as the avenue to effect change, it may be beneficial for all Asian Americans to identify, at least generally, with the umbrella term for the purpose of effective governmental advocacy.

11.2 Federal Understanding of Health Disparities in Racial and Ethnic Minorities

The health of racial and ethnic minorities became a federal concern after the publication of *Report of the Secretary's Task Force of Black and Minority Health* in 1985 (Heckler 1985). This "Heckler Report," named for Margaret Heckler, the Secretary of the U.S. Department of Health and Human Services (HHS) at the time, was the first major federal document to reveal that ethnic and racial minorities experienced different health outcomes than white Americans. Without naming the reasons for these health disparities, the Heckler Report called for more research and data collection.

A decade later, President Clinton commenced the *Initiative on Race* in 1998 to examine thoroughly how the American view of race had affected the country's history and aspirations of its citizens. Its health section, the *Initiative to Eliminate Racial and Ethnic Disparities in Health*, examined six specific areas: cancer, cardiovascular disease, diabetes, HIV/AIDS, immunizations, and infant mortality (Health Resources and Services Administration 1998). In 2000, HHS published

Healthy People 2010, the guide for the federal government and, thus, federal grant funding, to follow over the decade to gauge improvement in the country's health status (HHS 2000). It contained 28 health categories, each with objectives and targets to reach by the end of the decade. The six areas from the 1998 *Initiative* were included in *Healthy People 2010* as health areas to watch especially for disparate treatment and outcomes for racial and ethnic minorities. *Healthy People 2010* specifically rejected that genetics and other biologic characteristics alone were responsible for these treatment and outcome disparities.

In 2002, the Institute of Medicine (IOM), at the request of Congress, produced *Unequal Treatment: Confronting Racial and Ethnic Disparities in Health Care*, a report that stated that cultural bias and stereotyping affected diagnosis and treatment decisions by healthcare providers (Smedley et al. 2002). The report concluded that, even when access-related factors like insurance status and income were controlled, racial and ethnic minorities received a lower quality and intensity of healthcare than non-minorities and that this often led to poorer outcomes. With little quality research available at the time regarding the health status of South Asian Americans, *Unequal Treatment* only mentions the ethnicity with regards to their disproportionately high rate of being uninsured, 19%.

In 2008, the World Health Organization (WHO) published *Closing the Gap in a Generation: Health Equity through Action on the Social Determinants of Health*, which emphasized that health disparities are the shaped by the environments of people's daily lives—their socio-economic status, the foods they have access to and eat, the conditions of the air they breathe, the land they live on, and water they drink; opportunities for physical activity, access to healthcare, education level, housing, employment, social cohesion, exposure to crime, etc. (Commission on Social Determinants of Health 2008). In 2010, with the release of *Healthy People 2020*, federal focus was placed on understanding the role of social determinants of health in health outcomes (HHS 2010). The social determinants are categorized into six areas: Economic Stability, Education, Health and Health Care Access, Neighborhood and Built Environment, Social and Community Context, all of which demonstrate major impact on health status. *Healthy People 2020* has expanded to 42 health categories, each with a commitment to health equity, to reduce disparities and their causes, including provider bias and social determinants. Examples of categories added for *Healthy People 2020* include Healthcare-Associated Infections, Lesbian-Gay-Bisexual-Transgender Health, Sleep Health, Preparedness, and Health-Related Quality of Life & Well-Being.

11.3 In Pursuit of South Asian American Health Data

To understand the health status of South Asian Americans, to analyze whether they experience health disparities, and to determine how to improve health outcomes, relevant data must exist. Data are gathered most frequently from national governmental surveys, academic and foundation-funded studies, and community-based organization research. Ghosh (2003) examined both federal government grants and the published peer-reviewed scientific literature to discover that the scientific community at large had access to little relevant data with regards to Asian American health and that government grants were not targeted to fill the gaps in knowledge. From 1966 to 2000, only 0.01 percent of published research involved Asian American health. From 1986 to 2000, only 0.2 percent of federal grants included the study of Asian American health. Most of the studies and grants, as well as the 23 applicable federal health surveys, aggregated "Asian Americans and Pacific Islanders" (AAPI) as one group, so much of the data were useless to determine the health status of any of the numerous sub-populations within "AAPI." Although there were some studies and grants focused on specific subpopulations, no subpopulation's overall health status was studied enough to draw definitive conclusions and, subsequently, to create policies. Ghosh concluded the article with a warning about the need for data disaggregation: "Without more data, in 50 years…the medical community will be floundering over how to provide care for this group. If subpopulation analyses are not performed, the U.S runs the risk of creating a health policy on the entire Asian American and Pacific Islander population based upon data from a few of its subpopulations."

Also in 2003, the President's Advisory Commission on Asian Americans and Pacific Islanders investigated health disparities in numerous disease and social conditions, found a dearth of research and data, and called for a national strategic plan for improving the health of AAPI populations by understanding the diversity within the group.

These two significant admonitions roused the federal government and existing AAPI-serving organizations to focus on the stronger collection and analysis of health data about AAPI subpopulation communities. The HHS funded AAPI initiatives through its various agencies: Health Resources and Services Administration (HRSA), National Institutes of Health (NIH), Centers for Disease Control and Prevention (CDC), Substance Abuse and Mental Health Services Administration (SAMHSA), Center for Medicare and Medicaid Services (CMS), and Office of Minority Health (OMH) (See Fig. 11.1). That funding led to the creation of New York University School of Medicine's Center for the Study of Asian American Health and Temple University's Asian Tobacco Education, Cancer Awareness, and Research and the renewal of University of California Davis' Asian American Network for Cancer Awareness, Research, and Tobacco. The private W. K. Kellogg Foundation committed $16.5 million to study and eliminate AAPI health disparities. These efforts underscored that AAPIs experience disparities in areas including cervical cancer screening, hepatitis B infection and death rate, infant mortality, diabetes, smoking rate, osteoporosis, health insurance coverage, stomach and liver cancers, tuberculosis, and mental health.

Although the predominance of data still reflects East Asian cultures and "AAPI" or "AANHOPI" as a whole group, various academic and non-governmental organizations have placed emphasis improving the understanding of South Asian American

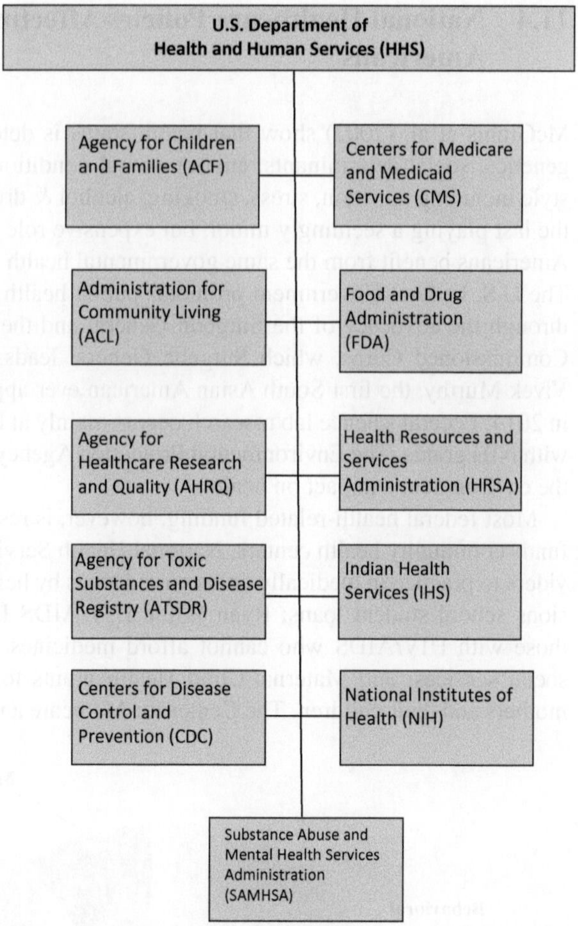

Fig. 11.1 Agencies of the U.S. Department of Health and Human Services

health. These include South Asian Public Health Association (SAPHA), Rutgers Robert Wood Johnson Medical School's South Asian Total Health Initiative (SATHI), Stanford University's South Asian Translational Heart Initiative, Memorial Sloan Kettering Cancer Center's South Asian Health Initiative, Sutter Health Palo Alto Medical Foundation's Prevention and Awareness for South Asians (PRANA), New York University School of Medicine Center for the Study of Asian American Health's Diabetes Research, Education, and Action for Minorities (DREAM) Project, and El Camino Hospital's South Asian Health Center. Focused on health issues pronounced in South Asian Americans, these organizations target coronary artery disease, diabetes, metabolic syndrome, obesity, cancer, access to culturally competent care, and mental health. Unfortunately, as AANHOPI research did a decade ago, South Asian health research lacks enough coordination to present a full picture of health status.

11.4 National Healthcare Policies Affecting South Asian Americans

McGinnis et al. (2002) show that health status is determined by the interplay of genetics, social determinants, environmental conditions, behavioral choices (lifestyle including nutrition, stress, smoking, alcohol & drug use), and healthcare, with the last playing a seemingly minor, but expensive role (see Fig. 11.2). South Asian Americans benefit from the same governmental health policies as other Americans. The U.S. Federal Government promotes public health through CDC activities and through the advocacy of the Surgeon General and the U.S. Public Health Service Commissioned Corps, which Surgeon General leads. The Senate confirmed Dr. Vivek Murthy, the first South Asian American ever appointed, as Surgeon General in 2014. Federal science lab research occurs mainly at NIH and at academic centers with NIH grants. The Environmental Protection Agency (EPA) oversees research on the environment's impact on health.

Most federal health-related funding, however, is reserved for healthcare. HRSA funds community health centers, National Health Service Corps, which brings providers to practice in medically underserved areas by helping pay their health professions school student loans; Ryan White HIV/AIDS Program to offer services to those with HIV/AIDS who cannot afford medicines, medical appointments, and social services; and Maternal-Child Health grants to promote the well-being of mothers and their children. The Center for Medicare and Medicaid (CMS) adminis-

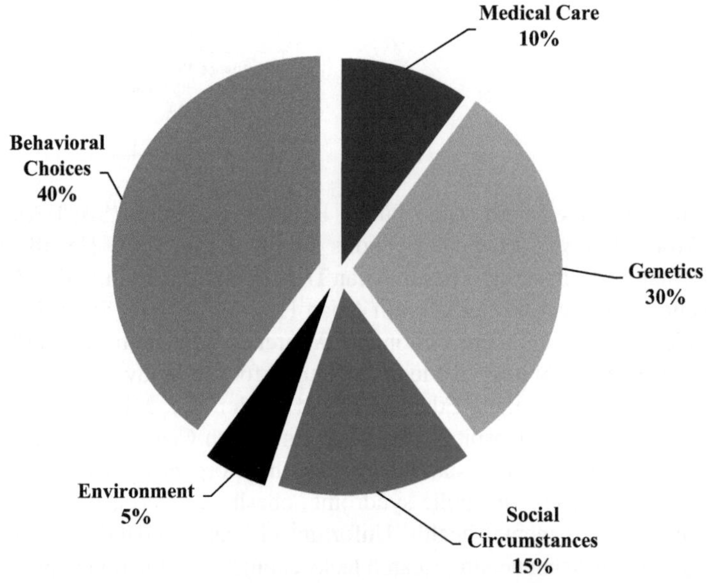

Fig. 11.2 Health determinants as a percentage of mortality (McGinnis et al. 2002)

ters the bulk of the healthcare funds through Medicare, Medicaid, and Children's Health Insurance Program (CHIP).

11.4.1 Medicare

Those aged 65 and older and who have worked and paid payroll taxes for at least 10 years will automatically qualify for Medicare, a federally funded program (CMS 2018). Medicare Part A covers inpatient hospital care after a deductible of $1,430 in 2018. Medicare Part B helps pay for private doctor visits. Enrollees pay a monthly premium (taken from Social Security checks) of $134 in 2018, a yearly deductible of $183, and 20% of Medicare-approved services. Medicare Part D is the pharmacy plan with a monthly premium, deductibles and co-pays that vary by plan; the average monthly premium is about $35. Medicare Part C, also known as "Medicare Advantage," is the section comprised of Medicare plans administered by private insurance companies. These plans combine Medicare A, B, and D and have monthly premiums over and above the standard Medicare premium. These private plans may offer more services than traditional Medicare and usually have a cap on expenses that beneficiaries must pay.

Per benefit period, Medicare pays 100% for days 1 to 60 in a hospital, requires $335 per day co-insurance (2018 rate) for days 61 to 90, and, after that, charges $670 per day co-insurance (2018 rate) for each "lifetime reserve day," of which there are 60 days over a lifetime. A benefit period continues until someone has been out of the hospital for 60 days. Medicaid will cover costs of a skilled nursing/rehabilitation facility if within the same benefit period and if a patient has been admitted to the hospital prior to the rehabilitation services for at least 3 days. While Medicare will cover hospice care, Medicare will not cover catastrophic illness, which usually requires extended hospitalization, or long-term elderly care. Although Medicare pays for most of the healthcare costs of the elderly, Miller et al. (2015) estimates that the typical elderly couple will still need an additional $220,000 to cover such costs throughout retirement.

11.4.2 Medicaid

Funded as a partnership between the federal government and each state, Medicaid is the program for those who live near poverty (CMS 2018). Prior to the passing of the Patient Protection and Affordable Care Act (ACA) in 2010, qualification varied state by state. Generally, the program covered families with children who earn less than the poverty level. The "working poor"—those who were employed but live just above poverty-- as well as childless adults at poverty, could not qualify for Medicaid. Since, generally, they could not afford to buy private policies either, they remained uninsured. When they would go to hospital Emergency Departments and could not pay the bills, the government would pay. ACA's Medicaid Expansion allows states to cover low-income individuals (no longer just families with children) by basing qualification solely on an income level up to 138% ($16,753 annual income for an individual in 2018) of the official poverty line. A family of four can make no more than $33,534 per year. This allows more Americans to gain the regular care of a primary provider. Instead of having to pay Emergency Department charges to treat these individuals, the government would pay the negotiated price of its cheapest healthcare program, Medicaid. The U.S. Supreme Court, however, ruled that not all states had to expand Medicaid. As of June 2018, only 34 states (plus the District of Columbia) had chosen to expand Medicaid, but this number continues to grow as states realize the financial advantages of doing so (see "The Patient Protection and Affordable Care Act" below).

11.4.3 Children's Health Insurance Program

The Children's Health Insurance Program (CHIP), also funded through a federal-state partnership, provides health coverage to uninsured children whose families earn up to and above 200% of the Federal Poverty Level ($50,200 for a family of four in 2018), too much to qualify for Medicaid, but too little to afford private coverage (CMS 2018). All states provide free immunizations and well-baby/well-child care.

11.4.4 Obstacles to Healthcare

While many governmental programs reduce the financial burden of healthcare for South Asian Americans, The Personal Responsibility and Work Opportunity Reconciliation Act of 1996 (PRWORA) affects new South Asian immigrants adversely. PRWORA prevents new legal immigrants from accessing federal welfare funds, including Medicaid and CHIP, for five years after arrival. As of 2018, The District of Columbia and 15 states, including the four states where 47% of all South Asian Americans live: California, New York, New Jersey, and Illinois (U.S. Census 2010), extend Medicaid-like coverage to new legal immigrants using state funds only. In 2002 and 2009 the federal government made changes to these rules to allow some federal funding for the healthcare of new immigrant children and pregnant women. Twenty other states chose to cover care for these groups with a combination of state and federal funds (Pew Charitable Trusts 2014).

Undocumented South Asian Americans, do not qualify for either Medicare or Medicaid. Hoefer et al. (2012) estimate that 240,000 Indians in the United States are undocumented. If any undocumented person has a medical emergency and seeks treatment at the Emergency Department of a hospital, that person would be treated, and the hospital could bill through the Emergency Medicaid program. This, however, is reserved for emergencies and not for primary care.

Twenty-one percent of South Asian Americans lack health insurance (Brown et al. 2000) and 40% of non-elderly South Asian Americans report that they lack a consistent healthcare access (Asian Pacific Islander American Health Forum 2006). These uninsured or underinsured may access HRSA-supported community health centers across the country. These centers, of which there are over 10,000 sites, provide quality, complete primary care without regards to ability to pay, insurance status, or immigration status. Community health centers currently provide care to over 25 million Americans yearly.

11.4.5 The Patient Protection and Affordable Care Act

Passed by Congress in 2010, The Patient Protection and Affordable Care Act (ACA), sometimes known as "Obamacare," represented the most significant change to America's healthcare system since Medicare was enacted nearly 50 years prior. Its major purpose is to decrease healthcare costs while increasing quality. The proposed changes align well with the development of healthcare systems in other developed countries and evolve logically from America's previous healthcare structure. Fig. 11.3 shows a flowchart of the step-wise changes that healthcare systems generally take as populations grow and become more urbanized, as countries become wealthier, and as political authority becomes more centralized.

The U.S. followed a similar trajectory (Starr 1982). Labor unions started to pool funds to create health insurance at the start of the twentieth century. Private insurance companies were established after World War I as were new federal health benefits for veterans. As more and more insurance companies entered the market and as medicine modernized, prices increased. The elderly and the poor, among the most medically vulnerable, were the first to leave private insurance because it was unaffordable to them. In 1965, Congress created Medicare and Medicaid to support healthcare for the elderly and poor, respectively. Despite the elderly and poor, the most expensive patients, now out of the system, private insurance continued to rise exponentially in price. In the 1970's through 1980's, Health Management Organization's (HMO) forced prices down by keeping patients in narrow provider and hospital networks. Tight control over testing and pharmaceuticals stabilized prices temporarily. Americans, however, revolted at the lack of choice and constraints on testing, so insurance companies loosened their hold on HMOs, driving prices up again. Kaiser Family Foundation (2011) found that, from 2001 to 2011, the price of insurance doubled and, subsequently, the uninsured rate jumped to 50 million, nearly one-sixth of the country. The high cost of healthcare was the main driver of personal bankruptcy. The health expenditure per capita in the United States was much higher, often nearly double, of other developed countries. Prices were high because, paid by the test and procedure, providers were incentivized to order extra testing and perform more operations, and patients express more satisfaction

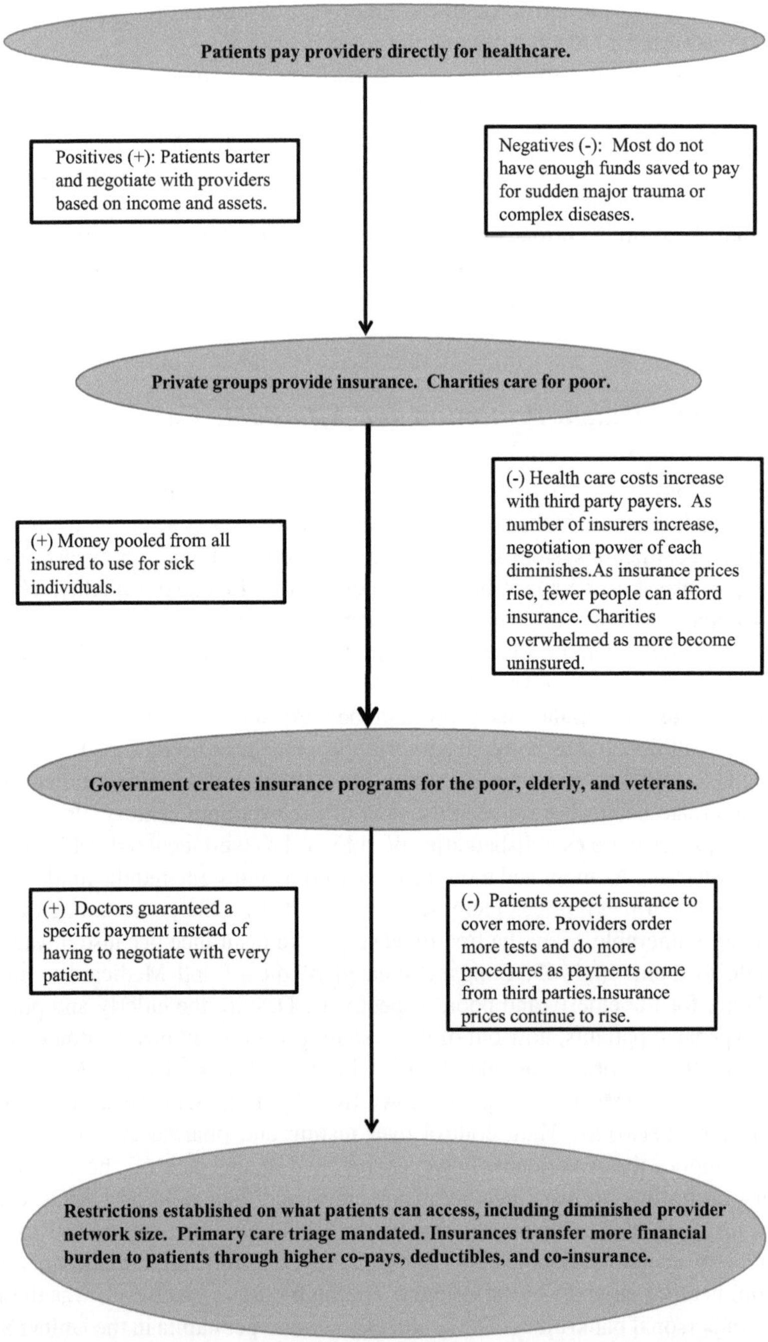

Fig. 11.3 The evolution of health care systems (Developed by Chandak Ghosh, based on review of international health systems. Used with permission.)
Historically, as countries become more populous, urbanized, wealthier, and politically centralized, they follow similar pathways with regards to their healthcare systems. With each step of the evolution, the negative outcomes drive movement to the subsequent step

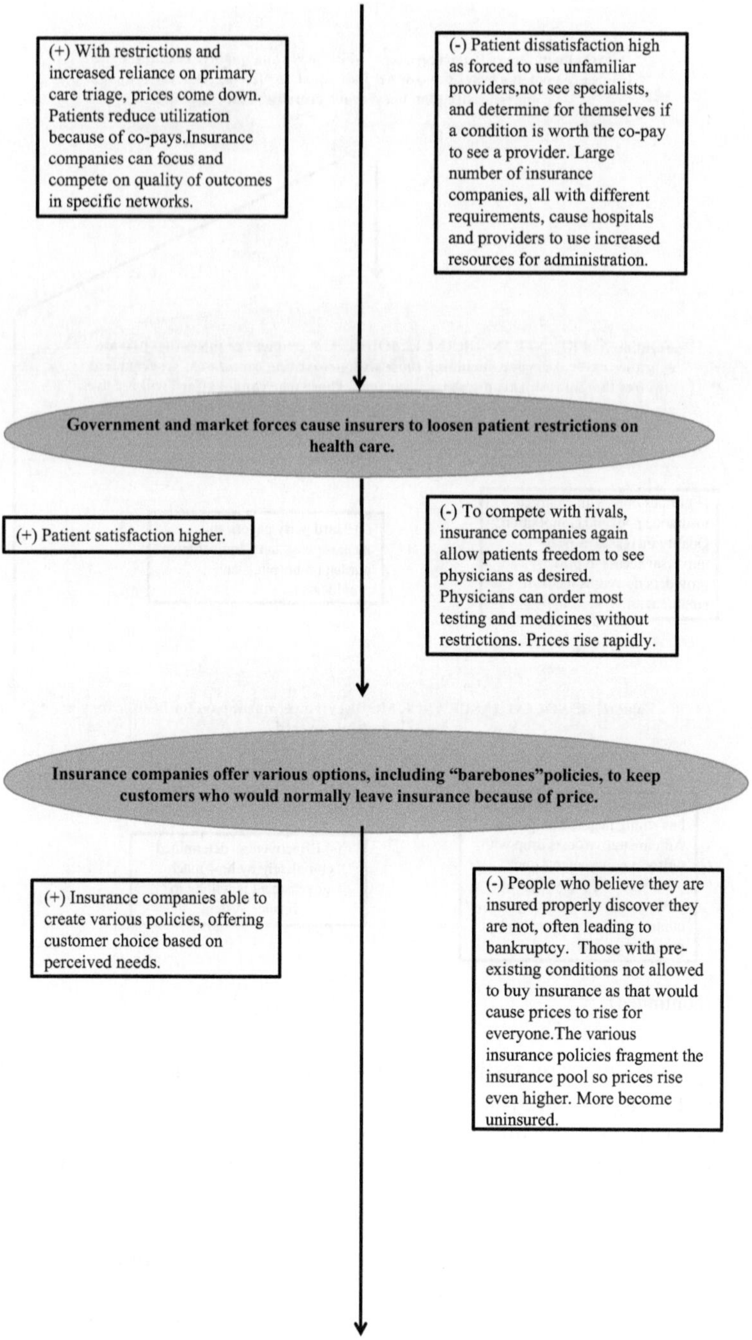

Fig. 11.3 (continued)

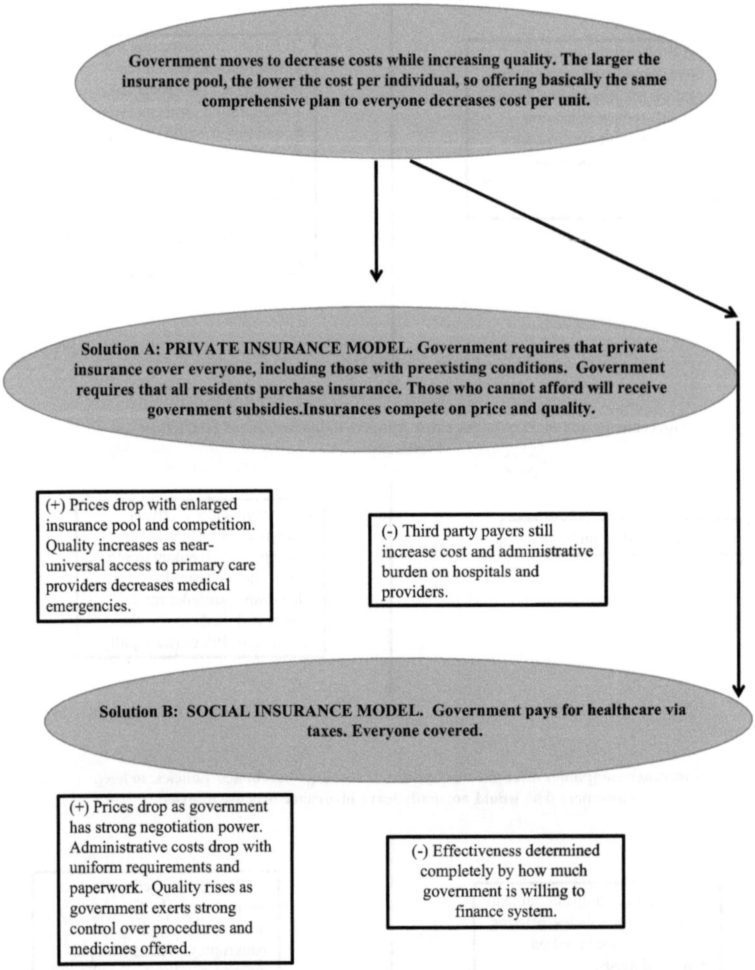

Fig. 11.3 (continued)

when they receive more testing; because Medicare Modernization Act forbid Medicare, the largest purchaser of drugs, from negotiating prices, allowing drug companies to charge ever-higher prices; because insurance company shareholders demanded constantly increasing profits; because the numerous insurance companies and their individual requirements created a massive administrative burden on provider practices and hospitals; among many other reasons. Finally, the federal budget was strained as Medicare, Medicaid, military health benefits, and healthcare for the uninsured were growing faster than any other part, particularly as the large "baby boomer" generation were just beginning to retire and using these programs (see Fig. 11.4).

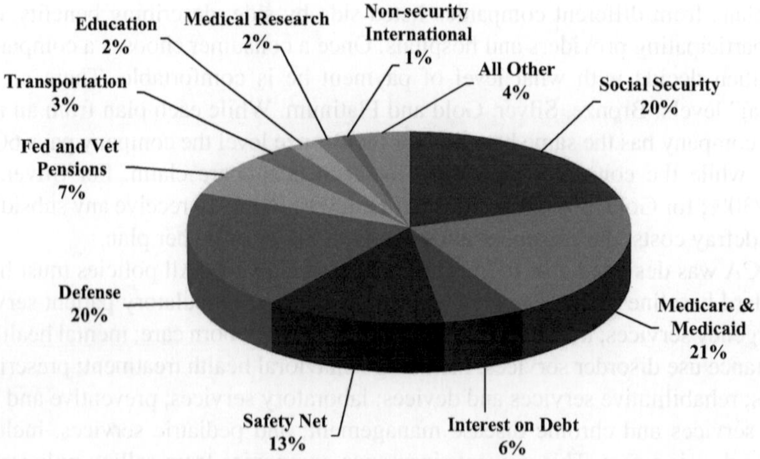

Fig. 11.4 U.S Federal Budget (CBO 2015)

The quality of American healthcare stood near the bottom of comparable countries because it was disjointed, inefficient, unequal, disease-centered, profit driven, and, often, dangerous. Wilper et al. (2009) showed that 45,000 excess deaths yearly are associated with lack of health insurance. Over 400,000 deaths are caused by preventable hospital errors (James 2013). The U.S. has ranked at the bottom with regards to the effectiveness of its healthcare system when compared to ten other western, industrialized nations for at least a decade (Davis et al. 2014). The United States was the last developed country in the world not to have a goal of universal healthcare. With this backdrop, the very complex ACA passed to fanfare and controversy.

ACA is a market-based solution to gain universal healthcare. Insurance companies would have to provide coverage to everyone regardless of age, health status, or pre-existing health condition. To maximize the size of the payer pool, which would bring down the prices of policies while still allowing insurance companies to profit, everyone would be legally required to purchase a policy. Those who cannot afford the prices would be given subsidies in the form of tax credits to use toward purchase. For insurance prices to fall and stabilize, all these parts would have to work simultaneously and properly.

Americans are fined if they refuse to purchase policies. In turn, they are protected from healthcare cost bankruptcy as out-of-pocket expenses are capped, in 2018, at \$7,350 for an individual and \$14,700 for a family (those for whom these amounts would cause bankruptcy qualify for Medicaid, which has few out -of -pocket expenditures). The 20% of Americans who will buy insurance directly from the insurance company instead of through an employer because they are, for example, self-employed, employed part-time, or unemployed can go to the online ACA Insurance Marketplace for their state to compare plans, choose the best plan and best cost sharing arrangement, and determine if they qualify for Medicaid. The Marketplace has plans from different companies listed side-by-side, describing benefits, costs, and participating providers and hospitals. Once a consumer chooses a company, he will then decide with what level of payment he is comfortable. There are four "metal" levels: Bronze, Silver, Gold and Platinum. While each plan from an insurance company has the same benefits, for the Bronze level the company pays 60% of costs while the consumer pays 40% for each healthcare claim. For Silver, is it 70%/30%; for Gold, 80%/20%; for Platinum, 90%/10%. To receive any subsidies to help defray costs, the consumer must choose a Silver or higher plan.

ACA was designed also to improve health care quality. All policies must have a standard baseline of 10 "essential" benefit categories: ambulatory patient services; emergency services; hospitalization; maternity and newborn care; mental health and substance use disorder services, including behavioral health treatment; prescription drugs; rehabilitative services and devices; laboratory services; preventive and wellness services and chronic disease management; and pediatric services, including oral and vision care. This prevents insurance companies from selling policies with few benefits but alluringly cheap premiums. Policies must also allow for preventive examinations and testing without co-pay so more people will take advantage. The 63 preventive services covered include annual physicals, mammograms, colonoscopies, vaccinations, and birth control. Birth control is included because it prevents unintended pregnancies, which occur at rates two to three times the national average in those already below the federal poverty level (Finer and Zolna 2016) and can be damaging to a woman's economic status and income (Chiquero 2010). Poverty is one of the strongest social determinants of poor health.

ACA gives financial incentives for distinct medical entities to join and form Accountable Care Organizations (ACOs). These networks aim to streamline patient care with primary care, specialties, testing and other procedures, and prevention counseling to reduce duplication and delays for care. ACA includes pilot projects--including financially incentivizing coordinated care, tying Medicare Advantage bonus payments to positive health results, and developing a seamless handoff from hospitalization to primary care-- to alter the payment model from quantity of testing and procedures to quality of outcomes. A companion law to ACA, The 2009 American Recovery and Reinvestment Act (ARRA) pushes doctors to computerize records to reduce testing duplication, transmit clear medical instructions to pharmacies, protect physicians from malpractice suits, and be reminded on screen of what standard testing and referrals should be made for specific diagnoses. A section of ACA known as the "Sunshine Act" requires pharmaceutical companies to report to HHS what payments, meals, and gifts physicians and teaching hospitals receive from these companies, which may influence the drugs doctors prescribe. HHS then makes these reports public in the hope that most physicians and hospitals will stop accepting favors from drug companies. ACA created Patient-Centered Outcomes Research Institute (PCORI), charged with comparing different drugs and procedures to determine the most effective. Insurance companies and Medicare may then apply the results when determining what drugs and procedures to reimburse. Within a few years of ACA's enactment, it showed success by causing the uninsured rate to drop. The uninsured rate was at an all-time high of 18.2% at the end of 2010 (Kaiser

Commission on Medicaid and the Uninsured 2015). By 2015, it was at 9%, the lowest ever recorded the National Health Interview Survey in its 50 years (Martinez and Cohen 2015).

Many newly insured Americans, however, began to complain that deductibles were so high that they could not afford paying them (Collins et al. 2015). ACA structured insurance rates to stay below the affordability threshold of 9.5% of income for those with access to employer-sponsored plans and 8.0% for those purchasing directly from insurance companies (Fernandez and Gabe 2013). In an effort to be fair, insurance policies are sold with low monthly premiums and high deductibles so that the insured only pay the larger amount when they actually need care. Also, high deductibles push consumers to comparison shop for the most cost effective procedures and tests for their conditions. Another problem is that most of the newly insured have a vague understanding of the complexities of health insurance, including how to choose a plan and provider from numerous competing plans and what cost sharing, including monthly premiums, deductibles, and co-insurance, entails. ACA also fails to control one of the most significant drivers of high healthcare costs: administrative costs. While most countries streamline administration by having one healthcare system, the US has five: (1) Medicare for the elderly, (2) Medicaid for the poor, (3) healthcare for the military (Veterans Health Administration, Tricare), (4) nearly 1000 separate private companies insuring the employed, and (5) self-pay or government grants/reimbursement for uninsured. Each has its own rules and paperwork. Hospitals and providers, in turn, must use one-third of their resources towards dealing with administration. Himmelstein et al. (2014) show that a single-payer healthcare system like Medicare-for-all would save the U.S. over $400 billion per year just in administration.

11.5 A National Health Action Plan

Ghosh (2010) described a potential National Health Agenda for Asian Americans and Pacific Islanders to gain funding and commitment to organize research efforts through strengthening capacity of existing local organizations, collecting subpopulation data at the national and community levels, developing investment strategies for funders, and supporting the collaboration of academic Asian-American Native American Pacific Islander-serving institutions and medical and public health professional organizations.

A similar National Health Action Plan for South Asian American Health would be an effective tool to understand health status, become aware of disparities and their social determinants, develop effective and culturally competent interventions, and optimize outcomes.

Such an Action Plan should include the following to be effective:

- **Collaboration.** Public health organizations, medical institutions, and provider professional groups should partner to develop and oversee the entire Action Plan.

This would support the inclusion of prevention and therapeutic principles. The Action Plan would contain both social concerns like cultural competence and access to prevention information and medical concerns like pharmaceuticals and surgery.

- **Reliance on Community-Based Participatory Research.** Because of the generally small South Asian American population and its concentration in specific urban centers, large federal surveys and national studies cannot register South Asian American health status effectively. Also, there are so many categories of people within "South Asian American" that national data samples may not reflect differences. For example, not only are there numerous countries of origin, but differing immigration status, diet, and socio-economic position to consider. Community-Based Participatory Research (CBPR) allows for the study of small, specifically-defined groups, with the possibility, but not requirement, that findings may be transferrable to other South Asian American groups in the U.S. Most such studies would investigate health status, availability of healthcare resources, and the results of interventions that disrupt social determinants of health. CBPR also supports the partnership of community researchers with academic mentors, who tend to have greater research experience and grant funding.
- **Sharing Results.** A consistent national meeting would bring together all those invested in South Asian American health improvement to present their work and exchange ideas. This would lead to a yearly health status report to include promising health practices and interventions based on meeting presentations and scientific literature published that year.
- **Advocacy.** Action Plan participants must advocate for government and private investment to build capacity of existing South Asian American health-focused organizations, support research and data collection, educate the public and policy makers about the Action Plan's progress and goals through media, and include information particular to the health and care of South Asian Americans in the curricula of health professions schools and health professional organization-sponsored continuing education.
- **Aligning with *Healthy People 2020 and 2030* goals.** *Healthy People* maps the country's goals for health each decade. To benefit from resources and investments that accompany the goals, the Action Plan should match South Asian American health needs to *Healthy People*'s objectives.
- **Becoming an Active Participant in "Asian American."** To gain notice, the larger and louder the group of constituents, the larger the influence. After decades of political and social advocacy, Asian Americans have established themselves as a significant voice among the racial and ethnic minority groups in the United States. South Asian Americans stand as a significant part of the Asian American population and the fastest growing. South Asian Americans must become part of a national movement for improved health for all Asian Americans. Joining "Asian American" will allow South Asian Americans to share an existing mature network of organizations, influence the directions they take, join a pipeline to positions that influence policy, and cultivate a movement to advocate for health policies that optimize South Asian American health outcomes.

11.6 Summary

Recognition that South Asian Americans experience unique health conditions and disparities is a recent phenomenon driven by the work of a few community-based organizations and academic centers. Federal and state governments generally lump South Asian American health into the overarching "Asian American, Native Hawaiian, and other Pacific Islander" category, making most of the research and data useless to understand and improve South Asian American health status. As South Asian Americans generally benefit from the same governmental health programs as other Americans, they should become familiar with community health centers, Medicare, Medicaid, Children's Health Insurance Program (CHIP), and the Affordable Care Act (ACA). South Asian American public health organizations and medical institutions must partner to institute a National Health Action Plan to focus research efforts on individual South Asian American communities. So that their health remains a research and political priority, South Asian Americans should become a stronger voice in AANHOPI.

References

Asian and Pacific Islander American Health Forum (APIAHF). (2006). *Health brief: South Asians in the United States*. https://www.apiahf.org/resource/south-asians-in-the-united-states/. Accessed 14 June 2018

Bijlani, J. (2005). Neither here nor there: Creating a legally and politically distinct South Asian racial identity. *La Raza L.J., 16*(2), 53–69.

Brown, E.R., Ojeda, V.D., Wyn, R., & Levan, R. (2000). Racial and ethnic disparities in access to health insurance and health care. Policy research report. UCLA Center for Health Policy Research & Henry J. Kaiser Family Foundation. https://escholarship.org/uc/item/4sf0p1st. Accessed 14 June 2018.

Center for Medicare and Medicaid Services. (2018). *Medicare*. CHIP: Medicaid https://www.cms.gov/. Accessed 14 June 2018.

Chiquero, A.N. (2010). The labor force effects of unplanned childbearing. Boston University, Department of Economics. http://www.unavarra.es/digitalAssets/141/141311_100000Paper_Ana_Nuevo_Chiquero.pdf. Accessed 14 June 2018.

Colby, S. L., & Ortman, J. M. (2014). *Current population reports: Projections of the size and composition of the U.S. population: 2014 to 2060*. Washington, DC: U.S. Census Bureau.

Collins, S.R., Gunja, M., Doty, M.M., Beutel, S. (2015). How high is America's health care cost burden?: Findings from the commonwealth fund health care affordability tracking survey, July–August 2015. The Commonwealth Fund. http://www.commonwealthfund.org/publications/issuebriefs/2015/nov/how-high-health-care-burden. Accessed 14 June 2018.

Commission on Social Determinants of Health. (2008). Closing the gap in a generation: Health equity through action on the social edeterminants of health. World Health Organization final report of the Commission on Social Determinants of Health. http://apps.who.int/iris/bitstream/10665/43943/1/9789241563703_eng.pdf. Accessed 14 June 2018.

Congressional Budget Office (CBO). (2015). *An update to the budget and economic outlook: 2015–2025*. https://www.cbo.gov/sites/default/files/114th-congress-2015-2016/reports/50724-Update-OneColumn_0.pdf. Accessed 14 June 2018.

Davis, K., Stremikis, D., Squires, D., & Schoen, C. (2014). Mirror, mirror on the wall: How the performance of the U.S. health care system compares internationally, 2014 update. The Commonwealth Fund. http://www.commonwealthfund.org/publications/fund-reports/2014/jun/mirrormirror. Accessed 14 June 2018.

Fernandez, B. & Gabe, T. (2013). Health insurance premium credits in the patient protection and affordable care act (ACA). Congressional Research Service. http://www.deesigned.com/wp-content/uploads/jwd-pdfthumbs/medical/obamacare/Premium%20Credit%20and%20ACA%20Law.pdf. Accessed 14 June 2018.

Finer, L. B., & Zolna, M. R. (2016). Declines in unintended pregnancy in the United States, 2008–2011. *The New England Journal of Medicine, 374*(9), 843–852.

Ghosh, C. (2003). Healthy people 2010 and Asian Americans/Pacific islanders: Defining a baseline of information. *American Journal of Public Health, 93*(12), 2093–2098.

Ghosh, C. (2010). A National Health Agenda for Asian Americans and Pacific islanders. *JAMA, 304*(12), 1381–1382.

Health Resources and Services Administration. (1998). *Health care rx: Access for all–the president's initiative on race*. Washington, DC: U.S. Government Printing Office.

Heckler, M. M. (1985). *Report of the secretary's task force on black and minority health.* Washington, DC: U.S. Government Printing Office.

Himmelstein, D. U., Jun, M., Busse, R., Chevreul, K., Geissler, A., Jeurissen, P., Thomson, S., Vinet, M. A., & Woolhandler, S. (2014). A comparison of hospital administrative costs in eight nations: US costs exceed all others by far. *Health Affairs, 33*(9), 1586–1594.

Hoefer, M., Rytina, N., & Baker, B.C. (2012). Estimates of the unauthorized immigrant population residing in the United States: January 2011. Policy Directorate. Office of Immigration Statistics, U.S. Department of Homeland Security. https://www.dhs.gov/xlibrary/assets/statistics/publications/ois_ill_pe_2011.pdf . Accessed 14 June 2018.

James, J. T. (2013). A new, evidence-based estimate of patient harms associated with hospital care. *Journal of Patient Safety, 9*(3), 122–128.

Kaiser Commission on Medicaid and the Uninsured. (2015). Fact sheet key facts about the uninsured population. http://files.kff.org/attachment/fact-sheet-key-facts-about-the-uninsured-population. Accessed 14 June 2018.

Kaiser Family Foundation & Health Research and Educational Trust. (2011). *Employer health benefits: 2011 annual survey*. https://kaiserfamilyfoundation.files.wordpress.com/2013/04/8225.pdf . Accessed 14 June 2018

Lam, D. J., & Palsane, M. N. (1997). Research on stress and coping: Contemporary Asian approaches. In H. S. R. Kao & D. Sinha (Eds.), *Cross-cultural research and methodology series* (Vol. 19. Asian perspectives on psychology, pp. 265–281). Thousand Oaks: Sage Publications.

Lin-Fu, J. S. (1993). Asian and Pacific islander Americans: An overview of demographic characteristics and health care issues. *Asian American and Pacific Islander Journal of Health, 1*(1), 20–36.

Martinez M.E., & Cohen R.A. (2015). *Health insurance coverage: Early release of estimates from the National Health Interview Survey, January– June 2015. National Center for Health Statistics*. http://www.cdc.gov/nchs/data/nhis/earlyrelease/insur201511.pdf. Accessed 14 June 2018.

McGinnis, J. M., Williams-Russo, P., & Knickman, J. R. (2002). The case for more active policy attention to health promotion. *Health Affairs, 21*, 278–293.

Miller, K., Madland, D., & Weller, C.E. (2015). *The reality of the retirement crisis. Center for American Progress*. https://cdn.americanprogress.org/wp-content/uploads/2015/01/RetirementCrisis1.pdf. Accessed 14 June 2018.

Pew Charitable Trusts. (2014). *Brief: Mapping public benefits for immigrants in the states*. http://www.pewtrusts.org/~/media/assets/2014/09/mappingpublicbenefitsforimmigrantsinthestates-final.pdf. Accessed 14 June 2018.

President's Advisory Commission on Asian Americans and Pacific Islanders. (2003). *Report to the president and the nation: Asian Americans and Pacific Islanders addressing health disparities: Opportunities for building a healthier America*. Washington, DC: Author.

SAALT. (2009). *Health care issues affecting South Asians in the United States*. http://saalt.org/wp-content/uploads/2012/09/Health-Care-Issues-Affecting-South-Asians-in-the-United-States.pdf. Accessed 14 June 2018.

SAALT & Asian American Federation. (2012). *A demographic snapshot of South Asians in the United States*. http://saalt.org/wpcontent/uploads/2012/09/Demographic-Snapshot-Asian-American-Foundation-2012.pdf. Accessed 14 June 2018.

Smedley, B. D., Stith, A. Y., & Nelson, A. R. (2002). *Unequal treatment: Confronting racial and ethnic disparities in health care*. Washington, DC: National Academy Press.

Starr, P. (1982). *The social transformation of American medicine*. New York: Basic Books.

U.S Department of Health and Human Services. (2000). *Healthy People 2010, second edition: Understanding and improving health and objectives for improving health*. Washington, DC: U.S. Government Printing Office.

U.S Department of Health and Human Services. (2010). *Healthy People 2020*. http://www.healthypeople.gov. Accessed 14 June 2018.

U.S. Census Bureau. (2010). *2010 Census. American Fact Finder*. http://factfinder.census.gov/faces/nav/jsf/pages/index.xhtml. Accessed 14 June 2018.

U.S. Census Bureau. (2016). *Profile America facts for feature: Asian/Pacific American heritage month, May 2016*. http://www.census.gov/content/dam/Census/newsroom/facts-for-features/2016/cb16-ff.07_asian_pacific.pdf. Accessed 14 June 2018.

Wilper, A. P., Woolhandler, S., Lasser, K. E., McCormick, D., Bor, D. H., & Himmelstein, D. U. (2009). Health insurance and mortality in US adults. *American Journal of Public Health, 99*(12), 2289–2295.

Chandak Ghosh, MD, MPH stands committed to the health needs of minority and underserved populations, particularly Asian Americans, Native Hawaiians, and other Pacific Islanders. A board-certified eye surgeon and Captain in the U.S. Public Health Service (USPHS), he has served three Presidential administrations in the Health Resources and Services Administration (HRSA), an agency within the U.S. Department of Health and Human Services. He contributed to the design and implementation of the Affordable Care Act and the development of the National Performance Review Protocol, utilized to improve all Federal health grantees, including hospitals, universities, and community health centers. The USPHS awarded Ghosh a rare Meritorious Service Medal, among its highest honors, for "influencing progress towards health equity on a national scale." He holds degrees from Yale, Medical College of Virginia, and Harvard School of Public Health.

Part V
Conclusion

Chapter 12
A Call for Healthy South Asian Americans: Need to Shape Intervention by Providers, Policies, and Prospects

Marisa J. Perera and Edward C. Chang

Emigration from South Asia was estimated to have increased from approximately 10 million in 1990 to 27 million in 2015, a nearly threefold increase (United Nations; Srivastava and Pandey 2017). Migration of South Asians to industrialized nations of North America accounts for a considerable amount of the total migration from South Asian to non-South Asian nations. In 2015, migration to North America accounted for nearly 14% of all immigrants from South Asian to non-South Asian nations. In the specific case of India, the largest South Asian nation, nearly 25% of Indian migrants immigrated to North America in 2015 (Srivastava and Pandey 2017).

Over 3.4 million people in the United States trace their heritage to the South Asian region, making South Asians one of the fastest growing ethnic minority groups in the U.S. (United States Census Bureau 2010; Hoeffel et al. 2012). The South Asian community in the U.S. is comprised of individuals with ancestry from the following nations: Bangladesh, Bhutan, India, Nepal, Pakistan, Sri Lanka, and the Maldives. Afghanistan is sometimes included in this list. South Asians from these regions have varied religions, customs, and immigration journeys, resulting in a rather heterogeneous community when considered together. Despite considerable cultural variation among individuals from these countries, individuals in the U.S. that descend from these countries have historically been considered together, or aggregated, as one homogeneous group in much of the research and prior knowledge concerning the health of Asian populations in the U.S.

M. J. Perera (✉)
University of Miami-Coral Gables, Coral Gables, FL, USA
e-mail: mperera@miami.edu

E. C. Chang
Department of Psychology, University of Michigan-Ann Arbor, Ann Arbor, MI, USA
e-mail: changec@umich.edu

M. J. Perera, E. C. Chang (eds.), *Biopsychosocial Approaches to Understanding Health in South Asian Americans*, Cross-Cultural Research in Health, Illness and Well-Being, https://doi.org/10.1007/978-3-319-91120-5_12

Data aggregated across Asian Americans, and often Pacific Islanders, can put the communities involved at risk of being underserved. Common errors associated with aggregation can leave the specific health needs of the aggregate groups unknown and unmet (Holland and Palaniappan 2012). Lower risk of coronary heart disease (CHD) in Chinese Americans has been incorrectly extrapolated as lower risk of heart disease for all Asian-American groups, including South Asian Americans, for instance. Yet, South Asian Americans are at higher risk for CHD than majority of other groups in the U.S. South Asians in the U.S. are affected by some chronic health conditions at rates higher than would be expected given their population size, including diabetes and cardiovascular disease, some cancers, and human immunodeficiency virus/acquired immunodeficiency syndrome (HIV/AIDS). Majority of these health conditions are preventable. Aggregation obstructs understanding of the health issues salient for South Asian Americans.

The intent of this handbook is to align with the movement to disaggregate "Asian American" by focusing specifically on the health of the South Asian community in the U.S. To holistically conceptualize health and inform practice for providers and researchers working with this population, all sections of this handbook applied elements of the biopsychosocial model of health. To synthesize current understanding of the biological, psychological, and sociocultural factors of health for the U.S. South Asian community, this handbook sought to gather information pertaining to the below four questions concerning South Asian American health.

1. How does South Asian American identity impact health?
2. What are South Asian biopsychosocial conceptualizations of "health?"
3. What is the chronic disease burden in South Asian Americans?
4. What are the barriers to promoting South Asian American health?

12.1 How Does South Asian American Identity Impact Health?

The intention of this question is to identify unique factors related to South Asian identity in the U.S. that also relate to the health of this group. Identity processes can impact an individual's perceptions of health factors, including significance of health stressors and effectiveness of health messages received. Identification with ethnic group membership is an aspect of how an individual defines him or herself, and this section considers how South Asian identity processes in the U.S. contribute to general health. Bhatia and Ram (Chap. 2) and Kaduvettor-Davidson and Weatherford (Chap. 3) describe identity-related stressors that have potential to impact health for South Asians in the U.S.

One major stressor is the contrasting discourses, or perceptions and stereotypes, of "South Asian American" that have contributed to the historical formation of South Asian American identity. Whereas one discourse depicts South Asian Americans as a group with high achievement and success, the other depicts this group as victim to pervasive racism in the U.S. The latter has been heightened following the September 11, 2001 terrorist attacks that fostered a perpetual foreigner stereotype. It is not uncommon for South Asian Americans to internalize pressures to be successful within the face of discrimination and racism, inherently resulting in stressful identity-related experiences.

Owing to the model minority myth, there is a prevailing idea in American society that Asian Americans do not experience poor outcomes, including health outcomes. Such a discourse obscures the magnitude of health disparities, and impacts the collection and interpretation of health data for this group. For instance, obesity prevalence in Asian Americans is lower compared with all other U.S. racial/ethnic groups (McNeely and Boyko 2004; Wang and Beydoun 2007), which has led to categorization of Asian Americans as low risk. Yet, obesity prevalence varies by Asian subgroup with the highest values in South Asian Americans. Despite high disease risk, South Asian Americans may be excluded from health policy conversations on obesity and from the allocation of resources and development of initiatives to address South Asian American health disparities.

Beyond the impact of these discourses, the experience of unpredictable and uncontrollable discrimination itself triggers negative health outcomes. Physiological responses of elevated blood pressure and cardiovascular activity, and psychological responses of anxiety, hopelessness, and fear are triggered (Dolezsar et al. 2014; Lazarus and Folkman 1984). When occurring over time, these responses negatively influence health, including increased risk of cardiovascular problems. Objectification as a foreigner is a unique stressor for South Asians born in the U.S. Identity denial can result when a person's core identity as an American is questioned and he/she perceives denied acceptance into their society of birth.

South Asians also face identity pressures and conflict within the South Asian community, resulting from interaction between the contrasting cultures of South Asia and America. Generally, South Asia and America are contrasted in that the former is collectivistic and the latter is individualistic in nature. Balancing family and community expectations with individualistic desires can produce stress related to identity conflict. In addition to stress related to navigating bi/multicultural identity, South Asians in the U.S. can experience stress stemming from expectations to conform to traditional patriarchal gender roles and pressure to attain high educational and professional achievements.

12.1.1 Recommendations for Providers

- Consider the role of aggregation when interpreting and generalizing literature on health data for Asian Americans.
- Recognition of the heterogeneity that exists within the subgroup of South Asian Americans.
- For immigrant patients, consider assessing pre-migration health status (diseases endemic in home country; exposure to disease in the U.S. less prevalent than

country of origin), health risks posed during the migratory passage, and duration of residence in the U.S.
- Consider factors generally contributing to the deterioration of health status following migration: dietary changes, substance use, commercial sex work, environmental health risks (i.e., crowded housing), unregulated work environments, and lack of access to health care services.

12.2 What Are South Asian Biopsychosocial Conceptualizations of "Health?"

The intention of this question is to identify elements of the South Asian American patient's belief system that concern health and disease and can influence health behaviors. This question is rooted in the notion that effective health care is delivered when the patient's belief system of health and disease is considered. An effective patient-provider interaction is a critical element of health care delivery, particularly for individuals who have frequent provider appointments to manage chronic disease. To apply a biopsychosocial understanding of South Asian conceptualizations of health, Kandula and Tirodkar (Chap. 4) review biological conceptualizations of health, Jilani, Chang, Lee, and Batterbee (Chap. 5) review psychological conceptualizations of health, and Sandil and Srinivasan (Chap. 6) review sociocultural conceptualizations of health. Health models and practices that originate from both South Asia and the U.S. are discussed.

12.2.1 Biological Conceptualizations of Health

Kandula and Tirodkar review the major models of traditional South Asian medicine, including Ayurveda, Siddha, Unani, and homeopathic medicine, and discuss their co-existence with allopathic practices in the U.S. The traditional models tend to involve holistic conceptualizations of good health as dependent on a balance of universal elements, and illness as resulting from disruption to the balance.

In Ayurveda, it is believed that the person inherits a unique mix of space, air, fire, water, and earth elements and that illness susceptibility results from an unbalanced mix of the body and environment. For instance, a strong mix of space and air is believed to increase susceptibility to heart disease, asthma, rheumatoid arthritis, and anxiety, whereas a strong mix of water and earth is believed to increase susceptibility to asthma, cancer, and diabetes. Like Ayurveda, Siddha recognizes the predominance of air, fire, and earth and water elements throughout the lifespan. Unani descends from Hippocrates and is consistent with a humoral theory of health where blood, phlegm, yellow bile, and black bile are four bodily humors whose balance determines health and illness. In the homeopathic tradition, symptoms of illness can be considered normal bodily responses as the body attempts to regain health. Often, the objective of the practitioner is to aid the natural forces of the body to heal itself and combat disease. Health factors that disrupt the balance of universal elements include a person's environment, climate, habits, activities, sleep, diet, stress, mental activity, and excretion/retention. Some of these indigenous systems have been supported by the Indian government and endorsed by major health organizations in South Asia. It is probable that South Asians in the U.S. have been exposed to and possibly hold some traditional, holistic conceptualizations of health.

A holistic understanding of health can contrast with biomedical, or allopathic, views of health. Although it is unclear if holistic explanatory models persist after immigration to the U.S., it is possible that South Asian American patients draw upon both traditional and allopathic medical systems when managing health issues, despite that medical training and care in the U.S. is primarily allopathic. Without provider awareness of medical pluralism, that is patient use of both indigenous and Western medical systems, the care of South Asian patients in the U.S. may be fragmented. For instance, a South Asian patient in the U.S. may supplement Western-prescribed treatment with traditional Ayurvedic medicines. Yet, Ayurvedic medicines are not reviewed by the Food and Drug Administration and can cause metal poisoning (lead, mercury, arsenic), and/or interact with prescribed medications. In addition, poor adherence to allopathic-prescribed treatment may result from different patient-provider conceptualizations of health and a proclivity for non-invasive care on the Indian subcontinent. Lack of awareness of use the patient's explanatory models of health and healing methods, including use of traditional products, contributes to fragmented care.

12.2.2 Psychological Conceptualizations of Health

Jilani et al. overview both existing Western-based models (The Health Belief Model, Theory of Planned Behavior, Health Locus of Control, and Transtheoretical Model of Change; refer to Chap. 5 for an overview of each model) and indigenous South Asian practices of health psychology. To promote health and prevent/manage disease, health psychology identifies individual health attitudes, beliefs, and behaviors that influence disease risk and are modifiable. This section identifies health attitudes, beliefs, and behaviors at the group level of South Asians.

When applied to U.S. South Asian patients with breast cancer, the Health Belief Model revealed a low perceived threat of being diagnosed with breast cancer, indicating the importance of psychoeducation to promote regular breast cancer screenings. In addition to beliefs about perceptions of threat, the Theory of Planned Behavior noted community attitudes of shame associated with certain medical conditions (i.e., HIV/AIDS; severe mental illness) as a barrier to prioritizing one's health condition and performing the healthy behaviors of health care utilization and treatment adherence. The Health Locus of Control noted a common cultural belief in fatalism, the belief that certain experiences are unavoidable, as manifesting as a belief that health concerns are unavoidable and as promoting reduced help-seeking behavior. By conceptualizing behavioral change as a continuum of stages based on motivation to change, the Transtheoretical Model of Health Behavior Change proffers suggestions to elicit higher rates of health behavior change. Collectively, these existing health psychology models indicate the importance of psychoeducation and health literacy to improve screening behavior, and of addressing community stigma and fatalism to improve disease self-management and treatment non-adherence for South Asians in the U.S.

Applying the Western-based models to South Asians in the U.S. also demonstrates potential discrepancies in applying them to South Asian Americans, including lack of a cultural component and poor conceptualization of navigating both Asian and American identities. Lack of adequate Western-developed model fit indicates a need to consider traditional South Asian conceptualizations of health attitudes, beliefs, and behavior to promote healthy behavior change. Traditional health-promoting practices are mindfulness, yoga, transcendental meditation, and prayer. Many of these practices have been modified by Western practitioners for health promotion and are prevalent throughout the U.S. Yet, there is limited empirical evidence examining sentiments toward and/or the usefulness of these modified practices for South Asian Americans. Despite that health behavior occurs at the level of the individual, health-related attitudes, beliefs, and behavior may be more socially conditioned and culturally embedded than isolated acts of an individual.

12.2.3 Sociocultural Conceptualizations of Health

Sandil and Srinivasan consider the influence of sociocultural values and experiences on biological and psychological conceptualizations of health. Religion, collectivism, morality, and gender are key sociocultural values that emerge in South Asian culture. These values relate to health on an individual basis and can be positive and/or negative. The positive impact of these values should be promoted; however, it is also important to identify the potential threats to health brought upon by negative impact of these values for disease prevention and risk reduction.

As aforementioned, religion can promote a strong external locus of control and sense of fatalism, which can promote lower likelihood of seeking health care in a timely manner for disease prevention. Collectivism is another sociocultural factor that can promote reduced healthcare-seeking behavior for stigmatized health conditions due to perceived threat to family honor. Influenced by traditional gender roles and a product of cultural values of morality and chastity, women are less likely to engage in sexual healthcare behavior (i.e., no monthly self-breast examination). They may also be non-adherent to treatment regimens that take time from household duties and other gender role expectations, and that may be construed as selfish. The South Asian American female patient with cardiovascular risk, for example, can be less likely to adhere to a prescription of increased physical activity given collectivistic obligation placed on family duty rather than "selfishly" taking time to engage in physical activity.

Intimate partner violence (IPV), acculturative stress, and racism are common sociocultural experiences that potentially influence health status. South Asians have high rates of IPV, and these rates may be underreported due to model minority expectations and varied cultural definitions of physical, sexual, and emotional abuse. IPV victims have overall worse physical health, including worse pain, sexual and sleep outcomes, and inhibited daily activity. Acculturation can result in temporary and/or long-lasting physical, biological, cultural, and psychological change and stress, often due to loss of family social support and occupational distress. As mentioned in Section I, racism and discrimination, when uncontrollable and unpredictable, are stressors that negatively impact health.

12.2.4 Recommendations for Providers

- Recognition that patients may not share your conceptualizations of health. Probe the patient's explanatory models of health to be optimally positioned to prescribe effective treatment to which the patient will be adherent. Probing can transmit holistic concern for the patient and open opportunities for psychoeducation, as appropriate. Probing questions (see Chap. 4 for more questions):
    - *What do you think caused your problem?*
    - *Why do you think it started when it did?*
    - *What do you think your sickness does to you?*
    - *What kind of treatment do you think you should receive?*
- Solicit information on the use of traditional healing products, including Ayurvedic products. If a patient is committed to using homeopathic dilutions, consider providing referrals for providers in your area who prepare the dilutions appropriately.
- To promote healthy behavior changes, probe for barriers to treatment adherence that manifest in health attitudes and beliefs. Elicit change talk and use a readiness to change ruler (Kivelä et al. 2014):
- *What makes you think you need to change?*
- *On a scale from 1 to 10, where 1 is "not at all ready to change" and 10 is "entirely ready to change," where are you right now?*
    - *What are the reasons your number is not lower?*
    - *What would it take to move from [insert lower number] to [insert higher number]?*
- When indicated, consider involving the family unit in the patient's healthcare given the salience of sociocultural values of collectivism and traditional gender roles, particularly for female patients.

- Awareness that sociocultural factors may impact health outcomes but may be underreported in this population, such as IPV.
- To address sociocultural determinants (i.e., limited English proficiency, education, and socioeconomic status) and stigmatized conditions, consider incorporating community-based outreach and opportunities for informal help seeking.

12.3 What Is the Chronic Disease Burden in South Asian Americans?

The intention of this question is to promote awareness of the patterns of chronic health disparities in this Asian subgroup to aid and inform conceptualizations of South Asian American health status. This section briefly reviews the chronic disease burden for South Asians in the U.S., specifically for diabetes and cardiovascular disease (Chap. 7), cancer (Chap. 8), and psychological comorbidity (Chap. 9). No chapter was devoted specifically to HIV/AIDS or autoimmune or gastrointestinal conditions in U.S. South Asians due to limited, variable, and inconsistent available data because of aggregation. Despite lack of comprehensive evidence, HIV/AIDS is a piece of the chronic burden profile in South Asia, and likely contributes to the profiles of South Asians in the U.S. (Chin et al. 2007).

As overviewed by Khan, Shah, Parikh, and Palaniappan in Chap. 7, South Asian Americans suffer disproportionately higher from type 2 diabetes mellitus (T2DM) at lower levels of body weight compared to the U.S. average. U.S. diabetes prevalence rate is 9.4% (CDC, 2017), and the South Asian American rate has been found to vary from 16–35% (Venkataraman et al. 2004; Rajpathak et al. 2010). Related to T2DM, South Asians in the U.S. are at heightened risk for heart disease because it occurs approximately 7–11 years earlier compared to the average of other U.S. groups. In Chap. 8, Gany, Hashemi, Ahmed, and Leng outline cancer risk, risk reduction, and screening and treatment among South Asians in the U.S. South Asians in the U.S. had a nearly twofold lower overall rate of cancer incidence compared to non-Hispanic Whites in the U.S. from 2006 to 2010. Cancer-related outcomes, however, may be poorer for this group due to delayed screening and/or treatment, likely due to modifiable psychological and sociocultural conceptualizations of health.

Chronic disease profiles are different for South Asians in the U.S. compared to South Asians in South Asia, highlighting the relationship between disease and environmental and social context. The prevalence of T2DM varies from 16–35% in the U.S. for South Asians (Venkataraman et al. 2004; Rajpathak et al. 2010), and varies from 5–14% in South Asia (Ramachandran et al., 2012). With more years spent residing in the U.S., cancer profiles change to more closely reflect incidence rates of the general U.S. population. Prostate and breast cancers are common among South Asians in the U.S. compared to cervical, oral, and breast cancers among South Asians in India (Mallath et al. 2014).

The exact causes of these changed risks are unknown, however changes to health behavior, including dietary changes and sedentary lifestyle, tend to occur after immigration to the U.S. Poorer health behaviors lead to greater obesity risk. Better understanding, and likely early intervention, is needed to understand the evolution of health behaviors post immigration, and their impact on cardiovascular, cancer, and HIV/AIDS risk in South Asian immigrants. The operant model of acculturation (Landrine and Klonoff 2004) predicts that health behaviors with a lower prevalence among low-acculturated minorities will increase in prevalence with increasing acculturation and have a higher prevalence among acculturated counterparts, and vice versa for health behaviors that have high prevalence among low-acculturated minorities. This model may be tested for fit with changes to South Asian American health behavior post U.S. migration to inform chronic disease risk reduction via health behavior change.

Chronic diseases are comorbid with psychological conditions such as depression and anxiety. Tummala-Narra and Deshpande explore the mental health of South Asians in the U.S. in Chap. 9 with a focus on the stress of immigration and acculturation processes. In the U.S., South Asians face challenges such as acculturative stress, language and communication barriers, family stress, trauma, and discrimination. These challenges are linked with greater depression, anxiety, and substance use, which impact an individual's management of his/her chronic disease. Patients with chronic disease and depression and/or anxiety have higher symptom burden, poorer disease self-management and treatment adherence, increased functional impairment, poorer adherence to healthy lifestyle behaviors, and more disease complications (Katon et al. 2004), indicating the importance of assessing for and treating psychological comorbidity in patients with chronic disease.

12.3.1 Recommendations for Providers

Awareness that statistics specifically for Asian Americans of South Asian descent are impacted by small sample size and have primarily been conducted with Asian Indian samples, as well as the limited number of overall studies with South Asian Americans disaggregated from other Asian subgroups. Available data on autoimmune conditions (rheumatoid arthritis, lupus, celiac disease, multiple sclerosis, type 1 diabetes, etc.) and HIV/AIDS in this group is limited and not included below.

- Obesity
  - 7–20% of adults in California (Wolstein et al. 2015; Jih et al. 2014).
  - Asian Indians
    - 46.7% overweight (23–27.4 kg/m^2) adjusted for age and sex using National Health Interview Survey (NHIS) data (Oza-Franket al. 2009).
    - 16.6% obese ($\geq$ 27.5 kg/m^2) adjusted for age and sex using NHIS data (Oza-Frank et al. 2009).

- T2DM
  - Prevalence range of 16–35% (Venkataraman et al. 2004; Rajpathak et al. 2010).
  - Asian Indians
    - Highest rate in every body mass index (BMI) category when age and sex standardized compared to Chinese or Filipinos from 1997–2005 (Oza-Frank et al. 2009).
- Cardiovascular diseases
  - 43.6% prevalence of 2+ cardiometabolic abnormalities (high fasting glucose, low high-density lipoprotein cholesterol, high triglycerides, hypertension) in South Asians from Mediators of Atherosclerosis in South Asians Living in America (MASALA; Gujral et al. 2017).
  - Acute coronary syndrome and overall cardiovascular mortality occur approximately 7–11 years earlier than average (Joshi et al. 2007).
  - South Asian migrants to high income nations have 1.5-2 times greater prevalence of coronary artery disease than age- and sex-adjusted European counterparts (Fernando et al. 2015).
- Cancer
  - Overall incidence of 216.8/100,000 in male (554.1 in non-Hispanic whites) and 212.0/100,000 in female (444.6 in non-Hispanic whites) Asian Indians/ Pakistanis.
  - Top 3 cancers for South Asians in the U.S.
    - Women: (1) breast, (2) ovarian, (3) uterine cancers.
    - Men: (1) prostate, (2) colorectal, (3) lung cancers.
- Mental health
  - Age-adjusted suicide rate of 4.8% in 2010 for Asian Indians (Kuroki 2016).
  - IPV prevalence of 21% in a community sample in Boston (Hurwitz et al. 2006).
  - Limited data on prevalence of clinical depression and anxiety due to aggregation and community stigma.
- Top 5 mortality causes in Asian Indians: (1) heart disease; (2) cancer; (3) stroke; (4) diabetes; (5) accidents/ unintentional injuries (Hastings et al. 2015).

- Cultural idioms of distress and emotional suffering can manifest as somatic symptomology more commonly compared to non-Hispanic Whites in the U.S.
- Psychological comorbidity is a negative prognostic factor for chronic disease. Consider referrals to mental health. Given cultural stigma around mental illness, a collaborative care model for common chronic disease and psychological comorbidity should be considered (i.e., diabetes and depression; Katon et al. 2004).

- Consider the role of modifiable psychological and sociocultural determinants of disease (delayed diagnosis; failure to seek treatment) on disease outcomes.

12.4 What Are the Barriers to Promoting South Asian American Health?

The intention of this question is to describe barriers to detection, treatment, and management of chronic conditions in South Asian Americans that promote poor prevention and treatment outcomes. Barriers can occur at the level of patient, provider, and policy/healthcare system. Factors that may serve as barriers at the individual and provider levels in health-related counseling in medical settings are reviewed by Ibrahim and Heuer (Chap. 10), while Ghosh reviews political and systemic factors (Chap. 11).

12.4.1 Patient

Barriers at the level of the patient primarily concern adherence to medical intervention. Known adherence barriers include health literacy, access to health insurance, and culturally- and linguistically-appropriate resources and care. Beyond known barriers, acculturation is a dynamic process that encompasses facets that can impact adherence. Of these facets are migration stress, loss of familial support systems, adaptation to U.S. culture and acceptance/rejection into the culture, and changes to lifestyle health behaviors that directly impact disease risk and complications.

12.4.2 Provider

A possible barrier at the level of the provider is overemphasis on the socially constructed meaning of ethnicity and race, which can lead to an overly homogeneous understanding of South Asians in the U.S., and application of generic cultural information that may not relate to an individual patient (i.e., the role of spirituality; somatization presentation). Assumptions of shared explanatory models of illness and health is another barrier that can contribute to marginalization of the relationship between culture and health, producing an under-emphasis on the patient's cultural health beliefs. Given strong connections between health beliefs and health behaviors, lack of attention to cultural health beliefs in the provider setting can lead to treatment with reduced effectiveness due to provider-patient mismatch in conceptualizing the patient's health. Lack of understanding of differences between Western and Eastern conceptions of the mind-body interaction can also influence the provider's interpretation of client symptom manifestation (i.e., emotional suffering manifesting as chest pain misconstrued as cardiovascular symptoms).

12.4.3 Policy

Ghosh details how South Asian American health has been "left out" of U.S. governmental health policies. Small population size and historical practice of aggregation have led to under-emphasis of South Asian American health concerns. Under the Obama administration, the Department of Human and Health Services established new data collection standards to disaggregate "Asian American and Pacific Islander" into subcategories, including a South Asian subcategory. These standards were set in 2011, emphasizing the recency of this movement and the nascent state of understanding South Asian health disparities in the U.S.

In recognizing that this group experiences unique health disparities, Ghosh puts forward a National Health Action Plan to better understand South Asian American health status, increase awareness of disparities and social determinants, and develop optimal interventions. The multifaceted plan calls for provider collaboration (professional provider groups, medical institutions, public health organizations) to comprehensively address sociocultural and biological concerns, reliance on community-based participatory research given the small and specifically-defined nature of this group, sharing of results in the form of a consistent national meeting, advocacy for government and private investment in the health of this group, aligning with Healthy People goals, and an active participatory role from South Asians themselves.

12.4.4 Recommendations for Providers

- Avoid overemphasis on the socially constructed meaning of ethnicity and race by acknowledging the heterogeneity of this group. Remain aware that generic cultural information may not apply to an individual South Asian patient, and avoid assumptions that knowing generic values of a culture of origin and typical health patterns will be applicable to all patients of South Asian descent.
- Assuming shared definitions and meanings of illness constructs across language and culture can contribute to marginalizing the impact of cultural beliefs of the patient. Awareness of differences between Western and Eastern conceptions of the mind and body when interpreting symptoms.
- Stereotypes about cultural groups can operate on an unconscious level and be enacted in the provider-patient relationship. Based on the type of health service provided, the provider may seek to increase awareness of his/her own cultural

assumptions and engage in self-examination of conscious and unconscious biases and assumptions (see Implicit Attitudes Test in Chap. 10) to enhance cross-cultural communication.

12.5 Towards a Biopsychosocial Approach to Address South Asian Health Disparities

Applying a biopsychosocial model to South Asian American health indicates attention must be paid not only to traditional clinical risk factors but also to psychological and sociocultural risk factors because they can impact disease-related outcomes. The modifiable nature of psychological and sociocultural factors can be harnessed to improve upon biological disease-related outcomes. In posing four general questions concerning South Asian heath in the U.S., this handbook sought to initiate the conversation on South Asian American health using a holistic, biopsychosocial lens. In considering the unique impacts of South Asian identity in the U.S. on health outcomes, the South Asians American patient's possible explanatory models of health and illness, this Asian subgroup's known chronic disease burden, and common barriers to promoting health, the hope is that this handbook can inform culturally-competent care to promote health, reduce disease, and maximize treatment outcomes. In calling for "healthy" South Asian Americans, the value of disaggregation of Asian American health outcomes is emphasized.

Disaggregated data is the most effective way to form evidence-based practice and policy around the distinct needs of this community. Whereas the aim of this book is to serve as a brief starting point in discussing the health of South Asian Americans and proffer considerations for providers working with this group, a comprehensive understanding of the health of this group is not wholly feasible at this time due to a history of aggregated data, recent understanding of unique health risks posed to this group, and limited available research with this Asian subgroup.

It is apparent, however, that an interdisciplinary, biopsychosocial approach is appropriate for this subgroup due to areas of poor fit with current conceptualizations of health and illness, as well as this group's historical and traditional exposure to messages of health as holistic. It is also apparent that U.S. South Asians have a different distribution of systematic health barriers (i.e., subject to racism and stereotyping as perpetual foreigners, pressure to be highly successful, cultural norms contrasting with U.S. culture, etc.) compared to U.S. Whites, indicating a need for future scientific efforts to not only modify existing health models but to also consider original conceptualizations of health that target this group's particular distribution of health barriers (Assari 2017). With culturally-sensitive intervention, holistic health conceptualizations can be harnessed to target this group's distribution of barriers and promote risk-reducing health behavior beliefs and change. The diversity that disaggregated data leads to can better create inclusion and equitable health policies for all Americans, particularly understudied and underserved ethnic/racial subgroups with nuanced health issues.

References

Assari, S. (2017). Unequal gain of equal resources across racial groups. *International Journal of Health Policy and Management, 6*(x), 1–9.

Centers for Disease Control and Prevention. (2017). *National Diabetes Statistics Report,* 2017. Retrieved from https://www.cdc.gov/diabetes/pdfs/data/statistics/national-diabetes-statistics-report.pdf

Chin, J. J., Leung, M., Sheth, L., & Rodriguez, T. R. (2007). Let's not ignore a growing HIV problem for Asians and Pacific Islanders in the US. *Journal of Urban Health, 84*(5), 642–647.

Dolezsar, C. M., McGrath, J. J., Herzig, A. M., & Miller, S. B. (2014). Perceived racial discrimination and hypertension: A comprehensive systematic review. *Health Psychology, 33*(1), 20–34. https://doi.org/10.1037/a0033718.

Fernando, E., Razak, F., Lear, S. A., & Anand, S. S. (2015). Cardiovascular disease in South Asian migrants. *Canadian Journal of Cardiology, 31*(9), 1139–1150.

Gujral, U. P., Vittinghoff, E., Mongraw-Chaffin, M., Vaidya, D., Kandula, N. R., Allison, M., & Kanaya, A. M. (2017). Cardiometabolic abnormalities among normal-weight persons from five racial/ethnic groups in the United States: A cross-sectional analysis of two cohort StudiesCardiometabolic abnormalities among normal-weight persons. *Annals of Internal Medicine, 166*(9), 628–636.

Hastings, K. G., Jose, P. O., Kapphahn, K. I., Frank, A. T. H., Goldstein, B. A., Thompson, C. A., … & Palaniappan, L. P. (2015). Leading causes of death among Asian American subgroups (2003-2011). *PLoS ONE*, 10.4 (Apr. 2015).

Hoeffel, E. M., Rastogi, S., Kim, M. O., & Hasan, S. (2012). *The Asian population: 2010. US Department of commerce, economics and statistics administration, US Census Bureau.* Retrieved from http://www.census.gov/prod/cen2010/briefs/c2010br-11.pdf

Holland, A. T., & Palaniappan, L. P. (2012). Problems with the collection and interpretation of Asian-American health data: Omission, aggregation, and extrapolation. *Annals of Epidemiology, 22*(6), 397–405.

Hurwitz, E. J. H., Gupta, J., Liu, R., Silverman, J. G., & Raj, A. (2006). Intimate partner violence associated with poor health outcomes in US South Asian women. *Journal of Immigrant and Minority Health, 8*(3), 251–261.

Jih, J., Mukherjea, A., Vittinghoff, E., Nguyen, T. T., Tsoh, J. Y., Fukuoka, Y., et al. (2014). Using appropriate body mass index cut points for overweight and obesity among Asian Americans. *Preventive Medicine, 65*, 1–6.

Joshi, P., Islam, S., Pais, P., Reddy, S., Dorairaj, P., Kazmi, K., & Yusuf, S. (2007). Risk factors for early myocardial infarction in South Asians compared with individuals in other countries. *Journal of the American Medical Association, 297*(3), 286–294.

Katon, W. J., Von Korff, M., Lin, E. H., Simon, G., Ludman, E., Russo, J., ... & Bush, T. (2004). The pathways study: A randomized trial of collaborative care in patients with diabetes and depression. *Archives of General Psychiatry*, 61(10), 1042–1049.

Kivelä, K., Elo, S., Kyngäs, H., & Kääriäinen, M. (2014). The effects of health coaching on adult patients with chronic diseases: A systematic review. *Patient Education and Counseling, 97*(2), 147–157.

Kuroki, Y. (2016). Comparison of suicide rates among Asian Americans in 2000 and 2010. *OMEGA-Journal of Death and Dying, 0*(0), 1–8. https://doi.org/10.1177/0030222816678425.

Landrine, H., & Klonoff, E. A. (2004). Culture change and ethnic-minority health behavior: An operant theory of acculturation. *Journal of Behavioral Medicine, 27*(6), 527–555.

Lazarus, R. S., & Folkman, S. (1984). Coping and adaptation. In *The Handbook of Behavioral Medicine* (pp. 282–325).

Mallath, M. K., Taylor, D. G., Badwe, R. A., Rath, G. K., Shanta, V., Pramesh, C. S., & Kapoor, S. (2014). The growing burden of cancer in India: Epidemiology and social context. *The Lancet Oncology, 15*(6), e205–e212.

McNeely, M. J., & Boyko, E. J. (2004). Type 2 diabetes prevalence in Asian Americans. *Diabetes Care, 27*(1), 66–69.

Oza-Frank, R., Ali, M. K., Vaccarino, V., & Narayan, K. M. V. (2009). Asian Americans: Diabetes prevalence acrossU.S. and World Health Organization weight classifications. *Diabetes Care, 32*(9), 1644–1646.

Rajpathak, S. N., Gupta, L. S., Waddell, E. N., Upadhyay, U. D., Wildman, R. P., Kaplan, R., & Wylie-Rosett, J. (2010). Elevated risk of type 2 diabetes and metabolic syndrome among Asians and south Asians: Results from the 2004 New York City HANES. *Ethnicity & Disease, 20*(3), 225–230.

Ramachandran, A., Snehalatha, C., Shetty, A. S., & Nanditha, A. (2012). Trends in prevalence of diabetes in Asian countries. *World Journal of Diabetes, 3*(6), 110–117.

Srivastava, R., & Pandey, A. K. (2017). Internal and International migration in South Asia: Drivers, interlinkage and policy issues. In *United Nations Educational, Scientific, and Cultural Organization (UNESCO)* (pp. 1–62).

U.S. Census Bureau. (2010). *The Asian population: 2010*. Retrieved from https://www.census.gov/prod/cen2010/briefs/c2010br-11.pdf

Venkataraman, R., Nanda, N. C., Baweja, G., Parikh, N., & Bhatia, V. (2004). Prevalence of diabetes mellitus and related conditions in Asian Indians living in the United States. *The American Journal of Cardiology, 94*(7), 977–980.

Wang, Y., & Beydoun, M. A. (2007). The obesity epidemic in the United States—Gender, age, socioeconomic, racial/ethnic, and geographic characteristics: A systematic review and meta-regression analysis. *Epidemiologic Reviews, 29*(1), 6–28.

Wolstein, J., Babey, S. H., & Diamant, A. L. (2015). *Obesity in California*. Los Angeles: UCLA Center for Health Policy Research, 2015.

MIX
Papier aus verantwortungsvollen Quellen
Paper from responsible sources
FSC® C105338

If you have any concerns about our products,
you can contact us on
ProductSafety@springernature.com

In case Publisher is established outside the EU,
the EU authorized representative is:
Springer Nature Customer Service Center GmbH
Europaplatz 3, 69115 Heidelberg, Germany

Printed by Libri Plureos GmbH
in Hamburg, Germany